Healthcare without Borders

Contemporary Cuba

UNIVERSITY PRESS OF FLORIDA

Florida A&M University, Tallahassee
Florida Atlantic University, Boca Raton
Florida Gulf Coast University, Ft. Myers
Florida International University, Miami
Florida State University, Tallahassee
New College of Florida, Sarasota
University of Central Florida, Orlando
University of Florida, Gainesville
University of North Florida, Jacksonville
University of South Florida, Tampa
University of West Florida, Pensacola

HEALTHCARE WITHOUT BORDERS

Understanding Cuban Medical Internationalism

JOHN M. KIRK

John M. Kirk, series editor

University Press of Florida
Gainesville · Tallahassee · Tampa · Boca Raton
Pensacola · Orlando · Miami · Jacksonville · Ft. Myers · Sarasota

Printed in the United States of America on acid-free paper

This book may be available in an electronic edition.

20 19 18 17 16 15 6 5 4 3 2 1

Library of Congress Cataloging-in-Publication Data
Kirk, John M., 1951– author.
Healthcare without borders : understanding Cuban medical internationalism / by John M. Kirk.
pages cm — (Contemporary Cuba)
ISBN 978-0-8130-6105-4
1. Medical assistance, Cuban. 2. Medical policy—Cuba. 3. Medical care—Cuba—Methods. 4. Public health—Cuba. 5. International cooperation. I. Title. II. Series: Contemporary Cuba.
RA390.C9K58 2015
362.1097291—dc23
2015013773

The University Press of Florida is the scholarly publishing agency for the State University System of Florida, comprising Florida A&M University, Florida Atlantic University, Florida Gulf Coast University, Florida International University, Florida State University, New College of Florida, University of Central Florida, University of Florida, University of North Florida, University of South Florida, and University of West Florida.

University Press of Florida
15 Northwest 15th Street
Gainesville, FL 32611-2079
http://www.upf.com

Contents

Tables

Preface

> For such a small nation, the number of doctors and nurses that Cuba is sending, as well as the speed with which the country has responded, is really extraordinary.
>
> Margaret Chan, director general, World Health Organization, September 12, 2014

In the fall of 2014, a deadly outbreak of Ebola swept through the West African countries of Liberia, Guinea-Conakry, and Sierra Leone. By mid-September, 5,000 people had been infected, over half of whom died, and just four months later the number of patients had risen to over 20,000, with more than 8,000 deaths recorded. Predictions about the total number of cases ranged from 20,000 to hundreds of thousands. Faced with an impending disaster, Ban Ki-moon, secretary-general of the United Nations and Dr. Margaret Chan, director general of the World Health Organization (WHO), appealed to the international community for help and stressed the need for doctors and nurses above all else. The first country to offer support was Cuba.

At that time the WHO had 170 medical staff working on this campaign but desperately needed more. (They had deployed some 500 specialists, but rotated them monthly due to the dangerous conditions, so that at any given time only about a third would be working in field.) Some international charities and NGOs had smaller numbers of medical staff working for short periods in West Africa, but others had withdrawn their members because of the dangers faced, and many healthcare workers had died as a result of infection. Some countries sent field hospitals and bedding, food, and medicine, while the United States provided extensive military support and others donated money. It was clear, though, that the greatest need was for medical personnel—a challenge ignored by most industrialized nations.

Cuba responded to the appeal within days by offering to send to Sierra Leone 103 nurses and 62 doctors, all of whom had volunteered to help. This was the first contribution of healthcare personnel by any country, and it is still the largest to date. Some context is appropriate here. At that time Cuba had more than 4,000 medical personnel already working in 32 African countries, and of these 2,400 were doctors. They chose Sierra Leone as the place to send the 165, since 23 Cuban medical personnel were already working there, and their program had been initiated several years earlier. The Cuban medical personnel who now arrived had an average of 15 years of professional experience, all had worked on missions in developing countries, and a quarter had worked in more than one. The Cuban commitment was to send their medical volunteers for a period of six months, after which they would reassess needs. Within a month the Cuban government had decided to increase the number of medical personnel, and it was announced that a further 296 would be sent to work in Guinea and Liberia.

The Ebola crisis in West Africa struck a nerve in North America and Europe, since some of their citizens who had worked in the affected countries also became infected. A Cuban doctor, Félix Báez, became infected with Ebola and was treated in Switzerland, where he recovered. He subsequently volunteered to return to work in West Africa. Several died after returning to their home countries, and there was debate about whether the virus could spread there. Many governments overreacted, and a certain level of panic set in. Cuba responded in an organized fashion, training its volunteers in a fastidious, methodical approach at Havana's prestigious Pedro Kourí Institute of Tropical Medicine in order to minimize the risks of infection.

Together with the WHO and the Pan American Health Organization (PAHO), they also organized an international conference in Havana to which hundreds of medical personnel came in order to better understand the significance of the Ebola epidemic and how to treat it. Given the traditional approach of preventive healthcare, it was not surprising when they trained 240,000 people in Cuba about treating the disease and sent public health personnel to bordering countries, as well as to countries in Latin America and the Caribbean, in order to provide information about how to avoid being infected by Ebola and, where necessary, how to deal with it. In this way they trained almost 13,000 people in Africa, as well as 66,000 in Latin America and 620 in the Caribbean. Most important of all, they sent their doctors and nurses, selecting them from the 15,000 medical personnel who had volunteered to serve in West Africa. The Cuban role—sending doctors instead of soldiers or money—was covered widely in the media, making many aware for the first time of Cuba's role in medical internationalism (MI).

While Ebola suddenly dominated media coverage and surprise was expressed at Cuba's leading role in the medical campaign against it, little was said about their medical contributions in dozens of countries around the globe. And yet there was much that could be said. In Guatemala, for instance, recent data show that the 468 Cuban medical personnel have saved over 292,000 lives there and given (at no cost to the patient) over 37 million medical consults since the medical mission was established in 1998. Bolivia has also gained significantly from Cuban solidarity. More than 30,000 lives have been saved by Cuban medical personnel, a large pharmaceutical production complex is to be built in order to provide essential medicines at subsidized prices, and 4,000 doctors have been trained in Cuba. Indeed, in Havana's Latin American School of Medicine, over 24,000 physicians from 83 mainly low-income countries have graduated since 1999, most without paying any tuition at all. Over 3 million ophthalmology operations have taken place through the Operation Miracle program now found in 31 countries—without any cost to the patients. In late 2013 some 11,400 Cuban physicians began working in underserved communities in Brazil, under the auspices of the PAHO. Cuban pharmaceutical products were being sold in some 50 countries in the Global South and at significantly lower prices than those charged by transnational drug companies. In sum, examples abound of different facets of Cuban medical internationalism being practiced, and yet most remain unknown.

This book studies the role of Cuban medical internationalism, examining key aspects of its many programs since 1960, when the first mission of medical *internacionalistas* flew to Chile in the wake of a major earthquake. The mission to West Africa in late 2014, although significant, is just the latest in a rich history of medical cooperation developed by Cuba for nearly six decades. It is a tradition that is not widely known and is often referred to as "medical diplomacy," the insinuation being that Cuba does this principally as a means of promoting its political agenda abroad. This is a simplistic, limited interpretation. Few are aware that, as the Cuban minister of public health, Roberto Morales Ojeda, pointed out in the joint press conference with Dr. Chan in September 2014, Cuba had 50,731 medical personnel working in 66 countries at that time. Of these, 64 percent were women and 25,412 were physicians. In the U.S. context this would be the equivalent of having a quarter of all doctors—over 200,000—working abroad in developing nations under extremely difficult conditions.

Morales gave precise data on the role of Cuba in the hundreds of medical missions in which Cuban medics had worked. Since that first contribution in Chile, Cuban medical personnel had served in 158 countries. They had performed 1.2 billion medical consults, attended 2.2 million births, and performed over 8 million surgeries.[1] In terms of medical assistance in natural disasters and medical emergencies, they also had decades of experience. In fact, they had offered to provide over 1,400 medical personnel to New Orleans in 2005 in the wake of Hurricane Katrina (an offer ignored by President George W. Bush).

At the same press conference, Dr. Chan said, "Cuba is famous throughout the world because of its capacity to train excellent doctors and nurses. It is also famous for its generosity and solidarity toward developing countries." This book does not fully agree with the first part of her claim. While the role of Cuba is indeed well known in developing countries, this is not the case in those of the industrialized North, where media coverage has been scant and poorly informed. The book seeks to show that, as the title suggests, since 1960 this small country of 11.2 million people has provided "healthcare without borders." Indeed, its prominent role in facing up to the threat of Ebola in West Africa is just the latest episode in a long tradition. The aim of this book is to present an introduction to this extraordinary tradition of basic humanitarianism and compassion, one that has also brought improved diplomatic relations. It is a story that deserves to be told.

Acknowledgments

This book has been a labor of love for almost a decade, one that started by accident and continued because of an ever-growing fascination for a topic that deserved to be told but had scarcely been touched. Many could argue that it had been deliberately ignored. Looking back now, it is clear that the long conversations on healthcare between Canadian premier John Savage and Cuban president Fidel Castro that I witnessed in 1994 and 1996, and that are the seed for this book, were extremely important. Since then, I have been fortunate to have met some extraordinary Cuban medical professionals whose conduct has consistently reminded me of the observation of nineteenth-century Cuban writer/revolutionary José Martí that "patria es humanidad" (All of humanity is our homeland).

Over the course of this long journey of discovery, I have interviewed hundreds of people throughout Cuba, especially *internacionalistas* who have returned after completing medical missions. They are the protagonists of this epic story, and I owe them all an enormous debt of gratitude. The Universidad Médica "Carlos J. Finlay" in Camagüey deserves special recognition, where I interviewed many members of the faculty who had served on diplomatic missions in developing countries. In particular I am indebted to Arturo Menéndez, who established a medical faculty staffed with Cuban professors in Gambia and later served in Venezuela. His sound counsel was always appreciated.

In Havana I met with numerous people responsible for the planning of medical cooperation. Drs. Jorge Delgado Bustillo and Yiliam Jiménez at the Unidad Central de Colaboración Médica (UCCM) and Néstor Marimón, José Portilla, and especially Víctor Manuel Rodríguez of the International Relations Department of the Ministry of Public Health (MINSAP) all gave generously of their time. A source of invaluable information on the Cuban public health system is MEDICC, and a tremendous amount of solid research is carried out there by Conner Gorry, Christina Mills, and Gail Reed. I am particularly grateful for their permission to use several tables that have appeared in MEDICC publications. All author royalties from this book are donated to support MEDICC's work. Particularly helpful in making contacts with individuals and institutions were the hardworking people at ICAP, especially Sandra Ramírez, Odalys López, and Esperanza Luzbert. Julio Medina, director of the Tarará program where the Chernobyl patients stayed, also provided insights into their experiences. I undertook several trips to the Latin American School of Medicine (ELAM) and am grateful to dozens of professors and students there for their assistance.

Many members of the medical profession throughout the island have been useful sounding boards, speaking about their own experiences on missions abroad or providing context for this project. They include Enrique Beldarraín Chaple, Rafael Llanes, Jorge Balseiro, Danay Saavedra, Pura Avilés, and especially Nicolás Garófalo. By expanding my understanding of the historical roots of medical cooperation, José Miyar Barrueco ("Chomi") enhanced my understanding of the significance of medical internationalism for Fidel Castro, whom he served for many years as a confidant in health matters.

The experience of accompanying Cuban medical personnel in Central America offered the opportunity to see Cuban medical cooperation firsthand. The support of Pedro Pablo Prada, Cuban ambassador to El Salvador, was particularly important, as was that of members of the Brigada Médica Cubana Salvadoreña Mons. Óscar Romero, especially Eduardo Ojeda and Mayra Fontes. I am grateful to the Brigada for permission to use tables located in chapter 11. Ronald Chávez and Jay Hartling provided invaluable insights into El Salvador and assisted me in making some key connections. In Guatemala the medical personnel at three Operación Milagro clinics that I visited and José Ramón Ruiz of the Brigada Médica Cubana provided insight into the large Cuban medical operation there. I am especially grateful to the many Salvadoran and Guatemalan graduates of ELAM who agreed to be interviewed and especially to Sandra Galdámez, an exemplary ELAMista.

Over many years of travel to Cuba I have been assisted by members of Cuba's diplomatic corps in making contact with medical cooperation officials and practitioners. A debt of gratitude is owed to Raúl Delgado, whom I met when starting my research on the topic. Carlos Castillo, Teresita de Jesús Vicente, and Julio Garmendía, all ambassadors of Cuba to Canada, have always been supportive of my research, and their assistance is gratefully acknowledged.

In Canada I was able to draw upon the advice of many colleagues and friends. Noni MacDonald, Leslie Ribeiro, Jessica Vostermans, and Chris Walker provided valuable feedback on specific chapters in areas where they all have a wealth of experience. Colleagues Michael Erisman, Lou Pérez, and Marguerite Jiménez in the United States and Antoni Kapcia in the United Kingdom read the manuscript and offered wise counsel. Tim Anderson in Australia was an invaluable source of Cuban cooperation in Timor-Leste. Similarly helpful were the conversations I enjoyed with colleagues and friends in Cuba, including many of the faculty at FLACSO-Cuba as well as Hal Klepak, Jorge Mario Sánchez, Rafael Hernández, Carlos Alzugaray, Jesús Benjamín, Alberto Roque, and Leonardo Padura.

I also appreciate the kind permission of Mexican colleague Edgar Zayaga, who allowed part of an earlier version of chapter 11, published in *El desarollo perdido* in 2011, to be used as the basis for my analysis.

Funding for the project for the past five years has come from the Social Sciences and Humanities Research Council of Canada (SSHRC), and their financial support has been fundamental to my carrying out research. Support in kind from colleagues at Dalhousie University in Canada is also greatly appreciated. The editorial staff at the University Press of Florida have been extremely supportive of this project, and I would like to thank Catherine-Nevil Parker for guidance in the preparation of the book and Elaine Durham Otto for her excellent copyediting.

Finally, I would like to thank two members of my immediate family who have been particularly helpful. Technical support (including patience with my limited computer skills) was provided by my wife, Margo. She has also been a superb companion over nearly four decades of research trips to Cuba. Our daughter Emily, a Cuba scholar in her own right, with excellent research on sexual health issues in Cuba, also deserves recognition. She read over much of my work and offered constructive and honest criticism.

All translations from the Spanish original are mine, and I accept full responsibility for their accuracy.

Introduction

Setting the Scene

> What other country can point to a record of greater selflessness than Cuba has displayed in its relations with Africa? Where is the country that has sought Cuban help and had it refused?
>
> Nelson Mandela, July 26, 1991

It is not easy to understand Cuba. This is a small country of 11.2 million that has the surface area of Virginia or Tennessee, yet for many years it has maintained an extremely high international profile. After four centuries as a colony of Spain, it gained its independence in 1898, and from then until 1959 it was heavily influenced by the United States in everything from politics to economic development, culture to foreign policy. In 1959 the revolution led by Fidel Castro occurred, and from then on a socialist revolutionary government has been in power. As with so many other aspects of Cuba, the country's foreign policy has been original, vastly different from what one would expect of such a small developing country. Yet as Nelson Mandela pointed out, it has had a major impact on many facets of life in Africa. The same can be said of Cuba's role in improving the health of millions of people in dozens of developing countries.

This book is about medical cooperation. It is a story that deserves to be told, because it has largely been ignored by media sources in developed countries, despite the fact that the contribution of this small island to global health dwarfs that of all other industrialized countries. Cuba maintains diplomatic relations throughout the developing world, where its medical internationalism policy has been in existence since 1960. The data about its role are clear-cut: in all, over 135,000 medical professionals from Cuba have worked abroad since then, and in March 2014 there were some 50,000 (including 25,000 doctors) working in over 60 developing countries.[1] Since then, several thousand more have arrived to work in Brazil at the request of the Rousseff administration.

Ban Ki-moon, secretary-general of the United Nations, visiting Cuba in January 2014, commented on how, in his visits to some of the most forgotten areas of the world, there was a common factor—the presence of either Cuban doctors or doctors from those countries trained in Cuba. He noted that many of the leaders in healthcare he met in developing countries had studied on the island and had incorporated lessons learned there into their own healthcare systems. He summed up the Cuban medical presence by saying, "They are always the first to arrive and the last to leave—and they always remain after the crisis. Cuba has a lot to show the entire world with its health system, a model for many countries."[2]

To a large degree Cuba's ambitious program can be carried out because of the extensive human resources that it possesses. World Bank statistics (for 2010) show that Cuba has 6.7 physicians per 1,000 people, approximately three times the corresponding figure for the United States (2.4) and Canada (2.1) and more than twice that of the United Kingdom (2.7).[3] More recent data provided by Cuban Minister of Public Health Roberto Morales Ojeda indicate that this has risen to 7.2 doctors per 1,000 people. He added that there were 19,000 students of medicine attending Cuban universities.[4] Not surprisingly, the delivery of accessible healthcare services, provided at no cost to the population, has resulted in a positive health profile. The Cuban government website maintained by the National Office of Statistics fleshes out data concerning the current medical situation in Cuba, one which has resulted in Cuba having a lower infant mortality rate (4.76 per 1,000 live births) than that of the United States (5.90) or Canada (4.78). Life expectancy for Cuba (78.05) and the United States (78.62) is similar, with that of Canada being slightly better (81.57).[5] The HIV prevalence rate in Cuba is one-sixth that of the United States, and the mortality rate for children under five is lower than in the United States (6 per 1,000 live births compared to 8).[6] Speaking in July 2014, Margaret Chan, director general of the World Health Organization, summarized the Cuban approach to healthcare: "Nobody should die nowadays of avoidable diseases simply because they are women or poor. If people do not have real access to healthcare, then we are not building a just world. Cuba has shown that it is possible to have health and well-being for all."[7]

Since the early days of the revolution, the delivery of accessible healthcare, available at no cost to the patient, has been a priority of the Cuban government. Indeed, the ability to export so many medical personnel is the result of this policy of training so many people in the healthcare field. Within Cuba in 2011 there were 78,622 doctors, 96,424 nurses and nursing assistants, and 12,793 dentists. This translated into a doctor for every 143 patients and a dentist for every 878. There were also 161 hospitals, 452 polyclinics, and, in line with Cuba's philosophy of preventive medicine, 11,486 family doctor offices (usually with a doctor and nurse team).[8] In terms of students of the six-year medical sciences program, there were 47,676 students registered in 2013–14, of whom 37,302 were Cuban and 10,374 were from abroad.[9] (This occurs in a poor country where average monthly state salary is around $25 and annual GDP is about $10,000 per capita.) In 2009, while Cuba spent $503 per capita on healthcare, the United States spent almost 15 times that sum: $7,410.[10] While many believe in "wealth before health" (with the delivery of healthcare being possible only after a country has developed economically), the case of Cuba shows that this is not always true. Political will and human capital are clearly more important.

Since 1960, Cuba has been involved in providing medical assistance to scores of countries around the globe, and more than 135,000 Cuban medical personnel have provided this medical collaboration. Significantly 69 percent of Cuban doctors have participated in at least one mission abroad as *internacionalistas*.[11] An analysis of the many reasons for their participation in these missions is provided later in this book. This support has often been paid scant attention by mainstream media, and at times it has been distorted. An example was a CNN report after the Haiti earthquake in January 2010 that referred to a Cuban doctor (wearing a Che Guevara T-shirt, speaking with a distinct Cuban accent, and identifying himself as Cuban) as being a "Spanish" physician. In general, most U.S. media outlets ignored Cuba's medical role in Haiti. In fact, Cuba's medical role in the developing world can perhaps be seen as the greatest story never told.

Cuba's role in providing medical assistance abroad is a remarkable story. The most recent example of this can be seen in Brazil where between late 2013 and spring of 2014, Cuba sent 11,400 doctors to work in underserved areas on three-year contracts. The government of Dilma Rousseff had earlier initiated a program, Mais Médicos, to provide healthcare for 50 million Brazilians living in rural and impoverished areas in the north. When few Brazilian physicians accepted the challenge of working in these difficult conditions, she appealed to the Pan American Health Organization for support. In all, 14,500 physicians were hired, with the Cubans representing 78 percent. Probably no other country in the world would be able to respond in this manner, yet little has been said about this significant role.

With this project I offer a corrective, comprehensive analysis of this medical cooperation program. This work complements my earlier book,

Cuban Medical Internationalism: Origins, Evolution, and Goals, written with H. Michael Erisman. But it goes far deeper than the original text, which focused largely on political aspects of the program. Instead, here I assess in detail the significance of this policy of medical cooperation (an expression consistently used by Cuba, which shuns the paternalistic term *aid*), both in general and with regard to specific aspects of the delivery of medical care. I consider an array of topics, from Cuba's medical support in Haiti to its rapidly increasing role in biotechnology joint ventures with developing countries, from its treatment of some 25,000 (mainly child) victims of the Chernobyl fallout in 1986 to the evolution of this program of medical internationalism (MI) as the major source of hard currency for the country today.

Little has been written in detail about Cuba's medical internationalism role. In order to provide a detailed assessment, the book consists of two sections. The first addresses general aspects and programs (such as the Operation Miracle eye surgery program that has operated on some 3 million people and is found throughout Latin America as well as in the Caribbean and Africa). The objective in this first section is to look at the "big picture" role of Cuba in a number of countries, often concurrently. This section examines the origins and development of MI, providing a basic framework and explaining the underpinning philosophy of the revolutionary government regarding internationalism.

The second section examines Cuba's contribution in specific countries (such as the evolution of Cuba's role in El Salvador after its initial support in the wake of Hurricane Ida in 2010, and in Timor-Leste, where it has trained almost 1,000 doctors). Venezuela is considered in detail, since Cuba has its largest MI program there and is involved in a number of public health programs. Cuba's role in Haiti is also analyzed in some detail, since it has been providing medical support (including the training of almost 1,000 physicians at no cost to that impoverished country) for almost two decades. The book concludes with observations on the evolution and rationale for this policy, assessing its role both traditionally and more recently under the government of Raúl Castro.

My research in medical internationalism developed out of a strong interest in Cuban foreign policy and in many ways was an accident of fate. While undertaking research in Havana about Cuban foreign policy over several years, I kept meeting medical personnel (ubiquitous on the island, since Cuba has more doctors per patient than any country in the world). When talking about research interests, I often encountered doctors, nurses, and technicians who had worked abroad in developing nations and were eager to share their views on experiences there.

On the international scene a significant development occurred in 2009 at the Summit of the Americas, held in Trinidad and Tobago, when President Barack Obama drew attention to the role of Cuba's medical cooperation program, even suggesting that Washington could learn from the cooperative approach used by Cuba in developing countries. Cuban teachers, engineers, and especially doctors and nurses, he noted, provided tangible support throughout the region—often at no cost to the recipient nations. Obama referred to this phenomenon at his closing press conference on April 19, 2009, following the Summit of the Americas in Trinidad and Tobago:

> One thing that I thought was interesting—and I knew this in a more abstract way, but it was interesting in very specific terms—hearing from those leaders who, when they spoke about Cuba talked very specifically about the thousands of doctors from Cuba that are dispersed all throughout the region and upon which many of these countries depend.

At the summit he witnessed both strong criticism of traditional U.S. policy in the region and widespread praise for Cuban medical support, including from traditional allies of Washington. Almost all of the region's leaders were concerned that the United States had blocked Cuban participation at the summit, which became even more of an issue at the following (2013) summit in Cartagena, Colombia. President Obama's intent to normalize diplomatic relations with Havana, outlined in December 2014, is therefore a positive step. One day it might even result in bilateral medical exchanges and research, from which both countries would benefit.

Understanding the context of recent events in Latin America, and Cuba's role in these, is needed in order to appreciate the political and moral influence of revolutionary Cuba. It is clear to most academics that Latin America has changed greatly in the last 15 years. Many indicate the election of Hugo Chávez in 1998 as a starting point for any analysis, although significant political currents were already reshaping the region. The decrease in U.S. influence in the region, growing opposition to neoliberalism and what was known as the "Washington consensus," and the disappearance of military regimes in the region all illustrated a major shift in the tectonic plates of regional politics. In this new political reality, Cuba's influence grew, particularly as several left-of-center governments were elected in Central and South America. An important strategic partnership resulted, involving Cuba's decades-long policy of MI and support for social programs paid for by Venezuelan petrodollars from the governments of Hugo Chávez and later Nicolás Maduro. This combination of Cuban human capital and Venezuelan financial support has proved a powerful mixture, from which many countries of the Global South have benefited. Cuba's role in the region has undoubtedly been enhanced by its commitment to medical cooperation since 1960, and Havana exercises significant moral influence—far more than a country of its size would normally hold. In boxing terms, Cuba punches way above its weight class.

President Obama's musings notwithstanding, it is clear that most commentators and politicians do not yet understand, much less appreciate, the full significance or extent of Cuba's medical assistance abroad. In my own case, in addition to meeting Cuban doctors in several Latin American countries, I have also read widely about their role since the first medical mission to Chile following an earthquake there in 1960.[12] Yet at that time I really did not grasp the significance of the enormous impact of Cuban MI on dozens of the countries of the developing world, much less the government commitment to the developing world.

Initially I had considered (erroneously, it transpired) Cuba's program to be mainly an extension of its foreign policy and a smart one at that. The term *soft power*, coined by Harvard's Joseph Nye (which is premised on the idea that it is possible to co-opt or influence a country or person with support and positive actions rather than to coerce them by using brute force and punishment) at first appeared to apply to Cuba's foreign policy strategy. It seemed logical to assume that to a large degree Cuba's approach was based on the application of soft power. Indeed, it could be argued that the Cuban approach was intended to win the hearts and minds of countries throughout the developing world, gaining their agreement for key United Nations votes or supporting Cuba's perspective at regional summits. As I researched the matter further, however, and as I met an increasing number of Cubans who had spent time under extremely difficult conditions in developing countries, my ideas began to evolve—and the idea for this book grew. I realized that the Cuban approach went far beyond the limits of Nye's interpretation of soft power. In essence, the Cuban approach was not based on the idea of co-opting a country's policy by offering medical support. While undoubtedly this aspect was factored into the analysis undertaken in Havana, there were many other considerations.

It is worth emphasizing the significant contribution of Cuban medical personnel in countries that have been extremely critical of its revolutionary process. After all, why share scarce resources with a country that condemns your model of development and supports your traditional (and self-declared) enemy, the United States? Yet in 1998 when Hurricane Mitch devastated Central America, hundreds of Cuban emergency specialists answered the calls for assistance from regional governments and flew to help, even though Cuba did not even have diplomatic relations with the countries that were most affected. An even starker example can be seen as early as 1972 when a massive earthquake destroyed the downtown core of Managua. Cuban doctors were among the first to arrive, even though Nicaragua's president, Anastasio Somoza Debayle, was a sworn enemy of the Cuban revolution, and at the time of the earthquake he went out of his way to cause problems for the Cuban doctors and planeloads of emergency medical support. Despite ideological differences, Cuba was among the first countries to send medical support to that beleaguered country as it suffered in the midst of a huge tragedy that killed 6,000 and left 250,000 homeless.

Several decades later, Cuba again ignored political differences in order to maintain a humanitarian mission in Honduras. When the democratically elected government of Manuel Zelaya, a strong ally of Cuba and member of ALBA (the Bolivarian Alliance for the Americas) was overthrown in a military coup, Cuban doctors remained at their posts, dealing with the poor and marginalized in Honduras, one of the most destitute countries in Latin America. They remain there still, despite major ideological differences between the governments of Cuba and Honduras. Cuba has also offered assistance to the United States, despite the fact that diplomatic relations have remained frozen since Washington broke them off in January 1961. When Havana offered the support of over 1,400 medical personnel to the people of New Orleans in the wake of Hurricane Katrina in August 2005, the administration of George W. Bush ignored the Cuban gesture, refusing even to recognize the offer. Two months later, when an earthquake occurred in the Kashmir region of Pakistan, Cuba sent 2,400 medical personnel to assist, established 32 field hospitals (later donated to Kashmir), and provided 1,000 medical scholarships to students in the affected region. And this despite the fact that diplomatic relations had lapsed and the Pakistani embassy had been closed for several years. The Cuban record of offering medical assistance where it is most needed has been consistent, and ideology has not played a particularly large role. Put simply, humanitarian solidarity has consistently trumped political considerations in the Cuban lexicon since 1960.

An important influence on my appreciation of the Cuban role in MI—but one which had remained dormant for many years—was a series of meetings I had by accident with Fidel Castro in 1994 and 1996. In both years I spent a week in Havana as the interpreter/counselor for Dr. John Savage, the premier of the Canadian province of Nova Scotia, in meetings with the Cuban president. Dr. Savage was a progressive family doctor who was renowned for his compassion, interest in international politics, and practical approach to medicine. He had worked as a volunteer with Medical Aid to Nicaragua, a Canadian NGO sending medical supplies to the first Sandinista government, and after retiring from politics he worked with the Nova Scotia Gambia Association, providing medical assistance to that country. The meetings between him and Fidel Castro were mainly focused on strengthening commercial ties between this Atlantic province and Cuba, and on both occasions Savage headed a large trade delegation. In private, however, the conversation between the two turned to questions of medicine and public health. Given the interests of the two politicians, this was natural, and I witnessed many fruitful exchanges of ideas. Castro spoke often about Cuba's MI interests, and it was fascinating to listen to them discuss questions of medical support for developing countries and express their support for access to universal, accessible, and free public healthcare in Cuba and abroad.

My approach to the question of MI remained somewhat limited, however, for years seeing it still largely as an extension of Cuban foreign policy. It seemed a particularly successful, well thought out strategy. For example, several of the countries in Central America to which Cuba had sent hundreds of medical personnel after Hurricane Mitch eventually normalized diplomatic relations with Cuba, as did Pakistan. This was in many ways a logical development, since for the recipients of Cuban medical assistance it was difficult to remain the enemy of a country that was saving the lives of thousands of their own citizens and at no cost to the government.

An illustration of Cuba's worldwide diplomatic success can be seen most dramatically in the annual vote at the UN to support a condemnation of the U.S. trade embargo (known in Cuba as the *bloqueo* or blockade), first imposed in 1960. In October 2014, for example, 188 nations supported Cuba's position with only the United States and Israel voting against it, and Palau, the Marshall Islands, and Micronesia abstaining. This was an embarrassment for Washington, and in fact it was the twenty-third time in a row that the United Nations General Assembly had voted against this aspect of U.S. policy toward Cuba. To no small degree this international support was due to Cuba's long-term vision of humanitarian cooperation. On one level, then, Cuba's approach could be interpreted as a masterful stroke in the application of Cuba's foreign policy and indeed of a Cuban variety of soft power. This, I gradually came to appreciate, was just one (albeit important) aspect of this multifaceted approach of Havana, a by-product of a commitment of over 50 years' standing.

Initially I failed to appreciate sufficiently the commitment of Cuba's revolutionary government to South-South cooperation, a major principle that it has applied in many of its programs of solidarity around the globe over several decades. The concept of internationalism had been in the Cuban priority list since the first days of the revolutionary process, and it came into its own in the 1970s with support in many spheres (from military aid to literacy programs, construction assistance, and advice in fishing and agriculture—and to dozens of developing countries). These programs had been implemented in many countries in Africa and Latin America, with a particularly large program (mainly military, but also with a substantial civil component) in Angola.

Another reason behind the internationalist nature of the Cuban revolutionary government was the nature and the influence of the *Comandante en jefe*, Fidel Castro. In late 2013 I interviewed José Miyar Barruecos, a physician and longtime confidant of the former president. Dr. Miyar (better known in Cuba by his nickname, "Chomi") had been the founder and director of the Cuban Rural Medical Service in the early years of the revolutionary process; the rector of the University of Havana; minister of science, technology, and the environment; and executive secretary of the Council of State from 1980 to 2009. The interview focused on Cuba's medical internationalism since the early 1960s, which according to Chomi was in large part due to a medical condition of President Castro. What was this condition, I asked. "Fidel has the *síndrome del sí*," he replied. I was perplexed and asked for further details about this medical condition, the "yes syndrome." Chomi then explained that the former Cuban president was often unable to turn down requests for cooperation from developing countries, and his charismatic style and occasionally impetuous nature resulted in Castro agreeing to provide medical support often when it had not even been requested.

In part my lack of awareness of Cuba's medical cooperation can be explained by the fact that traditionally so little had been said about it, either in academic studies or in the media. Referring to the "largest medical solidarity project ever known," José Manzaneda explains that there are two reasons for this lack of media and academic interest. First, he argues, the program depends on two countries with which the United States has poor relations, Cuba and Venezuela. In addition, the fact that MI "is not financed by any First World country, is not supported by World Bank funds, and neither does it count on the sponsorship of any business or private foundation" ensures that it will be overlooked in the media.[13] Sadly, this has been the case for many years. Gradually I came to realize that Cuban MI was not only an amalgam of international strategy as well as historical and ideological factors. It was also heavily influenced by the personal Third World vision and ideology of Fidel Castro. I also discovered that MI was even established firmly in the very constitution of Cuba, where a commitment to developing countries, particularly those of Latin America and the Caribbean, is stated with great clarity.[14] Internationalism is thus in the DNA of Cuban foreign policy as well as its history, its cultural roots, and its diplomatic and trade interests.

Throughout Cuban history, international cooperation—as early as the struggle for Cuba's independence from Spain in the late nineteenth century—has in fact exercised a significant influence on the government's philosophy. American Henry Reeve, after whom Cuba's emergency medical brigade is named, was a hero killed in battle in Cuba's first war for independence (1868–78), while the key military strategist in both that war and the 1895–98 struggle for independence was Dominican Generalísimo Máximo Gómez. In more recent times the very survival of the Cuban revolution after 1960 would have been unlikely without the support of the former Soviet Union and socialist countries of Europe, a process which lasted until 1990 and the implosion of the socialist countries of Eastern Europe. Of key importance was undoubtedly the philosophy of former president Fidel Castro. In an address in 2001 at the inauguration of the International School of Physical Education and Sports, Castro emphasized the value of the Cuban approach as developed throughout the revolutionary process for the basis of Cuba's *internacionalista* activities, comparing it to the strategy used by the United States: "In fact, a small country, a blockaded country that has yet to emerge from the Special Period [following the collapse of the Soviet Union], can do these things thanks to its human capital, because what costs them one hundred dollars costs us one dollar, because human capital cannot be bought with money, nor can all the money in the world achieve what can be achieved with human capital."[15]

Without a doubt, his vision of the need for unity of the Global South, and in particular of Latin America, was of paramount importance, as was his awareness of the development of human capital and *conciencia* (basically an amalgam of political awareness and commitment) in Cuba. Employing this long-term vision, the Cuban government offered medical cooperation programs to scores of developing countries, to allies as well as enemies, and clearly the strategy has succeeded. More important it has saved the lives of millions of people in the impoverished Global South. Speaking of the cooperation received in Bolivia, President Evo Morales noted how "Cuba is a country suffering a blockade, and yet is also the country that practices the greatest level of solidarity in the world. . . . There are countries that send troops to kill under the pretext of fighting terrorism—while there are other countries that send troops to save lives. Those are the Cubans."[16]

Perhaps another of the reasons why Cuban MI has been so ignored is that almost all those who have benefited live in the developing world, an area often ignored by First World media and governments alike. In addition, reciting the actual numbers themselves resulting from the numerous Cuban programs does little justice to illustrate how millions of people in poor countries have seen their lives affected by Cuban medical support. A common reaction of people in the developed world when they hear about the scope of Cuba's programs is one of disbelief. After all, how could a small and poor developing nation undertake such enormous initiatives in so many programs—and all around the globe?[17] This initiative is inconceivable to many of us in industrialized and "developed" countries, where we are simply not accustomed to such degrees of human solidarity.

Some examples are worth consideration at this point to illustrate the breadth of this vision and are developed more fully in this book. Cuba has established the Escuela Latinoamericana de Medicina (ELAM), the largest medical school in the world with over 24,000 doctors from dozens of Third World countries trained at no cost to the students. Together with Venezuela, Cuba is training another 60,000 doctors for Latin America and the Caribbean, clearly revolutionizing the delivery of public healthcare throughout the region. In addition Cuba has provided free medical treatment in Cuba to 25,000 survivors (mainly children) of the Chernobyl nuclear meltdown, and this occurred at a time when its own economy was falling apart following the implosion of the Soviet Union.

A report on the July 2013 graduating class in medicine provides interesting data. In all, 10,526 students from Cuba's medical schools graduated that year. Of that number 735 were international students, including 8 from the United States and 58 from China. The broader picture of graduates that year for all areas of medical sciences (including nursing, medical technicians, dentists, physiotherapists, and related fields) shows that 29,712 graduated (including 5,020 students from developing nations).[18] Clearly the Cuban government maintains a strong interest in developing large numbers of trained medical personnel, both to assist the local population and to export their expertise. It is worth noting in this regard that the export of Cuban medical services is now the largest generator of hard currency, bringing in over $8 billion annually, almost three times that earned through tourism.

Cuba has been involved in several spheres of MI. For instance, it has sent highly trained specialists in emergency medicine to several countries following natural disasters. As noted earlier, the title of this 2,000-strong contingent is the Henry Reeve Brigade, named after an American who fought and died in the first war of Cuban independence against Spain. The brigade was named shortly after the Bush administration ignored Cuban efforts to provide massive medical support after Hurricane Katrina ravaged New Orleans in 2005. In terms of South-South cooperation in technology transfer, Cuba has engaged in a number of joint ventures with developing countries ensuring the availability of medicines at affordable prices. In addition, medical schools have been set up by Cuban professors in Yemen, Guyana, Ethiopia, Uganda, Ghana, The Gambia, Equatorial Guinea, Haiti, Guinea Bissau, and Timor-Leste, and Cubans are teaching at over a dozen medical schools in the developing world. The largest medical school is in Venezuela, where in February 2012 the first graduating class of 8,000 medical students graduated (so far 20,000 physicians, specialists in integrated general medicine, have graduated, supervised by Cuban medical professors). Finally, Cuba has 25,000 doctors working abroad in the developing world, almost 30 percent of all practicing physicians in the country, ably supported by almost 30,000 medical personnel. Any one of these wide-ranging programs would be exceptional for such a small country—and indeed for a larger industrialized one. Yet when they are examined as a whole, this is a remarkable story.

This book is designed to offer some insights into this unusual approach to medical cooperation with developing countries. It provides an overview of this long ignored aspect of the Cuban revolutionary process, which has been five decades in the making and continues to evolve under Raúl Castro. In an article I co-wrote about Cuba's medical program in Haiti following the earthquake, we referred to this as "One of the World's Best-Kept Secrets"—and indeed it was.[19] But the same title could be used to describe the entire gamut of Cuba's MI programs, since so little has been written about this story of international cooperation, and it is the goal of this book to make a contribution to remedy this gap in the academic literature. It should no longer be kept a secret.

1

Origins and Evolution

From "Beggar's Helper" to a "White-Jacketed Army"

Of all the so-called developing nations, Cuba has by far the best health system. And their outreach program to other countries is unequaled anywhere.

President Jimmy Carter, interviewed in the documentary *Salud!*

Cuba initiated its role in medical internationalism (MI) in 1960, when a team of emergency medicine specialists flew to Chile following a devastating earthquake. Since then it has been involved in scores of medical missions, saving millions of lives. President Carter's comment is therefore pertinent, since no country has come close to equaling Cuba's humanitarian cooperation, particularly in developing countries. Yet surprisingly little is known about the extent of this contribution, given the extremely limited media coverage. Moreover, it strains the imagination to think that a poor country in the Caribbean could play such a major role in international medical cooperation.

Cuba is indeed a poor country. Gross Domestic Product per capita is an estimated $10,200 (compared with $15,600 in Mexico or $12,800 in Costa Rica). Exports are just $5.972 billion (2012 estimate), compared with $370.9 billion and $11.44 billion. For the other two countries, while reserves of foreign exchange and gold in Cuba are just $4.69 billion, compared with $167.1 and $6.85 billion (as of 2012).[1] The right-wing Heritage Foundation sums up Cuba's "socialist command economy" as being "in perennial crisis. The average worker earns less than $25 a month, agriculture is in shambles, mining is depressed, and tourism revenue has proven volatile."[2]

A more balanced (but still critical) analysis was done by Richard Feinberg for the Brookings Institution in 2011. Citing United Nations Development Program data, he noted that per capita national income on a purchasing power parity basis was $5,747—far below that of Chile ($13,651), Uruguay ($13,808), or Costa Rica ($10,870). Agricultural output in 2010 had just recovered to 2000 levels, ending a lost decade of food production. In terms of national investment rates, Cuba was also in the bottom 10th percentile in the world, while Cuban exports of $4 billion in merchandise goods were less than 10 percent of its annual output. The ratio of exports to GDP for Cuba was 20 percent (compared with 38 percent for Chile, 43 percent for Costa Rica, and 61 percent for Barbados). Moreover, Cuba had an external debt of $31.6 billion. Feinberg sums up his findings, noting that Moody's rated Cuba as a Caa1 level in terms of investment risk and concluding, "In short, Cuba is both illiquid and insolvent."[3] Clearly, government rhetoric aside, the Cuban economy was in poor shape.

Yet despite the statistics and the poor economic record, Cuba continues to provide an extraordinary example of humanitarianism. How can this be possible? How did Cuba's commitment originate and evolve?

This chapter seeks to provide a framework for the rest of the book and to offer a basis for an understanding of these fundamental questions. It does so by analyzing the distinctive periods of Cuban medical cooperation and by providing data and observations on the characteristics and significance of each phase. This will make it easier to understand both the rationale behind, and the extent of, the medical internationalism program that has developed over the past five decades. At the risk of erring on the side of being too simplistic, there appear to be four central periods when medical cooperation was particularly noticeable: in the early 1960s in the midst of revolutionary fervor, in the late 1970s (particularly in Africa following Cuba's major military role in Angola), in the late 1990s following two devastating hurricanes in Central America and the Caribbean, and after 2008, when Raúl Castro assumed the presidency of Cuba and the Communist Party of Cuba produced the *lineamientos*, guidelines to improve productivity that were later amended and approved by the Communist Party of Cuba.

Cuba and Internationalism

In the introduction, mention was made of the importance of international cooperation for Cuba, dating from the late nineteenth century, when volunteers from many countries came to support the fight for independence from Spain. Since 1959, government support for internationalism has been a constant, ranging from military aid in the 1960s for revolutionary struggles in several Latin American and African countries to civilian support, mainly in medicine, education, and construction, which developed apace in the 1970s and 1980s. To take one example, Cuba's literacy program "Yo, sí puedo" (Yes, I Can) is currently being used in 30 countries, and has taught more than 8 million to read and write. There was always a strong anticolonialist element in this policy, with Cuba's own history as a colony of Spain until 1898 not too distant a memory.

The civilian aspects of internationalism gradually outweighed the military aspects (not withstanding its significant military role in Angola and to a lesser extent Ethiopia), although this has not been sufficiently recognized. This book focuses specifically on medical cooperation, which reached its zenith in the 1990s. In his seminal work of 1989, *To Make a World Safe for Revolution: Cuba's Foreign Policy*, Jorge Domínguez summarizes the early years of Cuban internationalism, when the political aspects (and the struggle for survival) were of paramount importance: "The first rule governing this aspect of foreign policy [what he terms the Rule of Internationalism] is that Cuba supports revolutions in other countries." This form of military aid was common in Latin America, where Cuba provided military training, arms, and volunteers to several guerrilla groups. By the 1980s this policy focus had shifted away from military involvement with liberation movements, and Domínguez spends almost five pages (see 171–75) outlining the wide range of Cuban civilian cooperation that had developed by the mid-1980s. The figures were impressive: by that time 250,000 Cubans had served in Africa (in military or civilian functions); by 1987 some 24,000 students from 82 countries were studying in Cuba for free; 4,500 Cuban teachers were working in 20 countries (over 20,000 had already served overseas); and sports specialists were working in 18 countries. In addition, 3,044 medical personnel were working in 27 countries, representing 8 percent of Cuba's doctors, and Cuba had founded a medical school in South Yemen in 1976.[4] While these numbers pale in comparison with the number of Cuban medical personnel working abroad now, they illustrate the basis—over 30 years earlier—for the current approach.

In 1979 Cuba was elected leader of the Non-Aligned Movement (currently with 118 member countries), emphasizing its role as a force among developing countries, in many ways becoming the recognized leader of what was then called the Third World. (It was also elected to lead the movement from 2006 to 2009.) Cuba's increased role in sports and culture around the globe supplemented its military prestige following its military victories in Angola, and its medical and educational credentials had long been established. As a member of the socialist Common Market since 1972, and with support from Moscow, Cuba assumed a significant role on the world stage, both as an ally of the socialist governments and as a member of the Global South community. Starting in the 1970s, Havana now sought to normalize relations, particularly with governments in Latin America, rather than assist guerrilla forces in overthrowing them. The normalization of relations with several countries in the area gradually occurred, reversing the stormy years of the early 1960s when all countries of the Western Hemisphere (with the exception of Mexico and Canada) had broken diplomatic relations with Havana. Now was a time for rebuilding, a process in which cooperation and internationalism became important. Michael Erisman refers to the period of 1972–85 as being “the halcyon days of Cuban globalism,” one in which Havana developed an approach to counterdependency, while solidifying its burgeoning Third World leadership.[5]

If the first decade of Cuba’s foreign policy during the revolutionary process can be summarized as following a foreign policy of proletarian internationalism often accompanied by military aid for liberation and guerrilla movements, the 1970s saw a different strategy being implemented. In many ways, the execution of Ernesto “Che” Guevara in Bolivia in October 1967 symbolized the end of this approach, although some support did continue for liberation movements in Central America during the 1970s. While continuing to strengthen its role with the socialist community of Europe, an approach in which Cuba was supported financially by the Soviet Union, an improved relationship with Third World countries became the basis of Havana’s international strategy. The result, as Domínguez has indicated, helped to confirm Cuba’s rapidly emerging role on the world stage as a significant political actor: “Cuba is a small country, but it has the foreign policy of a big power.”[6] Humanitarian internationalism was a major facet of this foreign policy approach in this stage.

This commitment to international cooperation can be seen from a comparison with the United States development assistance at this time. In the mid-1980s while the United States sent abroad one Peace Corps volunteer or Agency for International Development (AID) employee per 34,700 U.S. citizens, Cuba sent one civilian co-operant for every 625 Cubans. In addition, whereas in 1984–85 some 7,000 university scholarships were provided in the United States to students from developing countries, Cuba had 22,000 scholarship students from 82 countries studying at high schools and universities.[7] Internationalism was increasingly ingrained into the Cuban body politic as a fundamental aspect of both foreign policy and government priorities. To this day it remains as part of the Cuban DNA.

In synthesis it is important to remember that the concept of internationalism, including sharing resources, developing mutually beneficial relationships, and strengthening ties among developing nations, is rooted in Cuban history and can be found throughout the distinctive periods of revolutionary Cuba. The sense of cooperation is also taught from preschool times, and these values are inculcated in all Cubans throughout their school years. As Michael Erisman has noted, "Such nationalistic aspirations to maximize the country's effective sovereignty are an integral element of the Fidelista ethos and have greatly influenced the Revolution's international agenda from the beginning: they are likewise deeply embedded in the larger society's political culture. This sentiment traces its roots to the earliest days of the independence struggle, and its resonance continues today."[8] Within this humanitarian internationalism, medical cooperation has been noticeable since 1960 and during four periods in particular.

The Early (Heady) Years: Revolutionary Romanticism

The Cuban revolutionary movement came to power on January 1, 1959, after President Fulgencio Batista (who had seized control in a military coup in 1952) was overthrown. Fidel Castro was the undisputed leader of the revolutionary process that resulted, a man who was able to channel the national frustration at the corruption and brutality under Batista into support for his nationalistic reform goals. While the honeymoon did not last long (resulting in 10 percent of the population eventually seeking exile), the level of support during that first year was unprecedented.

Sweeping legislation was passed, mainly benefiting those sectors of the population that had previously been exploited or ignored. Agrarian reform, the Urban Reform Law, reductions in electricity and telephone rates, the opening of universities to the underprivileged, legislation against racism, job creation programs, a reinvigorated cultural policy offering opportunities to all, support for women to provide training and job opportunities, the beginning of a national daycare program, the provision of food at subsidized prices, and a massive literacy campaign—all were needed, and most were initially popular. Societal polarization soon set in, however, as the revolution tilted leftwards, and many of these reforms were paid for at the expense of the traditional urban wealthy class, who now lost their extensive privileges. Private schools were nationalized, a national curriculum was introduced in schools, luxury taxes were introduced, private beaches were turned over to the population at large, businesses were expropriated, and the urban and agrarian reform laws came at the expense of losses to the elite and foreign investors (mainly American companies).

The almost universal support for the *barbudos* (literally "bearded" guerrillas) started to disappear as most of the middle class left for Miami, expecting to wait just months before Washington, incensed at the leftist rhetoric emanating from Havana, took steps to overthrow the revolutionaries now in charge. Several hundred people were executed, mainly for crimes against the 20,000 murdered under Batista's regime, and U.S. media railed against the new rulers, although they had largely remained silent on the widespread abuses under Batista. The societal polarization also had a devastating impact on health services. By late 1961 almost half of Cuba's 6,000 physicians had left, as had all but a handful of professors at Cuba's only faculty of medicine at the University of Havana. Yet Fidel Castro pressed on, convinced that the vast majority of the population still supported the necessary reforms.

Cuba's first example of medical internationalism occurred in the midst of this heady atmosphere of nationalism, sweeping reforms, substantial benefits for the underprivileged, advances in culture, societal polarization, increasing tension between Washington and the United States, and economic plans being composed often on the run. It was a time when the young brash nationalistic leaders seemed to believe themselves invincible and their dream of continent-wide revolution unassailable. In the midst of this mixture of revolution and radical reform, Cuba first volunteered its medical expertise abroad, after a major earthquake took place in Valdivia, southern Chile, in May 1960. It registered 9.5 on the Richter scale—the largest earthquake in the twentieth century—and between 2,000 and 6,000 people were killed. (In 1971 and 2010, Cuba also sent medical brigades to Chile following earthquakes there.)

At that time diplomatic relations between Cuba and Chile were strained. Jorge Alessandri, candidate of the right wing, had been elected in 1958, narrowly defeating the leftist opposition candidate Salvador Allende. During his presidency he supported a pro-business policy, limiting the government role in the economy and imposing wage restrictions. Closer ties with the United States resulted, and during his presidency (1958–64) the diplomatic relationship with Cuba chilled. Yet when the earthquake occurred, Cuba immediately sent a medical brigade to help, despite its own dwindling medical resources. Many years later, Salvador Allende remembered the Cuban role in helping his country: "I watched as Cuba mobilized . . . and beyond the (fraternal) attitude of the government, the obligation of its leaders,

I witnessed your attitude—the attitude of the people of Cuba. I saw the trucks rolling by [carrying] the anonymous generosity of people who gave what they needed for themselves."[9]

Cuba did not hesitate to share its scarce resources with the people of Chile. Ideology played no role in the Cuban government's analysis—or if it did, it was quickly overtaken by basic humanitarianism. The same approach was taken three years later in Algeria. In his study of Cuba's role in Africa, Piero Gleijeses has illustrated how the revolutionary government went out on a limb to help the FLN liberation movement, which was fighting for independence from France. In 1961 and 1962 Cuba provided arms and shipped wounded guerrillas, as well as Algerian orphans, to Cuba for medical treatment. In doing so, Fidel Castro risked the wrath of France's president, Charles de Gaulle—one of the very few allies that Cuba still had, since U.S. pressure to break relations with Cuba and isolate the socialist nation had increased.

Yet the revolutionary government remained a stalwart supporter of Algeria, led by Ahmed Ben Bella, who visited Cuba in October 1962 and outlined the multitude of challenges facing his country after the exodus of French professionals from their former colony. Fidel Castro, who had witnessed the same phenomenon in his own country as doctors fled to Miami, offered Cuban assistance. Despite the shortage of physicians in Cuba, he then invited Cuban medical personnel to volunteer their services in Algeria.[10] In the end 45 men and 10 women volunteered for the mission, including 29 doctors, 3 dentists, 15 nurses, and 8 technicians. It was headed by José Ramón Machado Ventura, later minister of health, who summarized their interpretation of the mission: "Really what we were offering was so little—just like a beggar who offers help. But we knew that the people of Algeria needed the assistance even more than we did, and we also knew that they deserved it."[11]

The impetuous, emotional response to the Algerian situation in many ways mirrored the somewhat chaotic, fast-moving tempo of developments in Havana at that time. For Fidel Castro the situation was straightforward: the newly independent North African country badly needed medical support and had requested Cuban assistance. Larger-scale concepts of geopolitics and the desire to refrain from alienating potential allies were pushed to the background, subordinated to the needs of a population that was desperately in search of something that Cuba could share in however limited a fashion. For the revolutionary government of Cuba at that time, the most pressing issues were international solidarity and the need for basic humanitarianism. Many Cubans could appreciate the situation of Algeria, since for decades both countries had been the victims of foreign domination and bore the scars of colonial rule. Both had suffered as opposition to the incoming revolutionary governments resulted in a brain drain of educated personnel. Moreover, both had been involved in a long war for independence and had paid dearly in that struggle. For the government in Havana, the picture was clear: Ben Bella had asked for Cuban assistance, and despite its limitations, Cuba could help, even if in only a minor way. Cuba was now benefiting from Soviet support following the rupture of diplomatic relations in January 1961 by Washington and the October 1962 Missile Crisis, and had some degree of financial and military security. For the revolutionary leadership, providing support was a moral imperative, and so the basis for Cuban medical internationalism was established.

In May 1963, a Cubana Airlines plane transported the medical delegation to Algeria. Preparations had been terrible. The volunteers had no idea how long they would remain in Algeria, where they would be located, or what they would be doing. They didn't even have passports—just sheets of paper from the Ministry of Foreign Relations in Havana. It was extremely cold when they arrived, and they were ill prepared. (They had been advised to bring short-sleeved shirts, since it was a tropical country.) They didn't speak the language or share the same customs or religion. They were regarded with suspicion by French and Algerian doctors, who could not understand why they had volunteered to come to Algeria, much less why they refused to charge patients for their medical services and treated women with such respect.

This was the first large Cuban medical delegation. The personnel stayed for just over a year, when they were replaced by a second mission in June 1964, which consisted of 24 doctors, 4 dentists, 24 nurses, and 9 health technicians, who helped to set up a national health system in Algeria. These early missions formed the basis for later medical internationalism operations by Cuba. In many ways this approach was based on spontaneous decisions made by the revolutionary government, with the medical staff launching themselves into the unknown and providing medical support on strictly humanitarian grounds. Pragmatism and careful planning were not part of the mission preparations. The medical personnel were there because they were needed. When viewed with the advantage of historical oversight, this experience also constituted the apprenticeship of much larger, more ambitious programs that developed in subsequent decades.

In the 1960s Cuba volunteered its medical cooperation to several other developing nations, mainly in Africa but also in North Vietnam, where specialists in surgery, orthopedics, anesthesia, and maxillofacial areas provided support. In the Congo (from 1965) Cuban medical staff worked alongside the guerrillas supporting Patrice Lumumba in the struggle against Mobutu Sese Seko. At the time of the arrival of the first Cubans, there were only nine doctors in the country for a population of almost 900,000.[12] The situation was made worse by an outbreak of polio in 1966. The Cuban government then sent Dr. Helenio Ferrer, head of epidemiology on the island, to plan a nationwide campaign to prevent the spread of the disease. As a result, vaccines were flown in from Moscow, and Cuban medical personnel were distributed in the three regions of the country to administer the polio vaccines. Some 61,000 Congolese children were vaccinated in Africa's first anti-polio campaign and indeed the continent's first mass vaccination campaign. In a February 2014 interview, orthopedic surgeon Rodrigo Álvarez Cambras, a participant in this mission, emphasized the far-reaching impact of the Cuban contribution and the difficult circumstances they encountered, since there were so few physicians in the country.

In 1966, a small group of Cuban medical personnel also arrived in Guinea Bissau, at the request of guerrilla leader Amílcar Cabral, who had visited Fidel Castro and requested assistance. They had come to help in a guerrilla-controlled territory of some 540,000 people. Prior to their arrival there had only been one foreign doctor for the entire population. Duties revolved around helping both the guerrilla army and the civilians, and since the need was so great, the Cuban doctors sought out talented Guineans and trained them in basic nursing skills for two months. Several of their trainees later pursued formal nursing studies in Havana. In Angola, the first wave of Cuban physicians pursued a similar apprenticeship program, teaching basic nursing skills to Angolan youth. This idea of training local students in basic medical procedures was an approach continued by Cuba in several developing countries—a practical, cost-effective solution to a desperate need.

A summary of the challenges faced by the Cuban medical staff during this period and in several African countries can be found in the collection of anecdotes edited by Hedelberto López Blanch. These range from multiple medical challenges to cultural difficulties. (In Angola, for example, some patients refused help from black Cuban doctors, believing them to be Angolan. Instead, they requested help from "the Cubans"—and were only convinced otherwise when they heard the accent of the physician.)[13]

Cuban physicians were soon working in dozens of countries, providing elementary medical care, largely in rural areas. Piero Gleijeses notes that Cuba's role in Africa, "was an act of true solidarity, which brought Cuba no tangible benefit, but which also came with a real material cost."[14] The importance of this particular mission resides in the fact that it was the first in a long history of medical cooperation missions.

Cuban Medical Internationalism from the 1970s: The African Experience

The second stage of Cuba's medical internationalism program can be dated from the mid-1970s, especially after its role in Angola grew. It derived great benefit from the experiences in sub-Saharan Africa after the late 1960s. This period lasted several years, involved the contribution of hundreds of medical personnel (tending to both military and civilians), and laid the groundwork for the expansion of Cuban medical cooperation throughout Africa. The original approach of providing medical support to a massive military mission soon evolved into a multipronged strategy. This involved sending large numbers of medical personnel to dozens of African countries in order to provide basic medical treatment in underserved communities (a program usually referred to by the Spanish acronym PIS, the Programa Integral de Salud or Comprehensive Health Program). In addition Cuba provided training in Havana to thousands of young people showing potential for medical studies and established medical faculties in several African countries. While Cuba provided medical cooperation in several areas of Latin America during these years, the role in Africa dwarfed those efforts. As Michael Erisman has shown, "sub-Saharan Africa was its main theater of operations. During the heyday of such activity in the early 1980s, for example, 40.8 percent of all such personnel were posted in Africa in 1981, and that rose to 47.3 percent in 1984."[15]

Cuba's military role in the Angolan struggle was important, helping to support the MPLA, which fought against two western-backed parties, UNITA and the FNLA, and to retain power as the national government. Between 1975 and 1991, more than 300,000 Cubans fought in Angola, while the 1987–88 campaign against South African troops involved 55,000 soldiers. What is not so widely known is that some 50,000 civilians also worked in Angola, principally in healthcare, education, and construction. In all, some 2,000 Cubans died fighting in Angola, a significant sacrifice made by Cuba, which was referred to with respect by Nelson Mandela, since it ensured the freedom of Namibia, and contributed to the overturning of apartheid.[16]

Mandela expressed his gratitude to Cuba on many occasions both for its role in helping to overthrown apartheid in South Africa and also providing medical cooperation throughout the African continent. He once noted that "Cubans came to our region as doctors, teachers, soldiers, agricultural workers, but never as colonizers. They have shared the same trenches as us in the struggle against colonialism, underdevelopment, and apartheid. Hundreds of Cubans have given their lives, literally, in a struggle that was, first and foremost, not theirs but ours. As Southern Africans we salute them. We vow never to forget this unparalleled example of selfless internationalism."[17] After he was released from prison, the first country outside Africa that he visited was Cuba. Moreover, at Mandela's funeral in December 2013, Raúl Castro was one of just six leaders invited to address the South African population, along with leaders from China, India, neighboring Namibia, Brazil, and the United States. This was a clear sign of respect for Cuba's internationalist role in southern Africa. He was introduced by African National Conference chair Baleka Mbete as a president of "a tiny island, a people who liberated us."[18]

The situation in Angola in some ways resembled the case of Algeria, in that the withdrawal of the colonial power (Portugal) and the granting of independence to the former colony in 1975 left a political and administrative vacuum. In 1975 an estimated 350,000 Portuguese residents departed, and at the lowest point of medical care there were only 14 doctors left in the country. They were joined by an initial supply of 200 Cuban medical personnel, and by 1989 hundreds of Cuban teachers had come to work in local schools, while 323 Cuban doctors—41 percent of the medical personnel in the government-controlled area—also worked there. By contrast, at that time according to one estimate there were only 230 Angolan doctors for the population of 9 million.[19] This second wave of Cuban doctors and nurses, most of whom arrived in the late 1970s and early 1980s, was far larger than the first stage of medical internationalism of the early 1960s, and their role was delineated in all of the African countries in which they worked. In practical terms this meant that in 1977 Cuba was providing between 45 and 84 percent of the physicians working in six countries in Africa, an extraordinary responsibility. Speaking in 1997 to an international medical conference, Fidel Castro summarized the basic philosophy of Cuba's contribution:

> Indeed, our Revolution is not a revolution of millionaires. Instead, it is one carried out by the poor, and is one which dreams of ensuring the well-being not only of our own poor, but rather all the poor in this world. And that is why we talk of internationalism—and we do not just talk about it. We also carry it out. And we have not just contributed material supplies—we have also shed our own blood.[20]

It is useful to bear in mind the domestic context of Cuba when analyzing this level of medical cooperation, since in the early 1970s the country was in the midst of major changes. Following the October 1967 execution of Che Guevara in Bolivia, the Soviet Union pressured Cuba to decrease its foreign military exploits, a policy with which Havana disagreed. In 1970 the failure of the "10 Million Ton" sugar harvest campaign meant that Cuba's attempts to lessen its dependence on the Soviet Union had failed. Instead the country then depended increasingly on Moscow for economic support and subsidies, and Soviet political influence grew as a consequence. In 1972 Cuba joined the Council for Mutual Economic Assistance (referred to by the acronyms CAME and COMECON), the trade association of Communist nations, cementing this alliance. In economics and to a certain extent also in politics it was a time of increasing orthodoxy, central planning, and pragmatism. Cuba was advised by Soviet leaders to reduce its military support and humanitarianism abroad and concentrate instead on making its economy more efficient.

Yet while Cuba listened to Moscow in terms of domestic economic policy, its foreign policy strategy remained distinctive from that of the Soviet Union, and in fact its role in some countries—such as Angola and Nicaragua—angered the Kremlin.[21] In general the 1970s and 1980s saw Cuba normalizing relations with countries throughout Latin America and the Caribbean and developing closer ties in sub-Saharan Africa, where its cooperation programs were particularly active. A study of Cuban developmental aid personnel abroad between 1977 and 1986 illustrates this. In the Middle East and Africa, for instance, there were 5,403 civilian workers from Cuba deployed in 1977, rising to a high of 9,435 in 1981, before falling to 8,540 in 1986. In Latin America and the Caribbean this increased rapidly from 190 in 1978 (mainly in Jamaica) to 5,420 in 1984.[22]

Cuban medical cooperation spread quickly in Africa after the Angolan experience, particularly in the countries of sub-Saharan Africa. According to Julie Feinsilver, over 30 countries in Africa were receiving Cuban medical support by late 1988, as were others around the world. These included Algeria (which began in 1963), Mali (1965), Congo (1965), Tanzania (1966), Guinea-Conakry (1967), Vietnam (1969), Democratic (South) Yemen (1972), Equatorial Guinea (1973), Laos (1973), Guinea-Bissau (1975), Sao Tomé and Príncipe (1976), Angola (1976), Guyana (1976), Cape Verde Islands (1976), Mozambique (1977), Benin (1977), Ethiopia (1977), Saharan Arab Republic (1977), Iraq (1978), Kampuchea (1979), Nicaragua (1979), Uganda (1979), Burundi (1980), Seychelles (1980), Ghana (1983), Kuwait (1985), Burkina Faso (1985), Zimbabwe (1986), Sri Lanka (1986), Maldives (1988), and Botswana (1988).[23] This was a humanitarian contribution that the industrialized countries could not come close to matching.

Medical cooperation under Raúl Castro is now a major source of income for the national economy. In the case of Brazil, for instance, Cuba deployed 11,400 doctors in 2013–14, and this exportation of medical services will bring in some $400 million to Havana. Significantly, however, most poorer countries in the developing world have traditionally received these services at no cost or at a heavily subsidized rate. Others that could afford to make a contribution for professional services did so. In the case of post-conflict Angola, for instance, Cuba charged the government $1,100 per month for the services of an experienced physician. By 1981 there were 686 medical personnel working there (335 doctors, 12 dentists, 174 nurses, 157 medical technicians and 8 support workers).[24] Angola has extensive oil reserves, and as a result the country was charged an agreed-upon rate, one that was low by international standards—yet helped to subsidize medical cooperation elsewhere.

Cuba has also been involved in training students from these regions back in Havana and in establishing medical schools in several developing countries. Cuba's interest in training medical students in Cuba during the 1980s continued to grow. By 1990, 16,700 foreign students had graduated from Cuban schools, including 5,800 at the university level. In terms of medicine, a similar level of support can be noted. By the end of 1984, Cuba was supporting 1,800 scholarship students from 75 developing nations who were studying to be physicians, medical technicians, or medical specialists. Feinsilver has noted that "1,523 foreign doctors had graduated prior to the 1987–88 academic year, another 355 doctors had completed postgraduate training, and 752 middle-level health technicians (including nurses) had graduated." She adds that in 1990–91 a total of 3,587 medical personnel (whose specialties were not defined) graduated, with most coming from the Americas (1,418), sub-Saharan Africa (1,507), and North Africa (517).[25] The Cuban government paid all costs of education for these students.

A parallel approach to training doctors in Cuba from the developing countries of Africa and elsewhere was to establish medical faculties in various countries. This was an important development, since in many ways it was a far more sustainable and cost-effective healthcare program for these countries than importing physicians. As a result, faculties of medicine, employing Cuban professors, were established in Yemen (1976), Guyana (1984), Ethiopia (1984), Uganda (1986), Ghana (1991), The Gambia (1999), Equatorial Ghana (2000), Haiti (2001), Guinea Bissau (2004), Venezuela (2005), and Timor-Leste (2010).

The Cuban model of healthcare since 1959 has always emphasized preventive rather than curative approaches, which are cheaper and more effective. This proved a challenge to most postcolonial governments in Africa, which have traditionally preferred to invest in hospitals, technology, and imported medicines, following the curative model promoted by the colonial administrations. Long accustomed to the systems introduced by their colonial rulers, it has often been difficult for developing countries to move to more innovative approaches. Some, however, have been able to adapt to more pragmatic strategies and have benefited from Cuban cooperation. The Cuban philosophy argues that South/South cooperation is essential, that it is important to pay attention to indigenous traditions and to cooperate with them, and that capacity-building and training of local talent to ensure its sustainability are all essential components of any strategy to improve a nation's health. The Cuban approach was unlike the accepted way of thinking. The countries named above also agreed with the Cuban philosophy and were able—with the support of professors from Cuba—to train their own physicians.

Cuba's experience in setting up a medical faculty in The Gambia is in many ways illustrative of its role during this second stage.[26] In April 1999 President Yahya A.J.J. Jammeh visited Havana, where he discussed with the revolutionary government the establishment of a medical school there. Things moved quickly after Fidel Castro agreed to the request, and the first medical classes were given in October 1999. The initial cohort of Gambian doctors, educated in their homeland, graduated in 2006. Working with the Royal Victoria Teaching Hospital, by 2004 the school (staffed by 12 Cuban professors) had 109 students enrolled. This facility was important in a country where life expectancy in 2002 was 54, where 82 percent of the population lived on less than $2 per day, and where there were only four physicians for every 100,000 people. In September 2007, the Cuban program was amended, and in March 2008 the New Program for the Teaching of

Community Doctors in Gambia was established in four locations, in which Gambian students were supervised by Cuban professors, working in clinics but also taking theoretical classes taught by Cuban medical professors. Thirty-five students passed the first year, supervised by 29 professors. This approach, similar to the hands-on model used in the Barrio Adentro program in Venezuela, seeks to increase the number of doctors in The Gambia, and the results have been encouraging.

The preparation for the curriculum to be taught illustrates the pragmatic Cuban approach to health education, employed in all of the medical programs established during this time. In order to determine the material to be taught, meetings were held between Gambian government officials, leaders from the West African Health Organization, the World Health Organization representative in the country, and the Cuban faculty. The objective was to decide upon the most pertinent medical training for the new faculty. The first Cuban director of the school, Dr. Arturo Menéndez Cabezas, noted the importance of community involvement and for practical training and "the need for general practitioners with skills in basic medical specialties, who were capable of working in difficult situations, as well as being prepared in disaster management."[27] His role was important in establishing a medical program that has saved thousands of lives.

This ability to serve in underserved areas, "working in difficult conditions"—often where there is no water or electricity, much less sophisticated diagnostic equipment—is a fundamental aspect of the pragmatic, hands-on approach favored by Cuban medical education. The objective is to train medical personnel who find themselves in underserved areas of poor countries, far away from middle-class urban areas and high-tech diagnostic supports. It is in the *barrios* and impoverished rural areas where the need is greatest and where facilities are often lacking. However, many directors of professional medical associations in countries where Cuban personnel are working have yet to come to terms with this approach. They criticize the Cubans' approach to medicine, yet their own training does not prepare students to work where they are most needed. This has been seen in Honduras, Ecuador, Venezuela, and most recently in Brazil, where the government of Dilma Rousseff has used the Pan American Health Organization (PAHO) to employ the services of some 11,400 Cuban physicians in rural and marginalized areas. When they arrived, the Cuban physicians were met by legal challenges from professional associations and even by threats and insults.

This period represents the coming of age of Cuban MI, with a concentration on cooperation with several African countries. The initial experience in Angola during the civil war was important in showing the potential that Cuba had in terms of exporting its medical services. In later years the focus has broadened to include Cuban medical workers providing primary care in dozens of African countries, as well as the training of African physicians both in Cuba and at several regional medical faculties.

During this time Cuban MI also continued to grow in Latin America, although not with the same intensity as in Africa. In her study *Healing the Masses: Cuban Health Politics at Home and Abroad*, Julie Feinsilver notes that by July 1991 over 1,000 Cuban doctors were working abroad and that more than 20,000 physicians and another 20,000 health workers had already served in over 26 countries. She shows that Cuba sent abroad proportionately more medical co-operants than the United States, the Soviet Union, and China, concluding that this had "made Cuba a world medical power in the eyes of many international organization officials."[28] Recent comments of the current president of the World Health Organization, Margaret Chan, and of the secretary-general of the United Nations, Ban Ki-Moon, show that this respect has only grown in the decades since.

By the late 1980s Cuba's medical prowess abroad had been established, largely because of its extensive cooperation in sub-Saharan Africa. The large number of medical graduates in Cuba from these impoverished countries, continued commitment to badly needed primary healthcare through the Comprehensive Health Program (PIS) in many developing countries, and the establishment of medical faculties in the region all helped to strengthen this reputation. Cuba was already contributing more to the health of the Third World than the wealthy nations. Events in Central America would soon conspire to encourage Cuba to move even faster and to dream larger in its approach to helping others.

The Year 1998 and the Mitch Factor

In 1998 the devastating impact of Hurricane Mitch in Central America and that of Hurricane Georges in Haiti resulted in a number of initiatives that launched Cuba's medical internationalism into a dramatically new stage. The PIS was now providing heavily subsidized medical care to 29 countries (including 20 in Africa),[29] but it was Cuba's role closer to home that soon became the focus of the government's efforts. Prior to this stage Cuban MI had focused largely on Africa. The role there continued, particularly in sub-Saharan countries, yet soon a new focal point for Cuban MI developed following two major natural disasters.

This is not to say that the role of Cuban medical personnel in Africa decreased; it continued, as table 1.1 illustrates. The efforts of thousands of Cuban healthcare workers had a major impact on the health profile of many countries in Africa. For example, the number of malaria cases in Gambia dropped from 600,000 to 200,000 between 2002 and 2004. Infant mortality also dropped in areas where Cuban physicians worked, from 59 to 7.8 per 1,000 live births in Ghana, from 48 to 10.6 in Eritrea, and from 131 to 35.5 in Equatorial Guinea. These services were offered to the population at no charge.

Natural disasters closer to home resulted in a new stage of Cuban medical cooperation. Hurricane Georges devastated Haiti in September 1998, causing over 600 deaths and $6 billion in damages. It was followed in October by Hurricane Mitch, the deadliest Atlantic hurricane since 1780, which wreaked havoc in Central America. Between 22,000 and 30,000 people were killed, and 2.7 million people were left homeless, mainly in Honduras and Nicaragua. In November the leaders of Central America issued an appeal for assistance, and by the end of December over 400 Cuban medical workers had arrived. This increased to 2,000 emergency medical specialists at one point before settling down to an average of 900, which remained constant for several years. The countries who suffered the brunt of the hurricanes had extremely poor relations with Cuba and were allies of U.S. policy in the region. Yet again, for the government in Havana the need for humanitarian support was more important than ideology.

Assisting the countries involved a two-track strategy. Cuba made the commitment to keep medical personnel in the areas affected as long as the governments there wanted them to stay. They remain to this day, although Cuba is now paid a modest amount for those services. In addition Cuba has trained over 2,000 physicians from the region in order to support a sustainable healthcare system. It is clear that in both countries the impact of Cuban MI has been significant.

In Guatemala, for instance, some 3,500 Cuban doctors had already served by 2009, mainly in indigenous communities, and at that time almost 400 remained. By 2009 Cuban medical staff had carried out 26 million medical consults, performed 144,000 surgical operations, and assisted at 70,712 births. In areas where they worked (17 of Guatemala's 22 provinces) infant and maternal mortality rates had been reduced by more than half. By this time some 470 Guatemalans had graduated as doctors from Havana's Latin American School of Havana (ELAM), with an additional 600 still studying in Cuba. In February 2014 a report was issued on the occa-

Table 1.1. Cuba's Comprehensive Health Program in 15 African nations, November 1998–June 2004

Country	Visits to doctors	Visits to pediatricians	House calls by physicians	Deliveries	Surgeries	Vaccinations
Botswana	98,275		583	560	2,831	1,648
Burundi	29,564	6,507	250	1,380	682	939
Burkina Faso	146,073	39,059	10,851	4,312	5,984	283,303
Chad	41,368	4,245			558	
Eritrea	305,575	67,702	3,261	935	3,707	
Gambia	3,757,036	1,235,492	221,851	220,794	40,074	328,812
Ghana	5,990,431	1,748,815	1,860,019	70,566	68,637	203,619
Equatorial Guinea	1,197,793		239,527	17,891	28,867	18,863
Lesotho	459,867			1,110	2,831	
Mali	748,867		42,240	33,090	6,449	98,125
Namibia	2,863,313	333,600	94,444	14,119	5,257	3,887,129
Niger	748,911	77,929	5,186	17,981	17,977	220,803
Sahrawi Arab PDR	12,573				317	
Tanzania	6,324				50	
Zimbabwe	3,115,085	808,080		21,169	58,315	
Total	**19,521,099**	**4,321,429**	**2,478,212**	**403,907**	**242,536**	**5,043,241**

Source: John M. Kirk and H. Michael Erisman, *Cuban Medical Internationalism: Origins, Evolution, and Goals* (New York: Palgrave Macmillan, 2009), 117.

sion of the arrival of a new coordinator of the Cuban medical cooperation program. It was noted that there were 427 Cuban health workers found in 16 provinces, and it estimated that Cuban medical personnel had saved the lives of 287,658 people.[30]

Honduras presented a similar picture in 2009, where some 300 medical personnel were working in the country's 18 departments. In all, 1,550 Cubans had served there. They had carried out 16 million medical consults, performed 455,000 operations and saved the lives of 236,000 people. In total 461 students had graduated from ELAM as doctors, while 1,200 remained studying in Cuba. Cuban medical staff had assisted at 85,000 births. In the regions where Cuban medical personnel worked, the infant mortality rate was just over 10 per 1,000 live births—compared to the national average of 37.[31]

The need for a sustainable healthcare system in these countries depended upon there being enough physicians to staff it. ELAM was established in November 1999 to meet this need, training students who were from the affected areas. Students with high school education from poorer backgrounds (who could not otherwise afford to pay for a university education) were chosen for the six-year ELAM program, since it was expected that they would be more prepared to return home and practice medicine in their own communities. In the initial years students from Central America represented a large part of the student body, as table 1.2 illustrates. Due to linguistic differences, Havana subsequently decided to train hundreds of Haitian students, as well as other francophone students from Africa, at a special medical faculty in the eastern city of Santiago de Cuba.

Two other key elements of Cuba's MI program were developed during this period. While Cuba's commitment to support the countries most affected by Hurricane Mitch was a focal point of their MI program after 1998, another key feature was the delivery of specialized emergency teams in response to natural disasters. As a result the government founded the Henry Reeve Contingent. While Cuba has provided this type of support since 1960, the development of this approach to natural emergencies into a nationwide contingent had not been established before.

Also significant during this post-Mitch period has been the development of Cuba's medical role in Venezuela. This is by far Cuba's largest medical cooperation program, with some 30,000 medical personnel working throughout the country at its peak. This was initiated with the arrival of Cuban personnel to work in the program "Misión Barrio Adentro," originally located in the underserved areas of Caracas. While this program continues,

Table 1.2. ELAM enrollment of students from Central America, 2004–2005

Country	Pre-med	1st year	2nd year	3rd year	4th year	5th year	6th year	Total
El Salvador	79	77	61	81	111	86	119	614
Guatemala	93	46	58	64	91	158	187	697
Honduras	84	54	46	66	96	150	215	711
Nicaragua	50	52	46	61	73	99	178	559

Source: John M. Kirk and H. Michael Erisman, *Cuban Medical Internationalism: Origins, Evolution, and Goals* (New York: Palgrave Macmillan, 2009), 128.

Cuban medical workers are also working in the hundreds of clinics, medical centers, and hospitals established by the Chávez government. Many are also involved in "Misión Milagro," the ophthalmology program that to date has restored the sight of over a million Venezuelans. A final plank in the development of a new approach to the delivery of public healthcare was the commitment signed by former presidents Fidel Castro and Hugo Chávez to train 60,000 physicians in Venezuela, using the experience of Cuban doctors and medical professors. There is no larger medical education cooperation program in the world than this model.

Also important was Operación Milagro. Some 3 million people from Cuba, Latin America, the Caribbean, and some parts of Africa have benefited from this program, which provides eye surgery at no charge, principally to people of limited means. Operación Milagro has now spread throughout Latin America, with dozens of clinics. As in several other public health initiatives, it revolves around two key components—Cuban human capital and financial support from the Venezuelan government.

One of the most neglected aspects of Cuba's medical internationalism is its role in treating almost 25,000 children (mainly from the Ukraine) following the explosion of the Chernobyl nuclear reactor in 1986. Cuba began to treat these children in Havana just as the Soviet Union was collapsing, taking with it some 85 percent of Cuba's trade. Despite the onset of the "Special Period" in Cuba that followed the implosion of the Soviet Union, as well as the belt-tightening and shortages that resulted, Cuba continued to treat the children at no charge until 2011, when the program concluded.

In many ways the decade starting in 1998 was key to the formation of the current MI profile in Cuba. It was during this time that medical cooperation programs expanded throughout Latin America and the Caribbean. To a certain extent this expansion was due to the strong personal commitment of Fidel Castro, whose ideas resulted in a number of extraordinary healthcare initiatives. At the graduation of the first cohort of students at ELAM, he outlined the basic philosophy of Cuba's MI. He first assessed the value of training a doctor—approximately $300,000 in the United States. Cuba, however, was currently training 12,000 doctors on the island (at a value of over $3 billion, using international data for medical education), and was planning to train 100,000 doctors from developing nations within a decade (a contribution to the poor countries of the world worth $30 billion). "What is the secret?" he pondered. "It lies in the solid fact that human capital is worth far more than financial capital. Human capital involves not only knowledge but also—and this is essential—conscience, ethics, solidarity, truly humane feelings, a spirit of sacrifice, heroism, and the ability to make a little go a long way."[32] This combination has been the hallmark of Cuban MI since 1960, and Castro's role in developing these initiatives is perhaps the single most important factor.

The Year 2006 and the Approach to Medical Internationalism of Raúl Castro

If Cuban medical internationalism during the previous four decades can be explained to a large degree by the personal initiatives of Fidel Castro, the direction since 2006 can be understood by analyzing the goals of his brother, Raúl Castro, and in particular his efforts to bring about economic reform within the socialist model. At first he assumed power as provisional president, but when it became obvious that Fidel would be unable to take up his position again because of health problems, his younger brother was elected president two years later. Under his guidance, while many aspects of MI have remained constant, there have been some significant changes.

Cuba has faced difficult challenges since Raúl Castro took power. Coming after such a larger-than-life figure as his elder brother in itself presents difficulties. In addition Cuba has been badly affected by a series of natural disasters. In 2008, for instance, three major hurricanes (Gustav, Ike, and Paloma) struck the island. Gustav was considered the worst hurricane in over 50 years, and 20,000 (of 25,000) homes on the Isle of Youth were destroyed. The three hurricanes together caused an estimated $8 billion in damage—almost four times the income from total annual tourist income. In addition Hurricane Sandy in 2012 caused an estimated $3 billion in damages, killing 11 people, mainly in the east of Cuba, and also added to economic difficulties for the government.

The backdrop to Raúl Castro's presidency has been an economy that has consistently underperformed, making a difficult financial situation worse.

The president has sought to turn the economy around, a herculean task given the entrenched bureaucracy that is fearful of losing its influence, the ongoing U.S. embargo, outdated machinery that is in poor condition, widespread low-level corruption, the legacy of the conditions of the Special Period, and a mind-set that is accustomed to top-down state management. Raúl Castro has been critical of the current situation in Cuba, bluntly noting that Cuba was living beyond its means and that it was necessary to bring in radical reforms to reverse the current process that was destroying the economy: "In summary, to go on spending more than the income we are receiving is the same as eating up our future, as risking the very survival of our Revolution. We indeed face some very unpleasant realities—but we refuse to close our eyes as we face up to them. We are convinced that we have to reject all forms of dogma, and we assume with firmness and confidence the continuation, which has already started, of our model to reform the economy."[33]

Given Cuba's new reality of facing up to economic challenges, of rejecting dogmatic solutions, and in particular of seeking innovative economic solutions, it is understandable that such a major (and expensive) program as that of medical internationalism would be scrutinized by the government. In April 2011 the Sixth Congress of the Communist Party of Cuba took place. Of key importance was the discussion of a series of *lineamientos*, or guidelines, on the future of Cuba that had been drawn up after nationwide discussions. Medical *colaboración* was discussed in several of the clauses, and it was decided (as guidelines 101–8 indicate) that this policy was important, particularly in terms of the Cuban economy—and increasingly as a major source of funding. In terms of basic medical cooperation, guideline 111 stipulated, "wherever possible, that compensation at least for the cost of humanitarian collaboration be considered." It was preceded by articles that stressed the need to evaluate carefully the economic cost of all programs of collaboration. New guideline 110 made this clear: "[We should] continue developing international solidarity through our programs of collaboration, *establishing the necessary economic and statistical data that will allow us to undertake the necessary analyses, especially of cost*" (emphasis added).[34]

The government has responded to the needed reforms in the country by introducing sweeping legislation to encourage Cubans to work harder and more efficiently, and in many ways Cuba today is based on a mixed economy. For example, approximately 1 million (out of a working population of 5.1 million) work in the private sector. This includes over 470,000 who are self-employed (up from 140,000 in 2009), and some 575,000 farmers who either own or lease their own land.[35] Being cost-effective is the new order of the day, with frequent reminders from Communist Party leaders that the "good old days" of extensive subsidies have long gone. It is now time to be efficient, to work harder, and to depend less on the state.

So what effect has this had on the medical internationalism program? In essence there are three modalities of international health cooperation, according to a March 2014 report of the Ministry of Public Health: a small nucleus of countries where Cuba assumes the major share of costs, others where the costs are shared with the host country, and a third group in which the countries pay (albeit at a cheaper cost than they would pay for medical services on the international market).[36] There has been a definite impact of the raúlista school of thought, in that the government weighs up each potential contribution of MI before agreeing to cooperate. A cost-benefit analysis ensues, with the *lineamientos* firmly in mind. At the same time, the government remains committed to providing cooperation when it is needed, as Raúl Castro noted in a February 2010 speech. He was talking specifically about Cuba's role in Haiti, but there was a general commitment reflected in his words: "I can assure you that the modest efforts of Cuban medical cooperation will remain in Haiti for however many years it is needed, providing that the government of Haiti wants this to continue. . . . Our country is the victim of a harsh blockade and has little to spare. Quite the contrary—we are short of everything. However, we are prepared to share our poverty with these nations that have even less."[37]

It is useful to measure these sentiments against the actions of the Cuban government since Raúl Castro came to power in July 2006. The costly missions of the Henry Reeve brigade, formed in 2005, illustrate the application of this dilemma. Cuba is the only country in the world where a brigade of several thousand specialists in emergency medicine is on standby. How has it been affected by the application of Raúl Castro's approach? In recent years the Henry Reeve brigade has acted in Guatemala and Pakistan (2005), Bolivia (2006), Indonesia (2006), Peru (2007), Mexico (2007), China (2008), and Haiti and Chile (2010). In May 2015, Cuba sent an emergency brigade of 49 specialists to Nepal, following the earthquake there.

In the fall of 2014 Cuba showed that, despite the increased importance of the exportation of medical services as a means of generating income, the government would also respond to those in need. In September, for example, Cuba sent six tons of medical supplies to Gaza following the 50-day conflict between Israel and Hamas that had killed more than 2,100 Palestinians. The outbreak of Ebola in several West African countries illustrates Cuba's support for developing countries in Africa. Cuba responded to an appeal by the WHO by sending 103 nurses and 62 doctors in early October to Sierra Leone, the largest contribution of health staff by any single country. Soon there were 256 Cuban medical personnel working in the Ebola campaign, with several hundred more being trained to join them. A reporter with *Science* emphasized the significance of this: "To put the numbers in perspective: The WHO has deployed about 500 foreign medical experts to the region. Because they rotate, at any one time about 170 of them are in the affected countries."[38] Cuba had committed to sending the element that was most needed and in fact was sending almost as many medical specialists as were working for the WHO in the area at the time.[39]

A commitment to solidarity, particularly for those in the Global South, remained a broad plank of Cuba's approach to medical internationalism. What was different under Raúl Castro was that countries and individuals who could afford to make a contribution to their medical support or training were now asked to do so. These changes can be seen in the Cuban government's approach to medical education at ELAM, in an effort to make the program more cost-effective. Since the first graduating class in 2005, more than 24,000 physicians from more than 80 countries have graduated, and it remains the largest medical school in the world. There are several estimates of the size of ELAM. In his March 2011 article, Don Fitz quotes the school's director of international relations, who claims that there were 21,018 students at ELAM and its sister campuses around the country.[40] A Canadian journalist put the number at 19,550, which is 12 times the number enrolled at the medical faculties of Harvard and the University of Toronto combined.[41] (On a visit to ELAM in December 2014, I was informed that the annual intake of students had been reduced to 750. I suspect that this is due to financial reasons). Meanwhile, Cuban medical professors have been training physicians in several schools. Most recently they have been active in Venezuela and Timor-Leste. The training of physicians has, in fact, increased. What is different now, though, is that students from countries whose governments can afford it are now charged on a sliding scale, following financial negotiations.

The pragmatism for which Raúl Castro has become famous can be seen in how these various programs are paid for. The same is true for Cuba's application of the dozens of in-country medical support programs, the Comprehensive Health Program (PIS). The approach now used is significantly different from anything found before, and the Cuban government applies a basic means test. If students, or their governments, can pay for the services, then they pay. If they can't afford to do so, then the Cuban government charges a nominal amount. The case of Haiti is a good example of the latter scenario, since Havana charges nothing for its medical services there or for training almost 1,000 physicians on the island. (To a large degree this is covered by financial contributions from the governments of Norway, Brazil, and Venezuela.)

In the past there was no charge for tuition at ELAM, but that too has changed—and once again the ability to pay is the key variable. For instance, students from El Salvador or Honduras do not pay for their tuition, whereas South Africa pays its students' tuition. This mosaic of differential fees has also been brought into play in countries which had previously been members of the PIS program. In several countries, when there has been an upturn in the economy, national governments have recently been encouraged to pay more for the Cuban medical services.

In October 2013 I spent a morning with an influential policymaker in the Ministry of Public Health. We went over a list of the approximately 60 countries to which Cuba provided medical collaboration. According to official Cuban statistics in 2012, there were 40 countries (12 in Latin America and the Caribbean, 22 in Africa, and 6 in Asia and the South Pacific) that paid a significantly reduced rate for the services of Cuban medical personnel. In 2013, however, the situation had changed, and half of these countries were now paying more for their services, again following a sliding scale that depended on their ability to pay.

Cuba is now following a path based closely on the *lineamientos*, in an attempt to provide medical support but at a less subsidized price whenever possible. Humanitarian services are still provided when needed, and heavily subsidized medical programs are offered to developing countries around the world. But increasingly the Cuban government is seeking to generate funding from this intellectual capital, as can be seen in one small way from its new corporation, Servicios Médicos Cubanos S.A., which offers medical services (ranging from hip replacement to neurological surgery) in Cuba at far cheaper prices than those offered in a developed country. Medical education and training in Cuban hospitals for foreign students are also increasingly available through this corporation.

A similar trend can be seen in the use of biotechnology under Raúl Castro. Cuba is producing medicines and vaccines for markets throughout the developing world. These are sold at a fraction of the prices charged by multinational drug companies. At the same time Cuba is now pursuing new directions. To a large extent this is the result of the foundation of BioCubaFarma in November 2012, a fusion of most of Cuba's research centers in the field of biotechnology. The new organization is seeking to expand its operations abroad and to work with foreign partners. In April 2014, for example, Agustín Lage, director of the Center for Molecular Immunology, was in Beijing, encouraging Chinese investors in biotechnology and pharmaceutical products to come to the new economic development zone at the port of Mariel and set up businesses there. In February that year an unusual partnership was announced between the Center for Genetic Engineering and Biotechnology (CIGB) and the French equity investment firm Truffle Capital (which had merged three French life sciences companies to form ABIVAX). The agreement tasked the CIGB with manufacturing the hepatitis B vaccine, which their French partner would then license for sale and market in Europe and Asia. As noted elsewhere, Cuba has made similar arrangements with companies in China, India, and Brazil, but this marks the first time that an arrangement of this kind has been made with a European company. It could well be the harbinger of a major shift in the field of biotechnology investment and exports for Cuba. With the agreement in principle of December 2014 to normalize bilateral relations, it is expected that U.S. investment in Cuban biotechnology will eventually be initiated and will then rapidly increase.

Under Raúl Castro, medical services (ranging from exclusive private medical tourism facilities in Havana to basic community medicine in Haiti) are all part of the offerings now provided by Cuba under the umbrella of "medical cooperation." Cost-effective collaboration is becoming a mantra in government circles. It should be pointed out, however, that even though Cuba does now charge many countries for their medical collaboration, the price is much cheaper than the international rates for the services of western physicians. Cuba does indeed continue to provide heavily subsidized healthcare to developing countries (e.g., Burundi or Niger), but this cost will be borne by the sale of medical services to wealthier countries (such as Qatar and Saudi Arabia). In addition, as the Cuban response to the Ebola outbreak in Africa showed, Cuba is prepared to assist when natural emergencies occur.

The sale of professional services—mainly medical and to a lesser extent educational—is now the largest source of hard currency for Cuba, bringing in $8.2 billion annually. Raúl Castro is aware of that as well as the potential income from the exportation of medical sources and biotechnology ($1 billion annually and growing). In many ways the challenge facing the Cuban government of developing the economy without losing sight of its traditional socialist, revolutionary base and traditions is reflected in the need to balance its five decades of humanitarian MI with the ever-increasing financial rewards from the exportation of medical goods and services. It remains to be seen how Castro—who has said that he will retire in 2018—will meet these challenges. Just as pertinent is the question of what will happen to medical internationalism in the post-Castro era.

Concluding Thoughts

Cuba has played a significant role in improving the health of tens of millions of people in the developing and underdeveloped worlds. Since 1960 Cuba has provided support through medical missions, as well as the training (both in Cuba and in their home countries) of tens of thousands of medical personnel, the establishment of medical schools, and the provision of inexpensive medicines to dozens of countries of the Global South. This has been a long history, based traditionally but not exclusively on humanitarian motives. Medical cooperation has evolved from the sending of a few dozen adventurous people into the unknown in Chile in 1960 to the current situation where there are over 50,000 healthcare personnel working in 60 countries. This story continues to unfold, now with a financial attraction, although the humanitarian quotient remains strong.

Not surprisingly the focus of this support in recent years has been the region that Cuba knows best and in which it plays a significant role—Latin America and the Caribbean. Yet at the same time, it has also made an important contribution around the globe. The multifaceted role in Timor-Leste on the other side of the world illustrates this. In Africa, too, it has made a major contribution to the continent's development. By June 2012, for instance, over 300,000 professionals had worked in Africa, while some 5,500 Cuban professionals (including 2,000 physicians) were working in 35 of the continent's 54 countries. Moreover, almost 40,000 Africans have studied in Cuba, and at that time some 3,000 were undertaking advanced studies on the island.[42] It was estimated that between 1999 and 2007 the Comprehensive Health Program, involving Cuban medical physicians in these countries, had saved 857,000 lives, given 36,290,000 consultations, performed 626,000 surgeries, and assisted at 549,826 births.[43]

A similar story was true in Latin America and the Caribbean. There, 3 million people could now see following eye surgery, while tens of thousands had benefited from the emergency response activities of the Henry

Reeve brigade, and over 40,000 new doctors trained by Cuban medical professors had graduated. Referring to the situation a decade earlier, Piero Gleijeses emphasized the contribution of the Cuban medical *internacionalistas*, living in poor conditions in the dozens of countries where they were stationed. He placed this role within the historical context, noting: "They represent a unique example: that of a poor country generously assisting other poor countries, just as Cuba has been doing for four decades—since the days when the first Cuban doctors left for Algeria."[44]

2

ELAM, a School for All Nations

> I know of no other medical school that offers students so much, at no charge. I know of no other medical school with an admissions policy that gives first priority to candidates who come from poor communities and know, firsthand, what it means to live without access to essential medical care. For once, if you are poor, female, or from an indigenous population, you have a distinct advantage. This is an institutional ethic that makes this medical school unique.
>
> Dr. Margaret Chan, director-general of the World Health Organization, Remarks at the Latin American Medical School of Medicine, October 27, 2009

The Escuela Latinoamericana de Medicina (ELAM) was opened in 1999 to provide a humanitarian response by Cuba in the wake of two natural disasters. From October 29 to November 3, 1998, Hurricane Mitch devastated several countries in Central America, and the previous month Hurricane Georges had laid waste to Haiti. The impact in Haiti was severe, with a death toll of 400 and 167,000 left homeless. The economic devastation was widespread, and 80 percent of banana plantations were destroyed. Even worse was the human toll throughout the Central American region, with thousands dead and disappeared. Infrastructure was destroyed, and the local economy was left in ruins. According to the Pan American Health Organization, by December 4, 6,600 people had died in Honduras, with a further 8,052 disappeared and presumed dead and 11,998 wounded. Nicaragua was also badly hit: 2,863 were confirmed dead, and there were 970 disappeared and 388 wounded. The total of dead and disappeared in El Salvador was 268 and 389 in Guatemala. The number of victims at that point was estimated to be 1,895,437.[1]

Fidel Castro responded to the calls for help from the Central American countries by sending large medical contingents. The immediate emergencies were resolved after several months of work. Afterwards, and with the agreement of the host governments, the Cuban medical staff remained, establishing Comprehensive Health Programs (or Programas Integrales de Salud). Cuba did so despite poor diplomatic relations with most of the

Central American countries. Relations with Guatemala, for example, were only restored in 1998, with Honduras in 2002, Nicaragua in 2007, and both El Salvador and Costa Rica in 2009. More pressing than the resumption of diplomatic relations, however, was the need for a sustainable approach to healthcare in the affected regions. Cuba identified the long-term need to train doctors from the devastated communities, so that they could provide badly needed healthcare for their own people, ultimately replacing the medical support from Cuba. In order to carry out this ambitious program, the Cuban government established ELAM, turning a large, sprawling complex west of Havana that for years had trained cadets for the Cuban navy into the largest medical school in the world.[2]

In November 1998 Fidel Castro outlined his plans for ELAM, rejecting the interest of Spanish investors in establishing a tourist complex there, complete with golf course. Instead it would be a place where, in President Castro's words, people would take "revenge" upon Mitch by training doctors to save more lives every year than had been lost in the hurricanes. The school was refurbished in record time, with the first students entering in February 1999, and since 2005 some 24,000 doctors from over 80 countries have emerged. Most have returned to their country of origin, especially to the countries of Central America, where they are gradually replacing Cuban physicians. The students at ELAM remain for the first two years on the Havana campus before being distributed throughout the island for a further four years of medical training at any of the almost two dozen training hospitals throughout the island. As of January 2014 there were over 11,000 students from 123 countries registered at ELAM. Included in this number were several dozen students from the United States, mainly from visible minority backgrounds. In his January 2014 visit to ELAM, UN secretary-general Ban Ki-moon congratulated Cuba on "the ingenious contributions of the school, for being leaders in South-South cooperation and in the forefront of international health" and referred to it as "the most advanced medical school in the world."[3]

This chapter, based on a half-dozen research trips to ELAM and dozens of interviews with people associated with the school—current students, medical graduates from a number of countries, professors and administrators at ELAM—seeks to analyze the importance of this experiment in practical medical education. It attempts to answer some of the fundamental questions raised about the value of this educational experience: what type of education do the students receive? What political influences do they receive in their training? How do they view their responsibilities as physicians? How well are the students prepared to provide medical care for their patients? What is the impact on them as doctors and as citizens?

The fundamental philosophy behind the medical training provided at ELAM is a blend of solidarity, humanism, ethics, and internationalism. The program instills in students the values inculcated in Cuban doctors over the last 50 years, with particular attention paid to those qualities which are believed necessary to transform communities and improve social conditions, especially for people in traditionally underserved areas.[4] The school selects students who are willing to improve the health of those most in need, seeing this as a humanitarian imperative. Access to public health is viewed as a fundamental human right for all, and this is emphasized throughout the medical training provided. Moreover, ELAM teaches the importance of commitment and personal sacrifice in the vocation of medicine, a concept of service that students are then expected to take back to their own communities while providing healthcare at no charge to their patients. This is brought about by instilling a sense of personal commitment and *conciencia*. (The Spanish term is difficult to translate, for there is no exact equivalent. In essence it is a combination of political awareness, commitment to the well-being of others, and a collective consciousness.) Needless to say, this represents a major challenge for those physicians trained in a traditional capitalist structure. ELAM graduates often encounter suspicion and hostility from medical associations (defenders of the traditional approach to medicine and the status quo) when they return to their countries and seek employment. For their part, leaders of the established medical associations—usually from traditional, wealthy families—look askance at the new breed of doctors who are prepared to work without charging for their services and who prefer to work in public service rather than in private practice. In short, the values taught at ELAM go against the traditional approach of medical school.

In order to communicate this philosophy effectively, the project also requires a teacher who understands the nature of this radically different form of education and is committed to impart this set of values. For this reason, almost all of the ELAM academic staff have worked in Cuban medical brigades in developing countries and therefore have a solid understanding of what they are asking the students to commit to in underserved and remote communities.[5] Often tutorial groups are organized clustering students from a particular country together with a Cuban medical professor who has previous internationalist experience in that country. This allows for the exchange of knowledge about medical challenges in that country. Throughout the training professors/mentors seek to develop in their students a series of humanitarian values that go far beyond the lessons learned at traditional medical schools, and in return they expect far more from their charges. As Cuban professor Leonardo Mauricio explains, "Real solidarity consists of sharing what you have with those who have less."[6] This commitment to serving the poor is a major theme which the Cuban professors teach their students at ELAM, and it comes from professors who have faced the challenges of living in extremely difficult circumstances during their internationalist duty. According to ELAM vice director Midalys Castilla Martínez, this vocation of service is of paramount importance: "The ideal professors will be excellent in scientific and professional aspects, but also it is vital that they will be ambitious educators. If they do not have a spirit of service then they will not be able to connect with the students."[7]

The experience of studying at ELAM is unique. The application process is different, as are the type of students who attend, the academic program itself, the underlying philosophy, and finally the medical training. The students are recruited through the Cuban embassy in their respective countries, and there then follows a process of consultation with local and Cuban medical staff as well as government authorities and local civil society representatives. All applicants must have graduated from high school with good grades, show aptitude for and interest in medicine, and pass an admissions exam. It also helps if they have been involved in community or progressive political activities or have made a significant contribution to local society through voluntary work. Afterwards there are interviews with the applicants to make sure that they are willing to return to their own communities (or others that are in equal need of medical personnel) upon graduation. It is worth noting that, of the students accepted, some 75 percent of them are children of workers or *campesinos*.[8] There have been some significant changes in recruiting students under Raúl Castro, with many from wealthier countries now paying tuition to study in Cuba, although the vast majority of students still receive their education without paying any tuition.

The ELAM students generally come from poorer socioeconomic backgrounds, from rural or underserved areas, and the vast majority would be unable to pay for a medical school education in their own country. They are also from a wide variety of racial, cultural, and religious backgrounds. (Christian and Muslim worship services, for example, are regularly held for the students.) In an interview at the medical school with an ELAM administrator in December 2014, I was informed that there were currently students from 98 countries studying at ELAM. This included 114 Americans. I was also informed that 3,000 graduates from ELAM had returned to Cuba to undertake further specialized training. They are mainly chosen from these underserved areas or backgrounds because it is understood that they are the ones who truly appreciate the necessity of medical care in their communities (often lacking in the areas from which they come) and are therefore more likely to return to help in those areas after graduation. Since they are aware that, without their education at ELAM, they would not be able to attend medical school in their homeland, these students are expected to be extremely committed to their studies. The approach is a clear alternative to the "brain drain," instead contributing to a "brain gain." Fitzhugh Mullan summarized this neatly: "Castro has removed the financial barriers and bet on motivation to overcome any educational liabilities that students bring with them to ELAM."[9] They graduate with an excellent medical training.

As a result of these factors, the students at ELAM generally possess an extremely well defined work ethic and understanding of the significance both of health needs in the community and their duty as healthcare providers. There are also enormous expectations placed upon them. They graduate debt-free, but are expected to return to their home community, or wherever the need is greatest, in order to pay back a debt to their society and ultimately to humanity. These heady concepts may well be alien to medical students in the developed world, faced with the daunting challenge of paying for their medical education and then scrambling to repay their debts, often ranging from $200,000 to $400,000. But in many ways this pragmatic approach constitutes the basis of medical education on the island for Cubans and foreigners alike.

The training they receive prepares them for—and expects of them—significant responsibility upon graduation. It is a very different form of medical training, and it is assumed that they will take on a variety of social and medical responsibilities after starting work. For example, they are not only expected to provide basic healthcare to their patients but also to contribute positively to the well-being of their community and indeed their country. They are responsible for undertaking research, collecting data, presenting health and sanitary-related information in community meetings, and teaching their patients methods of protecting and improving their own health. They are also expected to be leaders, contributing proactively to the health of their community, to live and work there. As two students at

ELAM have remarked, they are "taught that, as primary care physicians, they must play a dynamic role in leading their communities towards health, not just be stationary fixtures to come to at times of illness."[10]

In addition, their medical training prepares them to develop a close relationship with their patients, since all are members of the same community. They see each other socially, shop in the same stores, and their children participate in the same school activities. Unlike the traditional medical model that places them in a position of authority in a vertical societal structure, graduates of ELAM are trained to see themselves as the equals of their patients. Their extensive clinical training also prepares them to spend more time in clinical examinations and history-taking with their patients than is the norm elsewhere. They listen more actively to their patients and share knowledge about improving their health with them. They are trained to be active members of their community—to know and be known by members there. The term *duty* is the key to understanding their role in the community, and they live and work in Spartan conditions with a minimal amount of sophisticated equipment.

There are clear guidelines for medical school graduates, as can be seen from the parameters provided to students from Timor-Leste at ELAM and the expectations held of them. These concepts are instilled in all medical students of medicine in Cuba throughout their training, and the following core functions are seen as integral facets of their duties.

(1) In the area of health services provision: to provide comprehensive health services to individuals, families, communities and their living environment, through promotional, preventive, curative, and rehabilitative interventions undertaken at out-patient and hospitalized settings as well as home visits. Included here is also the duty to report and support actions on negative impacts of the living environment to the health of the individuals, families, and communities.

(2) In the area of teaching: to participate in pre-service and in-service teaching activities for health professionals, in his/her own self-education, as well as in the information and education of the target population.

(3) In the area of research: to apply in his/her daily professional life the clinical and epidemiological methods of diagnostic and problem-solving of health problems affecting individuals, families, communities, and their living environment. These include active

participation in the process of searching, evaluating on application of technical and scientific knowledge, as well as in the undertaking of research projects.

(4) In the area of health management: to perform administrative tasks in organizing work at health facilities, mobilization and effective use of available human, material and financial resources, as well as controlling and evaluating the progress of health programs under his/her supervision.

(5) Special functions: to participate, during situations of emergency and catastrophe, in the medical services to be provided to the affected people and the implementation of hygienic and into-epidemic measures to the target population.[11]

The role of this new breed of physicians was explained by former Cuban president Fidel Castro at the inauguration of ELAM, as he outlined their various duties: "The most significant, however, will be their absolute devotion to the most noble and human endeavor, that of saving lives and preserving health. More than physicians they shall be zealous guardians of what human beings appreciate above all else. They will be apostles and builders of a more humane world."[12] The doctors graduating from these programs clearly receive unusual training and develop a distinctive vision of their roles. One ELAM student articulated the nature of this patient-centered approach well: "We learn to practice medicine on the bases of altruism, honor, and sacrifice as a commitment to society. It is the patient that teaches us medicine; it is the hospital that sets the stage."[13] They also learn one of the basic lessons of the Cuban system, namely, that health issues are determined by a series of social, psychological, and environmental factors, and not just by medical pathologies. As a result, physicians do not concentrate solely on a particular medical condition of their patient. As one American ELAM student correctly noted: "You're taught to look at patients in that same integrated way. . . . Not just what diseases they have, but how they function socially, in their homes, in their work environments, schools . . . and how as doctors we can address all these things together."[14]

Critiques of the Cuban Approach

There are outspoken critics of the Cuban medical training. "Medical School Graduates from Cuba Deficient in Training, States University of Costa

Rica" and "Medical Graduates from Cuba Fail Exams in Chile" are two examples of articles from Latin American newspapers in 2012 that criticized the medical training provided at ELAM. In the former, the director of the Medical Faculty of the University of Costa Rica criticized the "grave deficiencies" in the academic training provided to students, noting that in the previous three years 138 students who had trained abroad (including 59 who had graduated from ELAM) had failed qualifying exams in Costa Rica. The situation was similar in Chile, where students who had studied abroad (mainly in Cuba) received noticeably lower scores in qualifying examinations, while graduates from Chilean medical schools fared significantly better, particularly in the case of graduates from private universities.[15]

Another complaint against ELAM concerns the politicized nature of the education. While ELAM officials, and indeed the vast majority of students interviewed, claim that students are taught medicine and not political propaganda at the medical school, others disagree. Journalist Jon Dougherty mentions a "requirement that students pledge allegiance to communism and the Cuban Marxist form of government." He also refers to ELAM as a "well-orchestrated piece of political propaganda" and quotes from a report, allegedly written by some ELAM graduates, that states, "Medical students who accept Castro's offer of free medical training may find themselves indentured serfs to Cuba's communism."[16] Based on my own interviews of about 30 graduates of ELAM in Central America and another 20 in Cuba (from a variety of countries), as well as reading comments of many others, it is clear that this claim is nonsense. (Indeed, another article, generally critical of ELAM, makes just the opposite argument, noting that several radical socialist students "felt frustrated when they couldn't carry out those same types of activities here.")[17] In fact, ELAM students are overwhelmingly supportive of the education that they receive there, and this should not surprise. Understandably they will be affected by living six years in a revolutionary, socialist society, influenced by the basic egalitarian spirit there. Students whom I interviewed at ELAM were impressed by the quality of the community-centric and accessible Cuban public healthcare system that surrounds them, as well as the dedication of their professors (who receive extremely low salaries), and will undoubtedly be grateful for the educational experience and opportunity to become physicians. The majority will not pay anything for their six years of medical training. That said, there is no such requirement "to pledge allegiance" to any political system. Rather than pledge allegiance to communism, they make a commitment to help humanity.

Other observers are less critical, and indeed many are fulsome in their praise of the level of medical education. WHO director Margaret Chan, who has been to Cuba on several medical missions, has also commented on the quality and nature of instruction at ELAM. In November 2008, while in Havana to lead the WHO Global Policy Group, she praised the level of medical education on the island and its pragmatic, hands-on focus, noting the need for an appropriate training of medical students in the world: "It is necessary to change the medical education system to be able to have highly qualified health specialists, and I am taking the Cuban experience with me."[18] José Luis di Fabio, the Cuba-based representative of the Pan American Health Organization (PAHO) supported the inherently practical approach employed at ELAM, and talked of his own role in "debunking some of the myths about its curriculum. Our reasoning is clear: the world needs doctors for primary healthcare, doctors who come from, and are willing to practice in, distressed communities and rural areas, and who are well acquainted with their own culture and respect others." He referred to the "resistance from some in the medical profession itself, particularly among specialists who were trained so differently. They don't understand these ELAM doctors who were trained in community settings and health facilities—something you don't see in many countries."

This combination of a fundamental philosophical divide and a different form of training (mainly in urban hospital settings instead of the community-based approach of ELAM) produces a gulf between the medical establishment in Latin America and the ELAM graduates. This helps to explain the bitter and at times insulting conduct of established physicians and medical associations in several countries where Cuban medical personnel and ELAM graduates have arrived in order to assist in underserved areas—regions where the traditionally trained sector prefer not to venture. This was the case in late 2013 when Brazilian physicians lined up to call recently arrived Cuban doctors "slaves" for working in poor rural communities—areas where the Brazilians refused to work. There are, in sum, two radically different approaches to medical training. In many ways, expecting students trained in the pragmatic, hands-on approach of the Cuban model to pass the qualifying exams designed for graduates from highly theoretical programs (which have fewer clinical hours and often none in underserved communities) is unfair. Instead, there should be recognition that both approaches are viable and have distinct, complementary qualities. A case can certainly be made, as the PAHO representative suggests, that the Cuban approach is more useful in the developing world.[19]

Table 2.1. Employment status of Haitian ELAM graduates, 2012

Status	Number	% of Graduates
Working with Cuban health team in Haiti	46	6.1
Working in Haiti's public health system	193	25.8
Completing social service in Haiti's health system	114	15.2
Working in private practice in Haiti	98	13.1
Total working in Haiti	451	60.3
Working outside Haiti	110	14.7
Unemployed	187	25.0
Total	**748**	**100**

Source: Conner Gorry, "Cuba's Latin American School," *MEDICC Review* 7, no. 5 (May 2005): 6.

One criticism that deserves to be leveled at ELAM is that in its original philosophical base it was overly optimistic in expecting physicians to find employment in their home countries. One example is Haiti, where by 2012 Cuba had trained 748 doctors, almost 40 percent of whom were unemployed or working abroad, as table 2.1 shows.

There are several explanations why there are so many unemployed medical graduates, and the Haitian situation is a microcosm of the challenges faced by ELAM graduates in many countries. As noted above, upon returning to their countries following their training, newly minted physicians often encounter opposition from traditional, and conservative, medical federations. There are often limited internship programs for all students, and stiff competition between ELAM graduates and those trained in national medical faculties ensues. Often the leaders of medical federations favor "their own," students trained in systems with which they are familiar and in which they also trained. At times, too, countries simply do not have the money to hire the ELAM graduates, even at extremely low salaries, as is the case in Haiti. This has led many graduates to return to Cuba to take further medical specialization, hoping that this will improve their employment possibilities at a later date. Significantly, however, as the number of ELAM graduates grows, and as parallel developments in Venezuela continue (with the establishment of a second ELAM and with the training by Cuban medical professors of an estimated 60,000 Venezuelan physicians), and finally while a "brain drain" of physicians from the Global South to developed countries also continues, the scales are slowly tilting in favor of the model found under the Cuban influence in medical training. This is the approach which the developing world needs and can afford—and which has proved to be a viable alternative to the scourge of the departure of medical talent to the Industrialized North.[20]

The (Different) Nature of the Medical Training

The goal of ELAM is clear: "to educate physicians primarily for public service in disadvantaged urban and rural communities, developing competencies in comprehensive primary care, from health promotion to treatment and rehabilitation."[21] Students usually study six months in a pre-medical foundations course, with non-Spanish speakers taking intensive language lessons, since all of their medical training will be in Spanish. Their first two years are spent taking courses at the ELAM campus outside Havana. After that, they are spread throughout the country in two dozen medical faculties, carrying out medical practicums in local hospitals. There they study and work alongside some 30,000 Cuban medical students who have taken courses at their own medical faculties. Significantly they will be exposed to a blend of clinical medicine and public health training designed to introduce them to the Cuban healthcare model, with its emphasis on preventive medicine. In addition, summer vacations are often spent in their home countries working on community health projects, strengthening their understanding of healthcare back home, and familiarizing themselves with the health challenges there.

The varying opinions noted above on the value of medical education at ELAM are similar to views expressed about the nature of the public healthcare system in Cuba. In essence it comes down to the fact that the Cuban model is totally different from anything encountered in any other country and often confusing to those trained in a traditional approach. An article in the *New England Journal of Medicine* put the challenge of understanding the unusual Cuban approach well and established a context to analyze it: "For a visitor from the United States, Cuba is disconcerting. . . . And the Cuban healthcare system also seems unreal. There are too many doctors. Everybody has a family physician. Everything is free, totally free—and not after prior approval or some copay. The whole system seems turned upside down. . . . Although Cuba has limited resources, its healthcare system has solved some problems that ours has not yet managed to address."[22] In synthesis, the Cuban approach is radically different from that found in any industrialized country and should not be seen through the filter of that society. The same could be said about the nature of medical education.

The differences between the Cuban medical training programs and those that follow a more typical or traditional training model are clear-cut. While the typical medical education model found in most industrialized countries has not changed greatly over the last few decades, the Cuban training models including that at ELAM as well as the New Training Model successfully being employed in Venezuela and a handful of other developing countries have undoubtedly pushed the boundaries of medical training. The "new doctors" who emerge from this training are capable of working in any circumstances, from hospital ERs to rural areas where there has been no medical care (much less advanced diagnostic equipment), and they are even trained to provide substantial medical support following disasters. They are trained to work not for monetary gain but rather for the benefit of the underserved. The essence of their medical training at ELAM has been summed up by Conner Gorry, a health reporter with *MEDICC*, who has lived in Cuba for many years: "Equal parts science and conscience, the ELAM adheres to a socially responsible curriculum that combines an evidence-based medical education with a humanistic understanding of health as a right for all."[23]

A major difference between the approach that Cuba employs in medical training and the typical international training model is the heavy emphasis on moral values. The students learn from the example of their professors, who have worked in difficult conditions in developing countries and who in Cuba are paid poorly for their work. Medical students can thus see for themselves their mentors' moral commitment to others at home and abroad. The students are reminded constantly that being a doctor is a privilege and an honor and that healthcare is a human right, not to be used for financial gain. This approach, set against the backdrop of Cuba training physicians for the developing world while facing its own nationwide hardships, probably influences young students spending six years there, as is illustrated by the views of two Pakistani medical students at ELAM. In a 2011 interview the students praised both the medical education that they were receiving and the value of the Cuban experience for their own country. The title of the article in the *Express Tribune* illustrates this clearly: "Medical Education: Inspired by Cuba, Students Hope to Overhaul Pakistani Healthcare."

In April 2010, a Haitian graduate, Dr. Patrick Dely, expanded on the value of ELAM's practical approach, but also explained why graduates faced criticism from the medical establishment when they returned to their home communities. He provided the hypothetical scenario of himself arriving back in Haiti after graduating and facing the reaction from an established doctor: "And I arrive from Cuba, extraordinarily enthusiastic to work anywhere I'm needed, to go to the most remote corner and serve in whatever conditions. This means I'm taking money directly from the [established doctor]. So we are seen as a threat and that's the first problem." A second problem occurs when many ELAM graduates—almost always from a lower social class—return to Haiti upon graduation: "Then all of a sudden there are these masses of humble young people returning as doctors, proving that they can be doctors too. . . . Once there is a larger supply (in this case doctors), it shifts the dynamic. We're a threat to that dynamic."[24] They do indeed represent the threat of a dangerous example to the established medical profession and the status quo.

Another difference is the actual methodology of teaching, since the teaming of theoretical and practical learning is heavily emphasized throughout the medical training. Rather than the learn-now-do-later model, the Cubans have instituted a learn-while-doing model. As a result of these teaching methods, doctors graduate from programs ready to work in extremely difficult conditions—often in areas where well-trained physicians from the traditional system will choose not to go. They are therefore able to transition easily from school to work, as well as being capable of working in various locations with either limited or significant access to sophisticated medical equipment.

The course material throughout their training is also unlike that taught elsewhere. In addition to learning about basic medical and scientific elements of healthcare, they are also taught about significant risk factors that contribute to the health of individuals and communities. Their coursework emphasizes that patients are largely influenced by their surroundings and that everything is interconnected in a biological, psychological, and societal web. Also noteworthy is the way in which students take courses that reflect problems they could face in their own distinct communities. Rather than learning about a disease they will likely never encounter, their training focuses in an extremely practical way on those issues and illnesses that will be present in the areas where they will be living and working. Students thus graduate prepared to treat specific and prevalent illnesses. Dr. Margaret Chan has articulated the pragmatic nature of the curriculum at ELAM, necessary in the developing world: "You are also privileged because the curriculum and methods of problem-based, hands-on learning are uniquely equipping you to meet the real challenges of medical practice in the twenty-first century. The greatest challenge today is not keeping up with the latest techniques using the latest high-tech equipment and procedures. Instead, the greatest challenge is to get essential care to the underserved."[25]

The ELAM Curriculum

The curriculum of ELAM is based on theoretical concepts and practical learning. Many students are required to take language courses as well as basic pre-med science courses. The objective is to provide a firm foundation for students from different cultural backgrounds and levels of scientific preparation. Successful completion of the pre-med courses thus allows all students to keep up with the rigorous academic program that lies ahead. The program itself lasts six years, with the first two spent on campus. Students participate in conferences, seminars, practical classes, laboratory practices, lectures, and independent study. Throughout the first two years of study on the Havana ELAM campus, students are also required to take courses in physical education, which is based on the theory that they must be fit in order to provide medical care to those in rugged mountainous or rural areas, since often they must travel by foot to reach their patients. There are three basic cycles of study for the six-year program. For the first three semesters, students take courses in biomedical and social sciences. In the fourth and fifth semesters, the focus is on clinical sciences, and this is followed by a development of their experiences in clinical sciences from the sixth through the tenth semesters. Put another way, there are two years of basic medical sciences, three years of clinical rotations, and one year of internship. This last year consists of a rotation of internships, known as "Pre-Professional Practice." The rotation includes internal medicine (10 weeks), pediatrics (10 weeks), obstetrics and gynecology (7 weeks), surgery (7 weeks), comprehensive general medicine (family medicine) (7 weeks), and medical licensing exams (4 weeks).[26] Common to the entire curriculum is an emphasis on the most frequent pathologies of the developing world, taught in a pragmatic, hands-on fashion.

An insight into this practical approach that is particularly helpful in developing societies was provided in 2007 by two ELAM students from the United States, Razel Remen and Lillian Holloway. They explained the emphasis placed on the need for a solid clinical diagnosis, based on a thorough medical interview with the patient and a physical examination. Significantly, imaging techniques and laboratory tests were to be used only to confirm the diagnosis and not as a matter of course, since in many

Table 2.2. Subject material taught at ELAM

Year 1, semester 1

Subject	Total hours	Number of weeks
Introduction to Comprehensive General Medicine	220	18
Morphophysiology 1 (Cell, prenatal development, basic histology)	124	11
Morphophysiology 2 (Osteo/articular and integumentary systems)	92	9
English 1	64	16
Physical Education	80	16
Lectures		21

Year 1, semester 2

Subject	Total hours	Number of weeks
Health Promotion	222	18
Morphophysiology 3 (Nervous system)	124	12
Morphophysiology 4 (Endocrinology)	84	10
Computer Science for Medicine	63	15
English 2	64	16
Physical Education	80	16
Lectures		23

Year 2, semester 3

Subject	Total hours	Number of weeks
Prevention	192	16
Morphophysiology 5 (Blood, haemolymphopoietic, and cardiovascular system)	100	9
Morphophysiology 6 (Respiratory, kidney, and digestive systems)	90	8
Research Methods and Statistics	63	15
English 3	64	16
Physical Education 3	80	16
Elective	80	2
Lectures		20

Year 2, semester 4

Subject	Total hours	Number of weeks
Community Medicine	144	18
Anatomy/Pathology	130	16
Medical Genetics	60	18
Medical Psychology 1	52	16
Microbiology, Medical Parasitology	129	18
English 4	64	16
Physical Education 4	80	16
Lectures		22

Year 3, semester 5

Subject	Total hours	Number of weeks
Preliminary Clinical Semiology	680	20
Pharmacology	26	15
Medical Psychology 2	44	13
English 5	64	16
Lectures		23

Year 3, semester 6

Subject	Total hours	Number of weeks
Internal Medicine	763	20
Pharmacology 2	56	18
English 4	64	16
Elective	80	2
Lectures		23

Year 4, semester 7

Subject	Total hours	Number of weeks
Pediatrics	764	18
Medicine for Natural Disasters	80	2
English 7	64	16
Elective	80	2
Lectures		23

Year 4, semester 8

Subject	Total hours	Number of weeks
Surgery	424	10
Gynecology and Obstetrics	514	12
English 8	64	16
Lectures		23

Year 5, semester 9

Subject	Total hours	Number of weeks
Psychiatry	212	6
Public Health	242	9
Comprehensive General Medicine	160	4
Legal Medicine and Medical Ethics	36	17
English 9	64	16
Elective	80	2
Lectures		22

Year 5, semester 10

Subject	Total hours	Number of weeks
Orthopedics	204	6
ENT	90	3
Ophthalmology	90	3
Dermatology	90	3
Urology	90	3
English 10	64	16
Medicine for Natural Disasters 2	80	2
Lectures		21

Rotating internship

Subject	Total hours	Number of weeks
Internal Medicine	608	10
Pediatrics	608	10
Ob/Gyn	416	7
Surgery	416	7
Comprehensive General Medicine	40	1
Optional Course	40	1
Lectures	2504	42

Source: ELAM, Primeros años de estudio e ingreso en la ELAM, http://instituciones.sld.cu/elam/primeros-anos-de-estudio-e-ingreso-en-la-elam/.

situations faced by ELAM graduates, these would not be accessible. As the authors note, "Students are encouraged to be creative in their thinking and their use of medical supplies. Indeed a favorite question that the Cuban professors love to pose to their students is 'What would you do and how would you make the diagnosis if you were working in the middle of the Amazon and did not have access to any diagnostic tests?'"[27]

Following the initial two years, students are integrated into 21 faculties of medicine and 444 polyclinics throughout the country's 15 provinces. It is largely at this time that Cuba's combination of practical training with theoretical instruction is seen. Students are obliged to attend classes but are also expected to learn from working alongside Cuban doctors in hospitals and polyclinics, where the overall student-to-patient ratio is about four to one at the medical school and two to one (students per bed) in practical classes in the hospitals.[28] The classes they take are also distinctive in that many are electives based on the countries they are from and in which they will be working, as well as classes in disaster management medicine. This is particularly useful in countries most affected by climate change and the natural disasters that result. There are also classes on alternative and indigenous knowledge-based medicines and region-specific diseases such as malaria and yellow fever and diseases related to altitude and poor nutrition, as well as classes in acupuncture, massage therapy, traditional medicine, and naturopathy.[29] Time is dedicated to traditional and natural medicine as many ELAM students will return to work in indigenous communities where shamans are often the trusted community health providers. Thus they learn not to oppose alternative medicines but rather to work with alternative healers and respect local customs, and to use local herbs with medicinal properties, thereby allowing them to provide healthcare to larger numbers of patients.[30]

It is also not uncommon for some advanced sixth-year students to return to their respective countries early to work alongside Cuban doctors in areas of greatest need or for what are termed "special missions." This allows the students to receive specialized training for the areas where they will be working upon graduation. In 2005, for example, some 350 of the 1,496 sixth-year students were sent on such missions. Among the students (accompanied by ELAM professors) were 150 Guatemalans who worked in 16 of the 22 Guatemalan districts, and 150 Hondurans who went to communities southeast of the Banana River where more than 1,400 indigenous Tawhoko settlers lived and were being cared for by Cuban medical brigades. They participated in these rotations in order to acquire a better understanding of the issues in the areas as well as to develop techniques that could be used to improve local healthcare after graduation.

A common theme emphasized throughout the six years of their medical training is the obligation for physicians to help wherever the needs are greatest. The earthquake in Haiti in January 2010 illustrates the degree to which this lesson had been absorbed. The ELAM central registry (a database on the activities of all students, including graduates) contacted 2,000 ELAM graduates to ask if they would be prepared to travel to Haiti to help their colleagues deal with the natural disaster. Approximately half stated that they could help, and eventually more than 700 of these doctors from 27 countries joined their fellow Haitian graduates and Cuban medical personnel.[31]

An illustration of the major components of the medical education given to ELAM students can be found in the huge two-volume textbook *Temas de Medicina Integral*, edited by Roberto Álvarez Sintes, which is based on the contributions of thousands of medical specialists. The preface talks of developing a "new paradigm in the training of health professionals, who need to provide integral care for the individual, the family, the community, and the environment; taking charge of health promotion in their community; leading a campaign in prevention of disease and other conditions that affect health; dealing with the major risk factors affecting illness and death; curing patients at the patients' bedside as a truly excellent physician; rehabilitating—in a physical, mental, and social sense—ill members of the community; and constituting the guardian of health of our people."[32] Volume 1 is used for the first two years of the program and again in the sixth year, while volume 2 is used during the clinical years. Specifically, the text focuses on understanding the Cuban approach to healthcare, which employs an intersectoral healthcare model.

The first volume provides the philosophical basis on which the entire training program rests, and it particularly emphasizes the social and environmental elements of health. Working within the community, promoting health education initiatives, and understanding the patient as a bio-psycho-social being, influenced and affected by many variables, are themes underlined with clarity. The need for personal communication with patients is stressed as being essential, as opposed to the "dehumanization of medicine" that has resulted from an excessive dependency on technology.[33] Dealing with the community in an effective, personal manner is extremely important, and primary healthcare is the key to achieving this: "Humans are social beings, and health concerns cannot be dealt with solely on an individual level. Rather, this has to be understood in the context of family and community variables. Without proper health of the community in general it is difficult to have good health for the family, and without proper family health the individual's well-being will always suffer."[34]

The 14 chapters in the first volume constitute the basis for the study of public health, as seen through the prism of the Cuban approach to public healthcare. After an initial chapter on the Cuban model, there are others that examine concepts of primary healthcare, the need for an integral, multidimensional understanding of health, the duty to work with the community and the role of the physician within it, as well as basic demography and epidemiology. The last five chapters act as a transition to the second volume and its focus on clinical medicine. Information is provided on academic training, research methodology, communication, and finally natural and traditional medicine.

Volume 2, with 22 chapters, is the essential companion for medical students' clinical training. The textbook emphasizes treatment of the most commonly found pathologies, since Cuban family doctors claim that they can generally identify 80–85 percent of the medical conditions of their patients through a proper medical examination and detailed history. As a result, one of the main thrusts of the clinical training is to examine the most common medical conditions that they would be expected to treat, hence the titles such as "Most frequently found infections," with the same being applied to ENT problems, as well as for respiratory tract, cardiac, vascular, mouth, digestive, urinary tract, gynecological, mammary gland, obstetrics, blood, endocrinology, ophthalmology, neurological, and finally limb and joints. The basis for the entire study of medicine, however, can be located in the foundation provided in the early chapters of the first volume, where the need for an "integral" approach to public health is emphasized, and advice is given to the students: "Consider always the unity of preventive and curative aspects of medicine, of both biology and social influences, as well as the conditions of the surrounding physical environment, all of which have a direct interaction with the individual and their society—and which conditions the process of health/illness. In order to fulfill their role, doctors need to undertake actions of promotion, prevention, restoration of health, and rehabilitation of the patient."[35] Most of the text is dedicated entirely to, or influenced by, community-oriented care and the role of the physician and the surrounding community. "You study the health of the community before the health of the individual," commented a Mexican student after his first two semesters at ELAM.[36]

While time is spent on subject competency, there is significantly more emphasis placed on the holistic approach of healthcare and by extension the framework within which physicians will be working in their respective communities. Noteworthy in the medical training is the fact that roughly 17 percent of all in-class hours in the six-year ELAM degree are dedicated to public health, compared with 14 percent of in-class time dedicated to primary care. The vast majority of training comes from working in the field alongside their professors or doctors rather than in the classroom. Moreover, throughout the first two years of medical school, the number of in-class hours dedicated to public health issues is more than double the class time spent on clinical skills, emphasizing the significance of working in the community.

In addition to the nature of the training and the time spent studying public health concerns, part of what makes the ELAM program so unusual is that the students have traditionally not been required to pay tuition. Moreover, the school provides monthly pocket money for all students, as well as covering all other living expenses including housing, food, and toiletries. Rather than using a business model of a university as a profit machine, the school only requires that the students sign a contract agreeing to practice in an underserved community upon graduation. This has changed in recent years, and students from some countries with the ability to pay are expected to contribute to their education. The majority, however, still pay no tuition.

The Students Speak

Since the first cohort of students at ELAM graduated in 2005, there is a significant body of material published in which their views of ELAM are given. Don Fitz, a professor at Washington University in St. Louis, is in an unusual situation since his daughter is a student at ELAM. He has written several articles on Cuban health issues, and in a recent piece he provides some useful insights into the experiences of students there.[37] He notes how students are the beneficiaries of free accommodation and meals, textbooks, medical services, uniforms, stethoscope, blood pressure cuff, and personal hygiene and laundry rations. For the first two years while they are on the ELAM campus they live under frugal conditions, with 8–14 students sleeping in a small dorm room. Personal space is a luxury, as is hot water. Discipline is strict: no alcohol is allowed on campus, and students are obliged to spend nights on campus during the work week. Cultural activities are actively supported, with students encouraged to cooperate in such activities with fellow students from their own country. Access to internet is limited—often to a couple of hours a month. Weekly room inspections take place, and physical education classes are mandatory. The challenging living conditions, emphasis on collective activities, obligatory physical education, and strict disciplinarian code of conduct are all designed to prepare the students for their work. For some, used to greater creature comforts at home, the discipline and spartan living conditions can seem excessive.[38]

Most students interviewed speak positively of the value of their education, the experience of learning from a radically different healthcare system, and their personal growth during the process. Understandably grateful for the opportunity to become physicians (since for most this would have been impossible in their home country), they are keen to put into practice the ideas and the ethos that they have learned. Particularly striking is their willingness to work wherever they are needed and to do so in a public system, accessible to all. While there are not published data on the post-ELAM careers of the medical graduates (although ELAM does keep its own set of records), there are many stories of disappointment. Often medical graduates, upon returning to their country, find that there are not opportunities for them, and occasionally they have to forgo their lofty aspirations and work part-time in private clinics. Many, too, have emigrated to countries where there are better prospects. Until its economic crisis, Spain was a common destination.

The academic evaluation of the students is also different. The exams and text evaluations are graded on a scale of 5 to 2 (2 being a fail). Should students fail, they are given extra time with any failing course and are able to retake the final exam twice. After the third failing grade, however, they are required to leave the program.[39] The quality of teaching is heavily monitored in order to ensure the competency and dedication of the students. Lectures, for example, are annually reviewed by a panel of two or three and must follow the outlined curriculum. Moreover, the progress of the lecturer's students is also closely followed.

The Role of Fidel Castro

Until the final years of Castro's role as president, it was often claimed that, because of his obsession with detail, overpowering personality, and tenacity, he ran everything in Cuba—from the strains of strawberries grown to the national steel quota. While there is some truth in the avid micromanaging on the part of the former president, it is only fair to concede credit for his role in the development of a host of initiatives in terms of public healthcare in Cuba, particularly in the field of medical internationalism. For Fidel Castro the role of doctors is of supreme importance, since in his words, "Graduating as a doctor is like opening a door to a long road leading to the noblest action that a human being can do for others."[40] His involvement with ELAM was particularly significant. In a speech on November 21, 1998, he spoke of the devastation of Hurricanes Georges and Mitch, the tens of thousands of people who had recently perished, and the need to assist the people of those affected areas.

Castro and colleagues analyzed the horrendous living conditions there. With the support of several hundred Cuban medical workers on the ground, he noted, it would be possible to reduce the infant mortality rates dramatically, and between 20,000 and 22,000 children could be saved each year. In the case of Central America he reflected on how people in the developed world were appalled by the death of 30,000 in the hurricane—yet paid little attention to the tragic reality that so many more avoidable deaths occurred every single year due to the lack of medical care for the impoverished. His famed attention to detail convinced him that a comprehensive health program provided by Cuban medical staff would save tens of thousands of lives.[41] He made an eloquent appeal to the industrialized countries, asking for medicines and offering human capital from Cuba to assist the devastated areas, although sadly his appeals to developed countries were largely ignored. While emergency assistance was appreciated, he urged them to think of those people who died every year in the affected regions because of a lack of medical care. A program of preventive healthcare was desperately needed in order to avert tens of thousands of deaths every year: "A hurricane worse than Mitch is causing terrible human damage. It is a hurricane that kills more people every year than this one. . . . [Twenty] years can pass without a Mitch and a million people will silently die in Central America without anyone taking notice."

Several hundred Cuban medical personnel were immediately sent to each of the affected areas. These he termed "doctors with the true spirit of health missionaries." But in addition to sending nearly 1,000 medical workers to the areas that had been devastated, the Cuban government decided to go a step further and to offer 500 medical scholarships a year for 10 years to students from the affected areas of Central America and Haiti. This basic idea came to fruition in the following year, as the first students from Central America and Haiti arrived, soon followed by hundreds more from throughout Latin America. When the official inauguration occurred, there were 27 ethnic groups represented, and an annual intake of over 1,400 students was established. (As noted earlier, this has been reduced to 750 students in 2014). Castro now saw clearly the need for an institutionalized approach to medical training, given the needs of the area. He placed the death toll of these natural disasters in the appropriate humanitarian context: "The television of images of thousands of bodies carried by the waters or partly covered by the mud shocked the world. Such are usually the days of generous offers and millionaire figures. But the shock fades away in a few weeks and soon everything is forgotten. The great promises are never delivered. Meanwhile, death continues to quietly take more lives every year than those caused by all the natural disasters together."[42] In his address the president noted that every year a million people from Latin America and the Caribbean died from preventable and curable diseases, a situation that was intolerable. His suggested solution was a new approach to public health, of necessity free and accessible and delivered by a new type of physician. The most significant quality of these graduates, he stated, would be "their absolute devotion to the most noble and human endeavor, that of saving lives and preserving health. More than physicians, they shall be zealous guardians of what human beings appreciate above all else. They will be apostles and builders of a more humane world. . . . They will be doctors ready to work wherever they are needed, in the remotest corners of the world where others are not willing to go. Such are the doctors who will graduate from this school."

Castro returned to discuss the foundation and goals of ELAM in several speeches and visited the school frequently to chart its success, meet with the students, and question faculty members about the curriculum. His was far more than a cursory interest in its evolution. At the first graduation of ELAM students in 2005, he recapped the goals of six years earlier—saving as many lives annually as had been taken by the hurricanes and progressively replacing Cuban medical staff with local doctors. He weighed the significance of Cuba's contribution to the developing world through the training of thousands of physicians, summarizing the humanitarian and highly ethical approach employed at ELAM.[43] He concluded his address in an unusually personal and emotional fashion, convinced of the enormous value of the Cuban role in this project, noting that "all the gold in the world cannot subdue the conscience of a true guardian of health and life, who is ready to go to any country where [their] services are required, convinced that a better world is possible!"

In Synthesis

The Latin American School of Medicine has produced over 24,000 physicians for the developing world and has imbued them with a radical new concept of their role.[44] It has also served as the staging ground for the more recent forms of hands-on medical training, seen most clearly in Venezuela, Timor-Leste, and The Gambia, where the physician/professor supervises small groups of local students in treating patients from the first year of their training, while they also take theoretical classes in a classroom setting from their Cuban medical professors. There are common features to both approaches, ranging from the core content of academic material covered to the humanistic philosophy in treating patients, from the role of the physician in the community to the very concept of access to healthcare as a fundamental human right. Cardinal Tarcisio Bertone, Vatican secretary of state, was able to appreciate this, commenting on "the solidarity with the poorest and the neediest" when he visited ELAM in February 2008. He was particularly struck by the emphasis placed on the humanistic Cuban approach to patient care, since "not only do they need a solid professional training, but also a 'training of the heart.'"[45]

Several features stand out when analyzing the impact of ELAM. The first is that since 1999 it has provided a free medical education to thousands of medical students from poor backgrounds who could otherwise never have been able to graduate as physicians. Since 2012, however, some students have been charged for their education, and a means test has been applied. "It is not a secret that Cuba is facing economic difficulties," noted the academic vice rector, Heidi Soca, "and to make this project of human solidarity viable we need finances."[46] As a result, for the first time in its history, ELAM is now charging some students for the general program and for specialized courses. Governments that are considered able to contribute are increasingly being asked to pay for the medical education of students. There are, for instance, 1,200 South African students at ELAM, and their government pays $60,000 per student for the six-year training program.[47] The second is the nature of the medical training itself, which is unlike that provided in traditional medical schools, either in developed or developing countries. The focus is on the community, on the analysis of a patient as a bio-psycho-social human being,[48] on the development of solid clinical skills that depend more on a solid physical examination than on technology, and on the need for preventive (and corresponding less on curative) approaches to public health.

"Old school" medical authorities look askance at this approach employed in the Cuban system. Trained in a system that emphasized curative medical strategies, and accustomed to dispensing medications to treat individual conditions, they see this approach to preventive healthcare, based on attending to the needs of the community, as an alien concept. Moreover, most are from fairly wealthy backgrounds, people who could afford to go to medical school and who in many cases have a limited understanding of socioeconomic conditions faced by the poor majority of their fellow citizens living in underserved *barrios* or distant rural areas. Most do not live in these districts and have little to do with these social strata. In addition, many work in private hospitals or clinics and make a living from charging people for their medical knowledge. For those trained in the Cuban approach to public healthcare, this is the antithesis of their beliefs. Indeed, ELAM (as well as the other Cuban medical programs employed elsewhere, most notably in Venezuela) is training doctors who do understand the public healthcare challenges of the poor, traditionally underserved majority, since most of these new physicians come from those same groups. They have been trained (for critics, brainwashed) to embrace a wholly different approach to medical care and have done so successfully throughout the developing world. They are prepared to work around the clock, to pay back their debt to humanity, and to provide medical care without charging their patients. Their numbers are growing rapidly (the Cuban program of medical training in Venezuela expects to graduate 60,000 within the next few years, and 20,000 physicians have already graduated). For the old medical guard, this is a growing danger, since they represent a significant threat to their status and their value system.

This chapter was introduced by a quotation from Dr. Margaret Chan, who began her career in public health in 1978. In an insightful address to faculty and students at ELAM on October 27, 2009, she praised the pragmatic nature of the medical training provided there. Students were being taught to deal with conditions in the developing world and to be full participants in their communities: "You are being trained to be engaged members of the communities you serve, and not just doctors in white jackets waiting for the problems to show up, preferably by appointment, in your offices." They were also specializing in a preventive approach to public health, to be active participants in their communities: "You are being trained to spot communitywide threats to health linked to living or working conditions, or lifestyles and behaviors, or what people eat, drink, or think." She approved strongly of this approach to medical training, so necessary for developing countries, and referred to their education in "the skills needed to help the underprivileged enjoy good health as a basic human right." This is exactly the humanitarian essence that the Cuban approach seeks to develop in its students.

Criticisms are leveled at the approach to medical training found at ELAM, usually by people who have received a classical medical education, often in private universities. While taking nothing away from their clinical skills, it is clear that their clients are very different from the patients of the ELAM graduates. At ELAM the students receive an education focused on meeting the needs of people who have traditionally been ignored and who consequently have received limited medical attention, if any. The ELAM graduates are prepared to work wherever and whenever they are needed—as was clearly shown by the participation of several hundred ELAM volunteers in Haiti in the wake of the 2010 hurricane and subsequent dengue epidemic. Since they and their patients are mostly from similar social backgrounds, they understand the conditions in which they live. Chan summarized with clarity the fundamental ethos of the ELAM approach: "You are being trained to correct an imbalance in the way medical care is distributed. You are being trained to return the practice of medicine to the basic values of people-centered, compassionate care, guided by need, and not by the patient's ability to pay."[49] The students at ELAM could not agree more.

3

Dealing with the "Handicapped" of ALBA

Setting the Balance Right

> They are not "handicapped." We need to eliminate that word from our vocabulary. The term [*minusválido*] implies something that is worth less. . . . They are our compatriots, people who are worth the same as us—because the efforts that they make, spiritually and physically, are a lot greater than what we have made throughout our life.
>
> President Hugo Chávez of Venezuela

> Being disabled is not a lack of ability. Rather it is part of the wonderful diversity that surrounds us.
>
> Vice President Lenín Moreno of Ecuador

> This was a Mission that committed itself to travel throughout the entire country, in the countryside and the cities, house by house, to every barrio, to help our brothers and sisters with any kind of *discapacidad*. . . . The Cuban doctors left their country, their homes, their way of life and made sacrifices, traveling along the dusty, forgotten roads in our countryside, in the cold *altiplano*, in our valleys, our tropical zones, and our plains.
>
> Vice President Álvaro García Linera of Bolivia

One of the areas of Cuban medical internationalism that has been least studied is the wide-ranging medical and social survey of people with physical and intellectual disabilities in a number of Latin American and Caribbean countries. This chapter analyzes the significance of the Cuban role in the three largest programs of assistance in this regard—in Venezuela, Ecuador, and Bolivia. The term widely employed in Spanish is *discapacitados* or occasionally *minusválidos*, both of which are inappropriate, since they refer to people being "handicapped" or "incapacitated," while *minusválidos* even hints at people with disabilities being of lesser value than those without disabilities. In this chapter every effort has been made to interpret the term in an appropriate fashion as the Cuban approach clearly shows and as Morales and Moreno note. In essence, scores of Cuban specialists led a nationwide campaign to survey the health of almost the entire population, to take the measure of those citizens with disabilities, and to draw up remedial actions to support them. In addition, Cuban medical personnel implemented a large genetic testing program that took place in five ALBA countries between 2007 and 2010 as a means of planning appropriate strategies to support them and their families. This was a door-to-door campaign designed to examine the health of the populations of Venezuela, Ecuador, Nicaragua, Bolivia, and Saint Vincent and the Grenadines. It was hoped that once this army of Cuban medical specialists (supported by local authorities and medical personnel in each country) had completed this detailed examination of the population, the governments involved would have a better sense of the degree of *discapacidad* in each community as well as the needs of their population at large. The argument was that, armed with this information, the government would then be able to draw up an appropriate plan to support their target population, allowing them to participate more fully in their society while simultaneously reducing societal stereotypes about people with disabilities. It was based on extensive interviews as the teams passed from house to house in order to determine the assistance required for the target population. It had never been done before, anywhere in the world—apart from in Cuba nearly a decade earlier.

Once again the Cuban model relied on specialized medical staff, prepared to travel throughout these countries and often in challenging situations. All of the Cuban participants had extensive experience working with patients who had physical and intellectual disabilities, and some had worked on more than one campaign, passing from one country to the next. Interviews with several of the participants in the various campaigns were conducted in Havana, and all subjects talked of the long hours and difficult conditions of work, many involving visits to isolated huts in the jungle and mountain areas, often meeting with families who had never even seen a doctor before. Many of the people visited were literally "undocumented," having never been registered or identified in a national census of any kind, and they lived entirely out of the reach of government programs or agencies. Nobody in authority knew that they existed. The process of the sweeping visitations then undertaken instilled in them a sense of dignity, ensuring that the questions of *discapacidad* would now be perceived in a different light. For the disabled, this "different light" revolved around their situation being improved, since they felt badly limited by the environment, society, and surrounding structure. To a large extent their condition has improved as a result of these programs.

The World Health Organization (WHO) has summarized *disability* in a fairly comprehensive manner:

> *Disabilities* is an umbrella term, covering impairments, activity limitations, and participation restrictions. An impairment is a problem in body function or structure; an activity limitation is a difficulty encountered by an individual in executing a task or action; while a participation restriction is a problem experienced by an individual in involvement in life situations. Disability is thus not just a health problem. It is a complex phenomenon, reflecting the interaction between features of a person's body and features of the society in which he or she lives. Overcoming the difficulties faced by people with disabilities requires interventions to remove environmental and social barriers.[1]

An estimated 15 percent of the world's population—approximately a billion people—live with some sort of disability. Sadly, questions of physical and intellectual disability are often swept to one side, ignored, and overlooked. This is particularly the case in developing countries, where there are more pressing day-to-day problems encountered and often little money to deal with them. People with disabilities are often hidden, made invisible, and therefore are not even on the radar of policymakers and governments. As a result their needs are often not considered. Significantly the WHO itself only issued its first global report on "disability" in 2011, a surprising oversight—but one which illustrates the tendency to overlook this important human challenge, and the millions of people affected directly and indirectly.

The basis for Cuba's initiative in these countries can be traced back to a program undertaken between 2001 and 2003 to ascertain the number of persons with physical or psycho-social disabilities there. This served as a prototype for the projects studied in this chapter. There were six basic criteria for inclusion in the study: physical movement limitations, visual impairments (ranging from limited vision to total blindness), hearing difficulties, chronic renal deficiencies (requiring dialysis or hemodialysis), mental health diagnosis (such as dementia or chronic psychosis, including schizophrenia and bipolar disorders), and intellectual disability. To carry out this program, an army of specialists and general practitioners spread throughout the country. Door-to-door inquiries in almost every home were made by teams of specialists, with follow-up home visits to the persons identified as having a disability by medical personnel and social workers, to both interview and provide a medical assessment of every single inhabitant. Initially there were three rounds of pilot studies undertaken to fine-tune the approach used, with the initial visit to each Cuban home being undertaken by two physicians, one a specialist in integrated general medicine and the other an educational psychologist. The first visit consisted of a general interview with all family members, followed by a more detailed meeting with subjects showing signs of intellectual or physical disabilities and a thorough clinical examination. If a more detailed consultation was needed, a team of professional specialists visited the home and, after obtaining permission from either the subject or the family, further genetic testing followed. When a person with developmental delays was identified, a team of professionals and technicians visited the family to devise a program to assist them.

One of the objectives of this interdisciplinary team was to identify the socioeconomic challenges that affected the patient, and the approach employed by the medical team was intended to improve their standard of living as well as make suggestions to support their medical condition. After two years of intensive medical work, 366,864 people were identified as having some form of impairment, resulting in an overall ratio of 3.26 per 100 inhabitants in the country. What is significant about the results is that the number of people determined to be impaired was almost three times larger than the number officially registered, underlining how badly understood the challenges faced by people with intellectual and physical disabilities were, even in Cuba. If this was the case there—with its high standard of public healthcare throughout the country and social participation—then understandably it would represent a far greater challenge elsewhere in the developing world, where often early intervention programs for people with physical and intellectual disabilities were both costly and infrequent. In the case of Cuba, the data showed that the age group with the greatest number of people with disabilities was those over 60 (7.8 for every 100 inhabitants), with the lowest being children under the age of 4 (0.6 per 100). The most common challenge was learning disability (140,498 or 38.29 percent of the persons identified), followed by those with poor motor skills (92,506 or 25.22 percent).[2]

In this nationwide survey, many causes were indicated to explain the physical and intellectual challenges encountered. Old age, accidents, violence, excessive use of alcohol, and exposure to chemicals were common causes of the subjects' impairments. Other causes such as malnutrition, extreme poverty, and the impact of natural disasters, particularly hurricanes, were also reported. These factors can be summarized in three basic groupings—sociocultural influences, genetic composition, and hygienic conditions. Cuban medical personnel noted various kinds of *discapacidad*, including paralysis (partial or complete), sight impairment, hearing loss, psychological challenges, organ (and in particular kidney) difficulties, and people who were deaf or blind. What became clear from the detailed examination at each home visit and, where necessary, follow-up genetic testing was that, despite the often excellent recordkeeping at the family doctor level, there was not an accurate picture of the number of people living with impairments. Consistently there was an underestimation of the numbers of those involved.

This two-year nationwide campaign by Cuban specialists, a detailed and meticulous strategy of door-to-door site visits, physical examinations, and follow-up specialized genetic testing provided the basic model for the massive campaigns employed in several countries that are members of ALBA (the Bolivarian Alliance for the Americas). These included Venezuela (where the campaign started on July 24, 2007, and finished on October 27, 2008), Ecuador (from July 1, 2008, until December 2010), Nicaragua (from October 8, 2009, to October 2010), Bolivia (from November 2, 2009, to August 13, 2010), and Saint Vincent and the Grenadines (March 1–26, 2010). The Cuban experience had shown both the need for such an exhaustive study and the strategy to undertake it. This led to several other member countries of ALBA (which had already received the benefit of Cuban medical cooperation) requesting this support. Cuban medical expertise and Venezuelan financial support prepared the way for the expansion of this program, one which had never been attempted before anywhere.

The same exhaustive, house-to-house approach that had been employed in Cuba several years earlier was again used in each participating country, with slight adjustments caused by the distinctive reality and geographical challenges of the various countries. Mass participation meant just that—the Cuban medical professionals numbering in the hundreds were clearly the inspiration and provided the ideas for the campaign. They were, however, supported by large numbers of local medical personnel, government officials, members of the military (needed for transportation to many of the rural locations that could be reached only with helicopters and amphibious vehicles), and civilians. The basic framework for this extensive work was closely based on the approach used in Cuba. Similar categories were also employed to determine the nature of impairment, such as physical/motor, visual, hearing, psycho-social, and level of mental delay.

Adapting the Cuban Approach to Latin America: The Mission in Venezuela

The first country to benefit from this Cuban model was Venezuela. This was understandable, since at the time there were already almost 30,000 Cuban medical staff spread throughout the country, particularly in marginalized areas. Not surprisingly these areas were exactly the regions with the highest level of people with physical and psycho-social disabilities, largely for socioeconomic reasons. The original idea for the study in Venezuela had allegedly come from President Fidel Castro, probably after suggesting it as a means of employing Cuba's large pool of medical capital while supporting his close ally. After it had proved successful in Cuba, he suggested it to his Venezuelan counterpart, Hugo Chávez. Already the highly successful Barrio Adentro and Operación Milagro programs had been established there. After it had proved a useful complement to the Barrio Adentro program in Caracas, the campaign to survey the population for potential intellectual and physical disabilities was then expanded. There were three stages to the approach used: diagnosis of the situation faced by Venezuelans with a variety of physical and intellectual disabilities, analysis of the needs to assist these people, and the design of a program to incorporate them into society. Cuban specialists participated in planning all three phases of this campaign.

As noted, the approach had proved its value in Cuba between 2007 and 2010, although it remained to be seen how it could be applied elsewhere. As was the custom in other countries where these programs were employed, an important symbolic name for the campaign was selected by the national government to illustrate its importance, in this case Dr. José Gregorio Hernández (1864–1919), a well-known figure in medical circles in Venezuela. He had studied in France, published on a variety of medical topics, and become renowned as a dedicated teacher. He had also studied for the priesthood (although he never became a priest) and was eventually canonized by the Catholic Church because of his compassion, generosity, and solidarity with the poor. In sum, he was a figure who had a broad appeal to the population at large. His selection showed that, despite the implementation of a Cuban program with the participation of Cuban specialists, this was in essence a Venezuelan project.

The program had a very simple goal: to discover the number of Venezuelans who live with physical and intellectual disabilities, in order to ultimately devise a strategy to provide them with better assistance. At the end of the first stage of the campaign (providing a summary of the numbers of Venezuelans with disabilities), detailed information was given to the Venezuelan public by Cuba's deputy minister of public health, Dr. Marcia Cobas (a specialist in this medical area). She emphasized the participation of Venezuelan professionals and volunteers (28,754) who had visited 620,105 homes, including in the most remote corners of the country. Later data showed a slight increase to 645,000 homes visited. It is generally accepted that, between subjects identified and family members, Cuban-Venezuelan medical teams interviewed or examined almost 4 million people. Of particular mention is the fact that over 5,000 Venezuelan medical students (most trained under Cuban medical professors) participated in the project, receiving hands-on experience as they came across areas of poverty and marginalization. A variety of specialists, Cuban and Venezuelan, took part in the Misión: geneticists, neurosurgeons, physiotherapists, neurophysiologists, and social workers as well as an army of medical students training to be comprehensive general physicians. The Cuban delegation consisted of 200 specialists in comprehensive general medicine (*medicina general integral*) and genetic analysis, 200 experts in education and special education, 17 specialists in clinical genetics, and a handful of specialists in neurophysiology, psychology, and pediatric neurology to support their colleagues with particularly complex cases. They were subsequently joined by physiotherapists, researchers, and computer specialists to help maintain records and undertake detailed epidemiological studies.[3] The latter were needed because, as is the case in the public healthcare system in Cuba, rigorous information gathering and accounting are widely used practices.

Medical professionals, social workers, and psychologists from both countries participated, as was the case in subsequent campaigns held in other ALBA countries. The Cubans provided the basic framework (to be adjusted to meet the needs of each country where it was implemented) and the key personnel in the process. In each of the countries where the programs took place, specialists and civilian volunteers supported their initiatives, forming the critical mass needed to adapt the model to the reality of the host nation. All of the campaigns emphasized the need to recognize disability as a social justice issue and not just a medical one. It is worth noting that each home was visited by a team of medical personnel (usually four or five people from different medical backgrounds) and not just one person. As a result, "all challenges of the patient, in terms of movement, sight, hearing, and intellectual—both genetic and acquired conditions—could be evaluated, as well as the possibilities of rehabilitation and therapy."[4] Follow-up visits were generally scheduled to evaluate complex cases, and if necessary, blood and urine samples were taken for analysis by geneticists in Venezuela and Cuba. Eventually a March 15, 2013, report noted that some 336,000 Venezuelans had been diagnosed with some sort of *discapacidad*, following visits to 645,000 homes in 335 municipalities of the country.[5] Marcia Cobas summarized the data that resulted from this exhaustive program:

- 128,836 people (including 9,311 children under 14) had difficulties of movement.
- 99,383 suffered from an intellectual challenge.
- 29,068 had hearing loss (including 2,080 children).
- 28,729 people were visually impaired (including 2,080 children).
- 22,661 had mental health difficulties (e.g., psychosis, schizophrenia).
- 22,256 suffered from more than one challenge (including 642 children).
- 13,478 had Down syndrome (including 5,660 children).
- 5,629 had chronic kidney deficiency (including 112 children)—important because it showed the extent of the need for dialysis.[6]

The next stage was to determine how the government could respond to these identified needs, and here the Cubans used their experience to support the initiatives of the Venezuelan government. Calculations were made concerning the number of facilities needed to provide special education, establish genetic testing and research centers, develop workshops to build prostheses, and improve the lives of those identified as having a disability. This had to be done with great sensitivity, given the high level of expectations among the people who had been visited and the wide media coverage that had been generated. Of particular importance was the need to determine which specific preventive measures could be taken to avoid further problems among those affected and how to improve their general living conditions. In the case of genetic conditions, it was also necessary to establish laboratories to test patients and to suggest programs for improved health. (It was shown in the same report, to take one example, that there were some 18,293 children between 5 and 19 who needed special education facilities.)

For people without arms or legs or living with a physical deformity, there was another clear need for practical support, and again the approach employed in Venezuela was based on the Cuban experience. As a result six laboratories for prostheses and for orthopedic support were built or modernized by 2013. However, there were not enough Venezuelan technicians to build prostheses, and training was also required for those working in the laboratories that had been set up. Again Cuba helped, and by September 2011, with the support of 18 Cuban specialists, 37 technicians graduated from the first course in producing prostheses, a first step in a nationwide program. By that time 1,358 Venezuelans had received prosthetic limbs, a process which has continued.[7]

Venezuela also needed a program of genetic testing in order to determine the causes of medical conditions, and by the following month over 10,000 consults with geneticists had been carried out.[8] To support this radically different approach, the nation's first national center for the study of genetics, as well as a master's program in genetic assessment, were established, with courses being taught by Cuban specialists. In addition, to support the 17,000 Venezuelans who lived with profound medical problems and were unable to leave their homes, more than 20,000 people were trained to care for them as personal attendants.[9] One perhaps unexpected aspect was the issuance of identity cards for some 12,000 people who, because they had profound physical and mental disabilities, had often been ignored (if not shunned) and were therefore virtually invisible. They were in essence nonpersons, without any basic legal rights. The Venezuelan government sought to remedy that situation, implementing a system to make them aware of their rights and to provide socioeconomic benefits to which they were entitled but which, because nobody knew of their existence, they had never received. This phenomenon was to be repeated in other countries, where tens of thousands of people were finally "discovered."

Venezuela consistently used the Cuban model as the basis for the various stages of the campaign employed throughout the country, adapting it to fit national characteristics. This practical adaptation of the Cuban model produced a prototype that served as a springboard for further campaigns in other ALBA countries. It illustrated the way in which Cuban medical staff could provide the basis for a pragmatic hands-on campaign, supported by local medical personnel as well as government bureaucrats and members of civil society. The mission was based on the concept of cooperating with local specialists and volunteers (while training them), which ensured badly needed continuity after the Cubans returned home.

The Misión Solidaria Manuela Espejo in Ecuador

The next country to take advantage of Cuban expertise was Ecuador, which ran its own program between 2008 and 2010 and produced similar results. In Ecuador the Misión Solidaria Manuela Espejo (named after a leading nineteenth-century feminist, writer, and supporter of the independence movement from Spain) was established as a result of the successful application of the Venezuelan campaign, the offer of support from Cuba (following meetings in Havana between Fidel Castro and the Ecuadoran vice president, Lenín Moreno), and recognition of the need for such a project by the Ecuadoran government.[10] In 2008 the government approved a new constitution that protected the rights of people with disabilities, a step that facilitated the Manuela Espejo Mission. With the advice and support of many of the people who had already implemented the program in Venezuela, the campaign was now launched.

An agreement was signed by the office of the vice president, the Ecuadoran Ministry of Defense (whose support was essential to provide logistical assistance, since many of the regions to be visited were often inaccessible), and the Ministry of Public Health in Cuba, as well as several other ministries and government offices. The objective was to implement the Cuban program while adapting it to Ecuadoran conditions. In all, 14 government ministries or bodies from the Ecuadoran government (ranging from the Ministry of Social Development to the Civil Registry) agreed to coordinate their support in the Misión Solidaria Manuela Espejo. Again the first stage was a detailed survey of the population, to determine the causes of the physical and intellectual disabilities faced by the population, bearing in mind biological, psychological, social, medical, and genetic factors. Societal factors as well as the individual medical variables were analyzed in depth. The final objective was to plan a program that could best support the needs of the affected population. The Cuban model, adapted in Venezuela, again formed the basic structure for the misión, although now it was adapted to better reflect the needs and idiosyncrasies of Ecuador.

The role of Lenín Moreno (vice president in the government of Rafael Correa from 2007 to 2013) was of key importance in the development of this campaign. Moreno was himself a wheelchair user, after having been shot in the back during a robbery. Described in an insightful article as being "the planet's most powerful wheelchair-using man," he resigned from his position in 2013, noting, "Power comes with a stroke of fortune and you should quickly leave it behind. But while you are in that space, you must take advantage of it to realize your dearest ambition. For me that was to promote the rights of the disabled."[11] State support for people with disabilities rose from a paltry $2 million to $150 million during his tenure, and many of those working in the vice president's office were themselves people with disabilities. This gave legitimacy to the program in Ecuador, since it was influenced not just by medical experts but also by people living with disabilities. He received many awards for his services and spoke at many conferences about the need for attention to be paid to all with disabilities, visiting 40 countries after 2007. With a spokesman as skilled as Moreno, and in such an influential position, the campaign of Ecuador was understandably very successful.

In September 2012 the vice president spoke about the successes of the Manuela Espejo campaign at a United Nations conference in Washington on the rights of people with disabilities, and he urged other countries to learn from the experience of Ecuador. In essence his message was that member nations needed to adjust their way of thinking. Services and programs for people with disabilities should be carried out not through a sense of charity but because of the need for human solidarity, for justice. True solidarity, he noted, "is given between equals, in a horizontal fashion, between people who are different but equal in both rights and duties."[12] He referred to his own situation, noting that being dependent on a wheelchair allowed him a different perspective, visually as well as physically. People able to walk generally looked to the front and upwards, whereas moving in a wheelchair obliged him to always look down: "There you discover a different reality—of people who are almost invisible in the eyes of the majority, a reality of human beings who that majority had wished to condemn to oblivion." As an alternative he offered the Ecuadoran experience in which both government and society needed to participate actively. While the government role had been important, so too had been the relatives of the intellectually and physically challenged, the media, public and private institutions, and society as a whole. In this way Ecuadorans with special needs were able to begin to recover their dignity.

In this mission the Cuban medical role was again significant. Some 229 Cuban specialists, together with 120 Ecuadoran colleagues and an army of volunteers, initiated the first stage of the program, providing a medical-scientific-social analysis of the situation of the population as a whole and seeking to discover and address the needs and supports of those living with disabilities. Again the time-tested model employed in Cuba and most recently in Venezuela formed the basis of the approach used in establishing a diagnosis of the health needs in Ecuador.

A team of medical specialists usually visited each home (some 1.2 million homes in total). The teams again consisted of four or five people—a specialist in general medicine, one or two specialists in psycho-pedagogy and clinical genetics, at times a community leader to encourage skeptical locals to allow themselves to have a medical check up, and a representative of the armed forces. The transportation, planning, safety, general logistical support, and mapping of homes and their locations were carried out by the military. Many of the homes visited were in inaccessible locations where various methods of transportation—including canoes, donkeys, and helicopters—were required. In all there were 70 multidisciplinary medical groups who were sent throughout Ecuador. In interviews held in Havana with participants in this mission, they explained to me the difficulties in reaching some of the most isolated areas, many of which could only be reached by canoe after long hours of traveling through dense bush. They also commented on the reaction of the people they encountered in such remote areas, since many could not understand why anybody, much less the government or foreigners, would take an interest in them. They were so accustomed to being ignored and abandoned that they were often initially at a loss to understand the idea that the government wanted to help them.

At each home that was visited by the medical team, all family members were interviewed. This was done to ascertain the health of the population and to see if there were any other members with disabilities. This was understandably an intimidating experience for many Ecuadorans, many of whom had never been able to afford a doctor and yet were being visited by a medical team (and foreigners at that) in their own home. Fortunately the presence of an Ecuadoran member of the national armed forces with each team was usually sufficient to convince them that this was an official government-supported program. The role of the general physician was extremely important in assessing the overall health of each person examined. A series of basic tests were employed by the psychologist in the team to measure the level of intellectual abilities of the family members and to ascertain if there were any people in the family with intellectual disabilities, after which the geneticist applied tests to measure clinical and genetic factors. If there were family members with a clear intellectual disability, a second visit with the geneticist was arranged, at which time blood and urine samples were taken and sent for testing. The objective was to determine the medical conditions and, after the diagnosis was made, to provide the appropriate treatment for the patient in order to improve their quality of life. In addition to these small teams there was also a larger team of Cuban specialists (general medicine, geneticists, physiologists, psychologists, ear, nose, and throat specialists, physiotherapists, cardiologists, pediatricians, and nurses) who were on call for assistance and with whom they consulted in complex cases.

The results were in many ways similar to those found in Venezuela. In total 1,286,331 homes were visited in all 24 of Ecuador's provinces and 221 districts (*cantones*), and 293,743 people with physical or mental disabilities were identified. The major groups were the 107,522 who had a physical impairment (36.6 percent), followed by those with an intellectual disability (71,417, or 24.3 percent), and 33,828 (11.52 percent) who had hearing impairments.[13] Further medical care was provided to another 825,576 patients who needed treatment for other conditions which had been diagnosed during the everyday course of visits. Moreover, there were 21,062 consults with geneticists (as well as 35,257 consults with other specialists), while 26,327 urgent cases of medical problems were indicated—and were dealt with immediately.[14] In many cases relatives of the persons identified also needed medical care, and some 144,336 people were treated after their relatives with disabilities had been helped.[15] The most frequent causes for many of the medical conditions encountered were related to the prenatal period or the first year of life, a situation which the government of Ecuador subsequently sought to remedy with a new program for infants.

There was a fundamental lack of awareness by both society and past governments of the situation of Ecuadorans with disabilities. Some research had been undertaken in the past, but remarkably little had been done to support the sectors identified. Many *campesinos* who faced particularly bad conditions had never even received minimal medical treatment and were often not listed in any government census. Added to this was the stigma imposed by society, which saw many people with disabilities as being virtually subhuman, preferring to ignore them and pretend that this sad reality never existed. Following the Manuela Espejo mission, however, the situation changed. It was now known who these people were, where they lived, what their needs were, and what their potential was. As was the case in Venezuela, many in the most distant areas had to have specific geo-references provided for their files, since they lived totally beneath any government radar. Again the role of the local armed forces was particularly helpful in this aspect. The Cubans had led the way by devising a program to discover these needs and offer suggestions, after which it was up to the government in Quito to decide how to improve their conditions.

The second stage in the Manuela Espejo program was the response of the government to the situation of people with disabilities. Following the nationwide campaign, Cuban and Ecuadoran specialists drew up a list of measures to meet their needs. Again, many factors came into play in pursuing an innovative strategy. Immediate support was given to those in the most precarious living conditions and to those where simple aids could make difficult living conditions more bearable. By February 2013, according to official data, hundreds of thousands had been assisted by the government: over 197,000 Ecuadorans with physical disabilities had received treatment, and some 430,000 had been provided with material support such as wheelchairs, walkers, canes, crutches, diapers, and mattresses. In addition almost 18,000 had received hearing aids, while 4,000 had been given prosthetic limbs, now made in Ecuador, avoiding the high cost of imports. In addition, 705,000 children had hearing tests, with 1,749 receiving hearing aids, while 1,400 health professionals were trained to administer the tests. For those who needed prostheses, three workshops, capable of producing 1,000 prosthetic limbs a year, were established in Quito, Loja, and Guayaquil, and mobile workshops were set up to reach rural areas.[16] More than $4 million was invested in these programs, and 4,606 Ecuadoreans received prostheses.[17]

The government response, designed to follow up from the findings of the Manuela Espejo Misión and to provide needed support, revolved around a new program known as the Misión Joaquín Gallegos Lara. It was named after the inspirational Ecuadoran writer, who had a physical disability. The objective was to provide support (both materially and financially) for those people who were in the greatest need. Those identified in the Manuela Espejo Misión were again visited, and a family member was registered as the person responsible for their care. Some 14,479 people benefited from this program, with a $240 monthly pension being given to their caretaker. The government also provided free medication and training in areas such as health, hygiene, nutrition, and rehabilitation, and life insurance (worth $500) was issued in the name of the person with the disability.[18] This follow-up mission also listed 115 medical conditions for which people experiencing these conditions would receive financial support from the government. In 2012 the government signed two executive decrees (1138 and 1284) to assist the beneficiaries. The first promised support to those with severe, "catastrophic," or complex medical conditions, while the second approved a financial aid package for young people living with HIV/AIDS. Among the "catastrophic" diseases or medical conditions covered were congenital heart diseases, all forms of cancer, serious kidney problems, cerebral tumors, any organ transplants, severe burns, and aneurisms. There were also 106 conditions for which Ecuadorans could qualify for a $240 monthly pension, ranging from serious anemia to fibrosis, autism to rheumatoid arthritis.

Given the high number of medical conditions that resulted in the first year of life, many of which could be avoided, a mass neonatal program was instituted under the slogan "Con pie derecho, la huella del futuro" (Right foot forward, footprint of the future). This consisted of taking a blood sample from a baby's foot soon after birth. This allowed geneticists to detect several basic conditions that could be treated immediately, avoiding potentially severe illness. These medical conditions are congenital hypothyroidism, phenylketonuria (PKU), galactosemia, and congenital adrenal hyperplasia. In industrialized countries these blood tests are taken immediately after birth in the hospital. In developing nations, however, access to hospitals can be difficult and expensive—and so there is generally a wait of several days before the blood samples can be drawn.

Cuban participants in this mission explained to me that when the blood test on one of the babies revealed medical problems, they were immediately treated by the specialists in that area. Speaking in August 2012, President Rafael Correa noted that in the previous months 149,643 newborns had been tested for these conditions, and it was hoped that the following year all 315,000 of the babies born each year in Ecuador would be tested.[19] The Cuban emphasis on preventive medicine was clearly a major influence in this program, and a formal bilateral agreement was signed to ensure Cuban technical cooperation. Support for the genetic testing was provided by Cuba in the form of specialized training for laboratory workers and technical advice on medical conditions detected. In addition, the Ecuadoran government agreed to buy from Cuba $900,000 for the reactive agents that allow technicians to detect the congenital malformations.[20]

Perhaps just as important as the immediate support provided to those with disabilities was, as in the case of Venezuela, a change in societal attitude toward this sector of the population which in the past had been deliberately hidden from public view. Now with the vice president himself using a wheelchair, it was time for a major shift in attitude. As was the case in Venezuela, identity cards were now issued to many people who in the past had been kept from public view. The government provided financial support for those with physical disabilities, visits by newly trained community doctors (many educated at ELAM in Cuba) were scheduled, and housing was distributed to those most in need. By August 2012 some 6,000 housing units had been provided, and plans were made for a further 9,000. (A critical article noted that the government had not lived up to its plans, since a need had been demonstrated for 13,295 houses, while only half that number had been constructed.)[21] Nevertheless, the government had taken an important step and had provided more support for the disabled than any had in the past. Vice President Moreno summarized this advance: "The most important aspect is that we have managed to make Ecuadorans with physical or mental challenges, and their family members, feel able to walk proudly on the streets. No longer are they kept in a dark corner, in a chicken pen, or even a rabbit hutch or a cave. They are no longer ashamed, and instead see their right to obtain happiness."[22] To ensure that Ecuadoran society was given the opportunity to participate in the follow-up to the program, many cultural and sporting events were held. The Juguemos sin Barreras (Let's Play without Barriers) Paralympics, the Choir of Silence, workshops in folk dancing and painting, the Circo Social (a social circus with the support of Canada's Cirque du Soleil), and the many Caminatas Solidarias (walkathons with special needs groups around the country, involving 180,000 people) illustrate this commitment. Given the importance of the work of this campaign and the need to maintain the dynamic of its application, in early 2013 the Ecuadoran government decided to change the "mission" into a full government secretariat.

Under Moreno, the government introduced a program called "Ecuador without Barriers," and it sought to sensitize people to the reality of the most vulnerable sectors of society that had remained basically forgotten and invisible for decades. Inclusion of all Ecuadorans was now a policy to be pursued rigorously. The government went a step further, mandating quotas of citizens to be hired in state offices as well as in large private corporations. The Organic Law of Public Service, passed in 2010, stated that 4 percent of all those employed in the public sector and 3 percent in the private sector had to be employees with disabilities. By January 2013 some 40,020 persons with disabilities had received employment as a result of this. The government instituted a program of visiting businesses to lobby for these programs, and in 2011 alone it inspected 3,750 public and private workplaces to ensure that the legislation was being respected. By 2013, between private businesses and public sector offices, government inspectors had visited 17,337.[23] Even civil servants received benefits from the Correa government, and Executive Decree 960, issued in March 2008, stipulated that all bureaucrats with disabilities had the right to travel accompanied by up to two people to assist them, including family members, and all would be paid a per diem for their work.

In many of the countries where Cuban doctors have worked for free or for relatively low salaries, there was a strong suspicion about the motives for their cooperation. Why would they do this? And why do so not for able-bodied people but rather for those with disabilities? Why were they not charging patients, as had traditionally been the case in Ecuador? Were they doing so to support the Correa government and promote socialism? In September 2009, the Ecuadoran daily *Hoy* published a long interview with Homero Arellano, former commander of the Ecuadoran navy, who was engaged to coordinate logistical aspects of the campaign. The reporter's questions to General Arellano revealed skepticism: Why was Cuba chosen to take the lead in the Manuela Espejo program? Arellano replied that Cuba had a well-developed public health system and had 860 geneticists in the country whereas Ecuador only had one. What guarantee was there that the Cubans would not become involved in politics, supporting the Correa government? He answered by noting that they were skilled medical personnel who worked exceptionally hard: "They leave early in the morning, have lunch, work, and at the end of the day have to produce a report of the work carried out. They are cautious and respectful of our internal politics. They are here exclusively to undertake a medical mission." And finally he was asked: Are they working to promote the Committees for the Defense of the Revolution? He replied: "I don't know why people are so afraid of the Cuban doctors. The work that they are carrying out has nothing to do with revolutions, and not with the CDRs or with ideology."[24]

While the Cubans were not participating in political activities to support the government of Rafael Correa (they were expressly forbidden to do so by Havana), there is no doubt that they were making an extraordinary impression in Ecuador. The eye surgery performed by the Operación Milagro ophthalmologists, the hundreds of Ecuadoran medical graduates from the Escuela Latinoamericana de Medicina (ELAM) who had returned to work in marginalized communities, the Cuban family doctors working through a bilateral agreement in many of the most underserved communities in the country—all helped to raise the profile of Cuba in an extremely positive way. Hugo Chávez also supported the work of the Manuela Espejo Misión, providing supplies worth several million dollars for the disabled community. Speaking in 2010, Vice President Lenín Moreno addressed the role of the Cubans: "We are extremely grateful to our Cuban brothers and sisters who have shown solidarity by sending us their medical *brigadistas*. As you can see, they work with such sincerity, and showing such solidarity, to show us how to do things better."[25]

An analysis of the website of the Cuban embassy in Ecuador reveals just how widespread the level of Cuban cooperation in the country has been, particularly in terms of medical collaboration. For 12 months starting in February 2012 a number of activities involving Cuban authorities were noted, such as plans for Cuban collaboration in higher education, the arrival of 56 literacy specialists to begin the second phase of the Cuban literacy program, "Yo, sí puedo," the graduation from the Cuban literacy program of over 5,000 Ecuadorans, and the visit of several commercial delegations. But without a doubt the common thread of Cuban-Ecuadoran relations was based on matters of public health. For example, Dr. José Fraga Castro, director of the major government biotechnology company LABIOFAM, visited just as the national campaign against dengue (using Cuban biotechnology products) was starting under the leadership of some 79 Cuban specialists in the province of Manabí (December 19, 2012). On December 12, 86 Cubans arrived as advisers. An agreement was signed on October 23, 2012, for Cuban assessors to implement a program to eliminate vectors in four provinces and five cities. On September 14, the Ministers of Foreign Affairs and Public Health visited two health centers and an ophthalmology center run by Cuban medical personnel, while on September 11, Minister of Health Carina Vance Mafla publicly thanked Cuba for the training of Ecuadoran health professionals. On June 21, Ecuador signed an agreement to buy 9,000 doses of the Cuban anti-diabetes drug Heberprot. In March 2012 a fresh cohort of medical students set off to study at ELAM (in September 2012 there were 1,700 Ecuadoran students of medicine at ELAM), while there was an extensive report on the three Cuban ophthalmology clinics in the provinces of Cotopaxi, El Oro, and Santa Elena that had undertaken 119,826 operations (mainly on cataracts and pterygium) since they had been opened in 2006. That same month the governor of the state of Napo, in the Amazon region, praised the Cubans for their extensive primary care role there. In February the minister of health welcomed 75 Cuban medical professionals who had arrived to train doctors in family and community medicine in the mountain regions and in Amazonia. That same month it was announced that 152 medical professors from Cuba would do the same in the Andean region of Chimborazo and the Amazon region of Napo.[26] As can be seen, there has been substantial medical cooperation in a variety of public health–related projects, of which the Manuela Espejo Misión is an important and often undervalued aspect.

The Misión Solidaria Moto Méndez in Bolivia

Clearly Cuban medical collaboration in these campaigns in both Venezuela and Ecuador had resulted in a major improvement for those sectors of the population with disabilities. The same is true in another ALBA country, Bolivia, where a large Cuban contingent employed the same strategy, adapted to meet the reality of that country. Prior to the beginning of the mission, and as was also the case in Venezuela, the Cuban medical brigade had been well established in the country. Speaking in La Paz on January 11, 2013, Cuban ambassador Rolando Gómez outlined the many aspects of medical cooperation that had been provided to date. In terms of medical centers, Cuban medical personnel were working in 32 community hospitals, 548 medical clinics (*consultorios*), and 6 ophthalmology clinics. In all of these installations since 2006 they had attended some 7,412,900 patients.[27] There was an extremely large Cuban medical presence there: 816 physicians, 305 health technicians, 68 support staff, and 8 dentists (with a further 11 assigned to the Moto Méndez mission). They were spread throughout the country, particularly in areas of greatest social inequities—in 79 of the 112 provinces of the country, providing medical coverage to 22.3 percent of the country's population.

In terms of the number of patients treated by Cuban medical personnel, again the data reveal a strong Cuban role: over 54 million patient visits had been recorded (including some 10 million in hospitals); 632,087 had been operated on under the Operación Milagro eye surgery program (2.1 million patients had been treated, with operations on those with greatest need); 30,718 babies had been delivered; 117,635 surgeries had been done, and 56,961 lives had been saved. In addition, Cuban technicians had carried out 471,725 X-rays, 784,827 electrocardiograms, 808,039 ultrasounds, 125,684 endoscopies, and 4,967,744 laboratory tests. Perhaps the most important data come from the training of Bolivians to replace Cuban personnel. In all some 265 Cuban professors of medicine were teaching Bolivian students in 191 clinics, while 4,302 Bolivians were studying medicine in Cuba. (An updated report from August 2013 noted how 800 medical graduates were returning from Havana, soon to undertake mandatory social service in rural areas of Bolivia, joining the 3,800 who had already graduated following six years of medical school in Cuba.)[28] As can be seen, there was a well-established tradition of Cuban medical cooperation in Bolivia, which definitely aided the implementation of the far-reaching campaign of the Misión Solidaria Moto Méndez.

The Cuban support for the Moto Méndez campaign lasted 10 months, following the same fundamental strategy employed in Venezuela and Ecuador, and supported by both Venezuela (with finances and equipment as well as medical aids for the patients identified) and Cuban medical practitioners. The objective from the Cuban perspective was to identify all those Bolivians with intellectual or physical disabilities based on clinical, social, and epidemiological analyses and to suggest future strategies to meet their needs. Under the government of Evo Morales, and in light of support from Cuba and Venezuela, this was an opportune time to identify the medical and socioeconomic challenges of the affected population and improve their conditions.

The same approach as noted earlier was employed in the field—a team of four was the norm: a geneticist, a social worker, a general practitioner (either Bolivian or a member of the Cuban medical brigade already in Bolivia), and a representative of the Bolivian armed forces who was in charge of logistics. Again the work of the brigade often took them "off map," or to regions that were basically inaccessible. In those areas Bolivians with disabilities were without any official support at all, largely because nobody knew of their existence. To put this in perspective, members of the Misión visited 101 communities that did not even appear on any maps, largely because they were so small and inaccessible. In these circumstances the role of the armed forces was crucial to ensure transportation and security and to provide a geo-reference for future support of any individuals identified. Moreover, given the decades-old presentation of the Cuban revolution as an extremely negative process, the presence of Bolivian military helped to assuage the fears of people visited, while strengthening the credibility and the role of the Cuban doctors and indeed of the entire project.

The original idea for Bolivia to participate in the project came at the summit of the members of ALBA in October 2009, when President Evo Morales requested support for the program. It was to be named "Moto Méndez" in honor of José Eustaquio Méndez, a Bolivian who had fought valiantly for the independence of Bolivia against the Spanish, despite having only one hand. Again the mission undertook an exhaustive study of the entire country in order to come up with a detailed list of those with disabilities in Bolivia. And again this was not intended to take just a sample of the population but to visit hundreds of thousands of homes. Again, in each of these home visits, the medical staff also treated any family members with medical needs and not just those with disabilities. Basic medical education was dispensed during this entire process, particularly important in explaining to family members the causes of any particular disability—how to support the individual and, where possible, how to avoid its cause in the future. The visit of several doctors to a house was unheard of for most Bolivians, for whom house calls were extremely expensive—as was access to medical services in general. For these people, who had rarely if ever visited a doctor, it was a shock to have a group of doctors visit them in their homes, seeking the best ways of helping the most neglected of their family members. The multidisciplinary teams were extremely helpful, since their presence allowed the family doctors to be able to draw on the expertise of specialists and therefore better assist the family members. It also made for a better understanding of the major causes of many of the physical and intellectual challenges, which specialists were in a better position to diagnose. By the time the Moto Méndez mission was completed, it had been supported by 97 Cuban specialists, 46 Bolivian doctors, 57 specialists in genetic assessment, more than 900 members of the Cuban medical brigade who were working in Bolivia, and 815 members of the Bolivian armed forces.[29]

Before the mission spread throughout Bolivia, it was decided to undertake a pilot study in three communities, Plan Tres Mil de Santa Cruz, Orinoca in Oruro, and El Alto, near the capital, La Paz. The medical brigade again employed the services of specialists in genetics, child psychology, nursing, trauma injuries, pediatric neurology, ENT medicine, and ophthalmology, although the majority of the staff were specialists in *medicina general integral* or comprehensive general medicine. The work took just under a year. By the end of it they had crisscrossed the entire country, visiting all 112 provinces in the country's nine departments, supported by the participation of people in 327 municipalities. In the end Cuban doctors had visited some 5.3 million people in 1.5 million homes, providing information on some 82,000 persons who were discovered to have physical or intellectual disabilities. They even helped to "discover" 101 communities that did not appear on any official maps. It is worth noting that, in addition to visiting persons with intellectual or physical disabilities, the medical teams also dispensed medical advice and supplies to all in the community who required it. While their objective was clearly focused on discovering Bolivians with disabilities, it was also important to help the community at large. As a result, health education and promotion was an important facet of their work in the community, as it was in each of the ALBA countries involved in these programs.

The results of the mission were in many ways comparable to those found in other countries in which the Cubans carried out similar missions. Following their door-to-door campaigns, they discovered 82,087 Bolivians with disabilities. Of these 18,429 had intellectual disabilities (although this probably also included mental health patients), while the remaining 63,658 suffered from various physical or sensory impairments.[30] A more detailed study of the data on Bolivians with intellectual disabilities identified the major causes of their impairment. In all, 6,338 people (34.39) had this disability because of prenatal factors, with 5,656 (30.69 percent) due to perinatal difficulties and 3,486 (18.92 percent) the result of postnatal problems. In terms of the proportion of patients with a minor degree of intellectual disability, in Cuba this was the case of 56.5 percent of all patients, whereas in Bolivia this was 20.12 percent. Conversely the percentage of people with profound intellectual disabilities was about 11.1 percent in Cuba, while in Bolivia this was almost double (21.02 percent).[31] Research by the medical teams revealed that the most common causes for this in terms of the prenatal group were arterial hypertension during pregnancy (28.01 percent of mothers) and alcohol consumption during pregnancy (21.62 percent). Not surprisingly, Cuban teams suggested education programs on the dangers of alcohol at this stage of fetal development and the need for frequent prenatal checkups for mothers. The most common factor for the postnatal group was sepsis, especially in the east of Bolivia with its tropical climate. Bacterial meningitis here was particularly high and resulted often in developmental disability. The study ended up recommending a program to teach medical genetics, both to reduce the impact of genetic diseases on health and also as a means of long-term strategies of health promotion and education in order to reduce the numbers of the population with intellectual disabilities.

Continuing the work undertaken in Cuba to prepare an accurate understanding of the numbers of those with developmental disabilities and to draw up a detailed strategy to support this population, the mission in all three countries studied here (as well as the others which followed an identical strategy) was successful. In geostrategic terms it was also a useful confidence-building mechanism among the countries of ALBA, which could not help but be impressed by Cuba's massive contribution in terms of health support and Venezuela's financial assistance, especially with the amount of goods provided to alleviate the difficult conditions of both the hundreds of thousands of people with disabilities who had been identified and their families. In the closing ceremony for the mission, the Venezuelan ambassador to Bolivia, Crisbelle González, summarized the enormous value of Móto Méndez: "This mission of solidarity, undertaken by the sister nations of ALBA, has no precedents in the history of humanity, our country, and our America—Latin America. This is why we are here today to celebrate the closing of one period—and to commit ourselves before the government of Evo Morales to continue our support as it is needed for the development of this new stage in this Mission."[32]

Once the results had been completed, the next challenge was to make use of the extensive data collected and, as had been the case elsewhere, suggest how Bolivians with disabilities could have a sustainable and dignified quality of life. As one Cuban participant noted: "Our objective in Bolivia, as is the case in Ecuador, Venezuela, and Nicaragua, is to make a contribution to improve the quality of life of people with intellectual and physical challenges, and to decrease the level of social exclusion which affects these groups."[33] Health promotion, popular education, the means to address preventable disabilities, and the social integration of people with physical and intellectual challenges were obvious needs. One of the first major projects to result from this was the Rehabilitation Center for patients with disabilities inaugurated in May 2010 at the Santa Bárbara hospital in the department of Chuquisaca, where local medical personnel had been trained by Cuban and Venezuelan rehabilitation specialists. The objective was to train Bolivians to staff 20 such centers.

Many initiatives resulted from Cuban involvement in the Moto Méndez campaign and especially the rehabilitation clinics. Again, Venezuela supplied medical equipment to assist and by November 2009 had supplied 12 tons of medical equipment. By August 2010, over 12,000 pieces of equipment (such as wheelchairs, canes, hearing aids, and mattresses) had been donated. The government also ran educational campaigns to explain the cause of many of the avoidable medical conditions. Down syndrome, for example, could be decreased if older women were encouraged to use birth control to avoid becoming pregnant, although for many this was clearly a controversial approach because of local cultural and religious factors. Likewise a reduced use of alcohol could avoid some of the key impairments that resulted, ranging from fetal alcohol syndrome to car accidents. Prenatal genetic testing and diagnosis were also becoming more common, particularly as Cuba trained a cadre of geneticists. Popular education was a particularly useful form of reaching the population, and members of Moto Méndez gave 20,000 presentations.[34] As was the case in Ecuador, the government also provided financial support for people with physical and intellectual disabilities, and those with major challenges received 1,000 *bolivianos*, a policy designed to assist some 13,400 people.

Concluding Remarks

Cuba's support for the three specialized programs studied here was successful in helping those sectors of the population often neglected—in wealthy developed nations as well as in poor developing countries. The basic difference lies, however, in the fact that developing countries scarcely have the funds to maintain the most rudimentary public healthcare systems, leaving little for disability supports and programs. As a result people with disabilities were usually forgotten when they were not stigmatized, ridiculed, and seen as being inherently less worthy.

Cuba had recognized over a decade ago that this sector of the population deserved to be treated with respect. As noted, however, and despite close medical support, medical practitioners were surprised to see just how many people with physical and intellectual disabilities there were. Cuba had designed and developed a successful public healthcare initiative to support people with disabilities and had implemented a major national campaign between 2001 and 2003. A viable model already existed in Cuba to undertake such a wide-ranging program, and the ALBA countries took advantage of this experience.

This occurred as the political scenario in Latin America as a whole was changing, particularly after the 1998 election of Hugo Chávez in Venezuela. The election of a dozen or so left-of-center governments and the formation of ALBA, the Bolivarian Alliance for the Peoples of Our [Latin] America, have been important in the development of a continent-wide identity. The original objective was inspired by Chávez, who sought a Latin American alternative to the FTAA (Free Trade Area of the Americas) proposed by Washington, and it was started as a bilateral agreement between Venezuela and Cuba in 2004. Since then several other countries have joined: Bolivia (2006), Nicaragua (2007), Dominica (2008), and Ecuador as well as both Antigua and Barbuda and Saint Vincent and the Grenadines (2009). Honduras joined in 2008 but withdrew following the military coup that deposed Manuel Zelaya. Suriname and St. Lucia were admitted in 2012 as “guest countries.” The creation in 2011 of the Community of Latin American and

Caribbean States (deliberately excluding the United States and Canada), consisting of 33 countries, also underlined the growing awareness of the need for stronger regional unity. Uruguayan president José Mujica summed up this newfound sense of identity: "We Latin Americans have never been so close. Never. I don't know if this is due to the sedimentation of the old struggles which have created a sort of fertility in our regional social soil. In the present context it can be seen in the views expressed by governments of different political stripes—yet all agree on certain key decisions about the region."[35] The financial support of Venezuela to several of the key social initiatives of the ALBA countries, the sense of unity among the countries of what José Martí termed "Our America," the influence of Fidel Castro (until his official retirement in 2008), and the potential of Cuba's medical capabilities—with decades of experience in dozens of nations since 1960—all coalesced in various healthcare initiatives, one of which was the support for people with disabilities.

While other chapters of this book focus on aspects of medical internationalism that cover the globe—such as Operación Milagro, the use of biotechnology support, or the provision of doctors to guarantee basic services in dozens of developing nations—this element of Cuban cooperation is no less significant. To spend so much time going door to door, visiting millions of homes, providing care to hundreds of thousands of people, and concentrating on those who traditionally had been excluded and ignored was a major development in public healthcare. It is a massive initiative that has never been undertaken by any other country, rich or poor. Yet a small (11.2 million) nation carried it to a handful of countries, some of which were larger (e.g., Venezuela, pop. 28 million and Ecuador, pop. 13 million).

Common to all three "missions" studied here was a determination not just to provide a census of regions of countries where there were people with disabilities but also to map out the situation of these populations in the entire countries and to offer remedies to improve their standard of living. With the exception of Cuba, no other country had ever carried out such a project. Using the technique of analyzing every individual as a bio-psycho-social being, medical teams of Cuban specialists and local medical staff fanned out to complete their task. In the three countries studied here, they faced substantial geographical obstacles, infrastructure challenges, and often situations where people could not comprehend what the Cubans were doing and were at times hostile.[36] People were not used to having medical personnel actually come to their homes and help them, especially at no charge. This resistance disappeared gradually as people realized that they stood to gain from this experience and that the Cubans were there to help.

The Cuban role was clearly important in providing the model, the personnel with the required specialization, and the experience. In addition to improving the medical and socioeconomic conditions of hundreds of thousands of people, their contribution also trained people so that their work could be continued. The old saying that nothing flatters like imitation was borne out by the fact that, following the successful campaign in Ecuador, specialists there who had been trained by Cuba then transferred their knowledge to the governments of Colombia, Guatemala, Peru, Uruguay, and Paraguay.

In August 2010, Fidel Castro welcomed back home 213 of the Cuban *brigadistas* after they landed in Havana. He thanked them for their cooperation in Bolivia and emphasized the enormity of their work there and that of their compatriots in the other ALBA countries. In Bolivia they had recognized over 82,000 citizens with disabilities. They had also offered more than 10,000 clinical genetic tests. A further 15,000 consultations had been provided by Cuban medical specialists. In these missions they had visited over 3 million homes in four countries and had identified 1 million people with physical and intellectual disabilities. Those 3 million homes were about the same number that existed in all of Cuba, he added. Their mission had brought support—and joy—to many families, he told the medical staff: "You have faced truly severe cases, such as those human beings born blind and deaf and dumb, people who have never seen a sunbeam or have never heard a single sound. In other words they have never had any real contact with life, despite having been born. These two simple examples that I have given are enough for them to feel happy, to sing, communicate with other people—simply, to live."[37]

Clearly the government leader in the best position to speak about people with special needs is the former vice president of Ecuador, Lenín Moreno, who took on the Misión Manuela Espejo as an extremely personal initiative. Given his own disability and the contribution that he had made to Ecuadoran society, he felt empowered—and indeed obliged—to speak to the issue of disability. In a December 2011 meeting with fellow Latin vice presidents he spoke about the need to change the situation: "We have placed barriers . . . that limit our dreams and, what is shameful, the enjoyment of our rights. It is time to eliminate these barriers, without exception. . . . The worst are the mental barriers, those which make us believe that others are not my neighbor and, when they are different, that they are inferior."[38] In

Table 3.1. Results of disability study in ALBA countries, 2013

Variables	Cuba	Venezuela	Ecuador	Nicaragua	Bolivia	St. Vincent	Total
Homes visited	—	814,328	1,286,331	179,039	1,529,8760	11,116	3,820,684
People with disabilities	366,864	338,545	293,743	126,316	82,087	2,195	1,207,472
Intellectual disability	140,489	100,124	71,417	32,741	18,429	497	363,191
Other disabilities	226,375	238,421	222,326	93,575	63,658	1,698	844,281
Genetics consultation	41,885	38,972	21,062	27,134	10,231	489	139,772
Consultation from other specialties	—	15,676	35,257	37,063	15,874	231	104,101
No. of consultations to others during study	—	605,395	825,576	203,457	326,256	7009	1,967,693

Source: Ministry of Public Health (MINSAP) in Cuba, "Estudio psicosocial, pedagógico y clínico-genético de personas con discapacidad," provided to the author in February 2013.

many ways he sums up accurately the goal of the medical teams in these missions in all five countries. Despite political will, none of the countries possessed the medical talent, much less the ability, to undertake such wide-ranging missions. Fortunately Cuba had the detailed experience of its own "missions," as well as the technical expertise and the human resources to channel these desires into reality. The hundreds of thousands of citizens of these five countries now enjoyed a far better life than they had before, thanks in no small part to the contribution of Cuba.

4

Operación Milagro

Bringing Vision to Millions

> Operation Miracle is humanity at its best. It is something that has never happened before in the world. It is an incredible gesture of international solidarity. Its impact on the region has been spectacular . . . and has touched the needs of the people directly.
>
> Ralph Gonsalves, prime minister of St. Vincent and the Grenadines

Being blind in a developing or underdeveloped country is much more of a challenge than it is in an industrialized one. Often the parents will have limited funds to spend on educational opportunities for their children, and what little is available will be spent on "able-bodied" siblings, since they are more likely to contribute to the family's precarious finances. Access to special education, braille machines, and guide dogs will be severely limited and often impossible to access, much less afford. As a result, most blind people in the developing world will be illiterate, poor, and unemployed. They often contribute little to the economic development of their country, as well as to their families. In addition, life expectancy of the blind is usually half that of someone with eyesight. Finally, because most blind people in underdeveloped countries are unable to find work, they are frequently an economic burden for their family and must be cared for, thus reducing even more potential family income.

By contrast, people who are cured of their blindness can become functional members of society. They develop self-respect, need little or no extra care, and can participate more fully in group activities. They can now work in the fields or city, collect water or firewood, attend schools, and learn to read (which also opens many doors to employment). According to the World Health Organization, there are 285 million people who are visually impaired worldwide, of whom 39 million are blind and 246 million have low or badly reduced vision. Significantly 90 percent live in developing countries.[1] It has been estimated that there are 3 million people in Latin

America who are blind, while between 7 and 10 million suffer from poor vision. The major causes of visual impairment are cataracts (50–60 percent), diabetic retinopathy (15 percent), and glaucoma (15 percent).[2]

Much of the blindness encountered in underdeveloped and developing societies is avoidable, since it is often caused by poor living conditions, contaminated water, malnutrition, and accidents, factors made worse by poor access to healthcare. Even more troubling is that many of resulting diseases that result in blindness, such as cataracts, glaucoma, and corneal opacities, can be resolved easily by surgery that takes but a few minutes. Cataracts, for instance, can be removed in a simple 15-minute operation. Tragically, these operations are usually beyond the financial means of the people affected by these medical conditions—and as a result they continue to live in darkness.

For most North Americans and Europeans, having cataract surgery is a relatively easy (and affordable) process, costing anywhere between $1,000 and $3,000, while in countries with a national health plan the operation is free. The surgery is quick and straightforward. Sadly, this relatively affordable charge is impossible for most living in the underdeveloped world, even when it costs just $100 or $200. Recognizing this need, the Cuban and Venezuelan governments initiated the Operación Milagro (Operation Miracle) program in 2004, seeking initially to contribute to the restoration of sight (and dignity) to the poor in Venezuela and subsequently to other countries in Latin America and the Caribbean.

A quick Google subject search of "Operation Miracle," or its subsequent development in Venezuela, Misión Milagro, results in hundreds of articles detailing the medical cooperation of Cuba in its ophthalmology program being provided in over 20 countries (although still mainly focused on Latin America and the Caribbean). A few examples will suffice to illustrate the extent of this medical cooperation. In no particular order there are articles on 45,000 eye surgeries having been completed by Cuban ophthalmologists in Uruguay since 2007; over 61,000 Jamaicans have been examined and 7,000 operated on by Cuban specialists; over 32,000 Africans and 1 million Venezuelans have received eye surgery; 37,000 Argentines have been operated on in Cuba and Bolivia; 15,000 Paraguayans have received eye surgery from Cuban ophthalmologists; the same is true for 93,000 Ecuadorians, 650,000 Bolivians, and 61,000 Nicaraguans; in February 2010 it was reported that Cuban specialists had performed almost 6,000 eye operations and treated 26,000 people in Suriname; more than 10,000 Salvadorans had benefited from the program between 2006 and 2010; in the Mexican state of Zacatecas some 4,800 patients were operated on by the Cuban ophthalmology team between 2007 and 2011.[3] The list goes on. All of these surgeries—on some 3 million patients—have been carried out at no cost to the patients themselves, with Cuba providing most of the medical expertise and Venezuela the financial support.

Origins and Evolution of "Operation Miracle"

Cuba, supported by Venezuela, seeks to restore sight to 6 million of the estimated 39 million blind people in the world and to date has made a major contribution. Conner Gorry notes that in Latin America and the Caribbean there are 2.8 million blind people and 11.2 million who are visually impaired.[4] Of these, two-thirds could have their vision problem reversed with simple surgery. For instance, conditions such as cataracts, glaucoma, diabetic retinopathy, and childhood blindness are easily treated. The problem has been that, until Cuba and Venezuela decided in 2004 to attack the problem with this innovative program, few leaders in the region had shown any interest or political will in dealing with vision problems, to no small degree because of the cost and lack of skilled medical personnel. Operation Miracle has changed this scenario.

Operation Miracle started almost by accident. As Cuba and Venezuela strengthened ties following the election of Hugo Chávez in 1998, a number of bilateral initiatives developed. One was a successful literacy program, "Yo, sí puedo" ("Yes, I can) that has been used in some 30 countries and has taught basic literacy to over 8 million people. During the course of the implementation of this literacy program it was discovered that many of the students were unable to progress—not because of any learning disability or intellectual challenge but because they could not physically see to make out the letters. This clearly defeated the purpose of the program. According to the director of the Pando Ferrer Ophthalmology Hospital in Havana, the Cuban president visited him late on July 9, 2004, to discuss this significant challenge for "Yo, sí puedo" and proposed the need for a wide-ranging ophthalmology program to resolve the situation. And in somewhat typical fashion for Fidel Castro's often spontaneous medical initiatives, a blueprint for Operación Milagro was drawn up the following day.

This program is now found throughout Latin America and the Caribbean, but it became increasingly important during Cuba's contribution to the Barrio Adentro program in Venezuela, when Cuban doctors discovered patients with treatable ophthalmology conditions (largely cataracts) who could not afford to pay for simple operations. For Cuban physicians used to accessible and free public healthcare, this was an unusual occurrence, and they requested support from Havana to resolve the medical condition.[5] (Strictly speaking, the terms "Operación Milagro" and "Operation Miracle" refer to the same ophthalmology program devised by Cuba and practiced both on the island and in a number of countries in Latin America, the Caribbean, and Africa, and are used interchangeably. Misión Milagro refers to the program situated specifically in Venezuela, providing ophthalmology treatment both to Venezuelans and to others from a variety of countries in the Latin American and Caribbean regions who are operated on in Venezuela. Some confusion has set in, however, and the terms are often interchanged.)

As is the case with several initiatives in MI, the basic concept and the enthusiasm (as well as the political will and the direction) came from the Cuban president, with Venezuela supplying financial support. In August 2005, the "Sandino Commitment" (so called because it was signed in the municipality of the same name in the western province of Pinar del Río in Cuba) was agreed to by presidents Castro and Chávez. This document fleshed out the basic commitment and agreed to expand it considerably. The goal was to provide ophthalmology treatment for 6 million people, improving their vision. Accordingly, after September 2005 Operation Miracle was further expanded—to a total of 15 Latin American nations and 69 clinics, using the same technology as was used back in Havana's major ophthalmology hospital, Pando Ferrer. Such an ambitious and far-reaching medical program had never been attempted before.

Several key ingredients contributed to the resulting program: Cuba had an abundance of medical talent, Venezuela was flush with petrodollars (and could pay for services rendered by Cuban medical staff), both leaders had a clear interest in providing expanded healthcare within the region, and there was a clearly identified need.

During the first year of Operation Miracle, 14,000 patients were operated on, mainly Venezuelans in Cuban hospitals. In the second year of the program, it was expanded significantly, with patients from 20 countries receiving surgery in Cuba. The first stage of Operation Miracle was centered on surgery provided at the large Pando Ferrer ophthalmology hospital in Cuba, with Venezuela paying to fly all patients—at no charge—to Havana and subsequently to other Cuban cities, where they stayed in hotels provided by the government. This expansion to other cities occurred as the numbers grew, and the Pando Ferrer's capacity was rapidly filled. The first operations took place in July 2004, after patients who had been screened in

Venezuela by Cuban medical teams were flown to Havana. In terms of the patients who were the initial focus of the treatment, there was an interesting evolution. Emily Kirk has shown how the program was originally intended for Latin Americans, principally Venezuelans, whose need was greater than that of the Cuban population, long accustomed to available healthcare services. However, after waiting times for Cuban patients increased, given the large numbers of Latin Americans who continued to arrive and be treated by Cuban specialists, a decision was taken to include them as well.[6] Cuban patients thus received the same treatment as that given to foreigners.

The initial phase of the program was impressive, largely because nothing of this magnitude had ever been attempted. It is also important to note how it has continued to grow, and within eight years more than 2 million patients (mainly in Latin America and the Caribbean) had their sight restored at no cost to them. To put this in context, this would be the equivalent of the U.S. government paying to offer free eye surgery to 60 million poor people from Latin America and the Caribbean, both in U.S. hospitals and in the region—and having Washington pay all the costs of hospital care, travel, and accommodations.

The country to benefit most clearly from the project in terms of the number of patients who received treatment was Venezuela. In many ways this was not surprising, since the Chávez government was paying Havana for the use of Cuban professional services. Significantly the Venezuelan president, like his Cuban counterpart and mentor, saw the delivery of accessible and free healthcare as a basic human right. During this first stage, the rapidly increasing Cuban medical program in Venezuela set about selecting patients for simple eye surgery, while Cuban medical teams also visited isolated communities throughout the country for the same purpose. Rather than wait for patients to approach the clinics, the Cuban ophthalmology teams went out to look for them. The idea was to develop a list of patients, so that they could be summoned on a particular day to have their surgery, thereby maximizing the efficiency of the operation.

Most patients could not afford to pay for surgery. Most had never left their home region, let alone flown to a foreign country. To assist them in this traumatic journey and surgical experience, a family member or close friend usually accompanied them, and their costs were also paid by the Venezuelan government. They were housed in local hotels, resulting in occasional travel advisories to tourists that their hotels were not available, having been occupied by Venezuelan patients and their accompanying family members. As the size of the program increased, patients from Latin

America and the Caribbean also started to arrive, with their expenses paid by the Venezuelan government. On several occasions I have visited some of these hotels where Operation Miracle patients stayed in order to interview patients. Although the government built accommodations especially for this purpose, most patients stayed at regular hotels.

Meanwhile, in Cuba there were significant changes under way to better prepare for this ambitious program. In November 2005 the Cuban Faculty of Ophthalmology was established, offering postgraduate specialized programs, with the clear objective of training a rapidly increasing number of specialists. Significantly, this is the only postgraduate faculty specializing in ophthalmology in all of Latin America. A website and electronic journal for the Misión Milagro program were also set up to share specialized knowledge on ophthalmology, as well as one for the Cuban Society of Ophthalmology.[7] In 2009 there were an estimated 800 ophthalmologists in Cuba, with an extra 1,000 being trained.[8] As the program expanded throughout 2004 and the thousands of patients were flown in from abroad, it became necessary to employ other hospitals in addition to the flagship Pando Ferrer, and eventually 24 other Cuban hospitals participated.

In most cases, after basic pre-op tests were carried out, the operations took place, followed by a period of convalescence (usually a week) and follow-up medical exams. By the end of 2004, some 14,000 Venezuelans had had their sight restored, and this rapid growth in the number of patients continued.[9] While this medical humanitarianism was understandably appreciated in Venezuela, it was often a different story in Cuba, where many people were disturbed by having to wait longer for their own surgery. As one Cuban noted, "First the plane full of Venezuelans arrives, then they all get their operation and leave—and after that yet another plane arrives."[10]

This process of waiting for Cubans only became worse when, in the later stages of Operación Milagro, the number of Cuban medical personnel working abroad increased, a process that also increased waiting times for Cubans. There are now an estimated 30,000 Cuban medical staff working in Venezuela, about 10,000 of whom are physicians. In actual fact the delays experienced by Cuban patients were not inordinately long, but they had been accustomed to having rapid access to a wealth of doctors, and for many the delays they now encountered were a major inconvenience. (In many ways the Cuban concerns, while understandable, were exaggerated. To put this in the appropriate context, Cuba has 6.7 doctors per 1,000 inhabitants, compared with 2.7 in the United States.)

Although some Cubans never accepted fully the presence of Venezuelans taking advantage of the arrangement, most reconciled themselves to the fact that this was a necessary development. And while Cubans faced longer waiting times for medical care, they also received more than 100,000 barrels of oil daily at significantly reduced prices. Living conditions on the island improved: power blackouts ended, and the government coffers were replenished as a result of Venezuelan payments for medical services. Indeed the exportation of medical services was soon generating more funds for the Cuban economy than tourism, mining, and remittances combined. Relief eventually came years later for Cuban patients through the training of extra personnel and the decision to focus on the exportation of ophthalmology services rather than transporting large numbers of foreign patients to Havana. This freed up hospital space for Cubans, although many remained unhappy at the presence of so many medical personnel abroad.

Before these changes occurred, however, the expansion of Operation Miracle continued apace. In 2005 Havana began extending benefits to other countries in the region. The Venezuelan government, promoting the benefits of ALBA, agreed to support these costs. Several governments in Latin America and the Caribbean took advantage of this offer, and soon patients from Jamaica, St. Lucia, and Dominica were arriving for eye surgery in Havana. I interviewed several of them at one of their hotels and at the Pando Ferrer hospital. The patients were delighted to receive quality treatment that they could never afford in their own countries, although many remained perplexed about Cuba's motives. How could Cuba manage to do this for so many people?

This noticeable growth of patients understandably caused an increase in the workload of ophthalmologists. This was compounded soon by the decision to send trained specialists to various Latin American and Caribbean countries. The director of the Pando Ferrer hospital, Dr. Reynaldo Ríos Casas, commenting on the hectic early days of Operación Milagro, noted that eye surgeons worked in three shifts, with the operating theatre being used 24 hours a day to deal with the thousands of foreign patients who arrived. At times a surgeon would carry out 40 operations in a single shift. He noted, however, some significant improvements that had occurred since those heady days in 2004: the budget had increased tenfold, the training of extra staff increased exponentially, and state-of-the art equipment had been purchased for the hospital's 34 operating theaters.[11]

In 2010 I spent a day at the Pando Ferrer, interviewing staff and patients. The "Pando," which is an international reference hospital, is impressive, with cutting-edge equipment, and a capability for almost clockwork-like operating precision. Sitting in the control room and watching the many monitors showing operations being carried out in the various theaters was fascinating. On average 40,000 surgeries are conducted every year. The hospital consists of a four-building complex, the largest having eight floors. The website (www.pando.sld.cu) notes that there are 140 specialist ophthalmologists on staff, 14 residents and 22 other specialists, as well as 218 nurses. It also has a major teaching function for medical students in Havana.

Most of the equipment is European and Asian, since the U.S. trade embargo makes it difficult to import equipment made in North America. It includes expensive HRT-II diagnostic devices (to carry out topographical studies of the optic nerve and retina, particularly useful in the early diagnosis of glaucoma), OCT-3 (for optical coherence topography, necessary for early detection of macular conditions), phacoemulsification capability (for surgery using ultrasound micro-incisions), Confoscal microscopes (to determine problems in different cornea structures), and the Excimer laser (used in refractive surgery for myopia, hypermetropia, and stigmatism). This could not have been possible, however, without financial support from Venezuela and the increasingly close ties between Havana and Caracas.

By late 2006, a new phase of the program had been established, this time revolving around the exportation of Cuban medical skills to countries that had requested ophthalmology assistance. In all some 204,000 people were treated in Cuba, according to Manuel Pacheco, coordinator of the Misión Milagro program in Venezuela.[12] It was now time, though, to move to a new phase of the program, providing increased service—but delivering it in a different manner. Put simply, the demands outstripped the potential for the services to be offered in Cuba, and the costs of transporting and housing tens of thousands of people were becoming prohibitive. At the same time there was a large enough body of Cuban medical professionals to carry out the necessary operations, and so it was clearly more cost-effective to provide these ophthalmology services in places where the patients were located. As a result, in the second stage of Operación Milagro the focus became the supply of medical services in the countries where they were most needed. For the Cuban government this was not a major problem, since it had a surplus of ophthalmologists, and the Venezuelan government was paying Havana for the medical services provided.

Since October 2005 Venezuelan hospitals have also become increasingly involved in receiving patients there, and in all 26 hospitals have received patients. As was the earlier case, patients did not come only from Venezuela. Indeed this is truly a Latin American initiative, mirroring the work carried out in Cuba. Patients with limited financial resources from 25 countries have been operated on in Venezuela, with the greatest numbers coming from Ecuador, Colombia, El Salvador, the Dominican Republic, Brazil, Paraguay, Mexico, Surinam, Guatemala, Nicaragua, Chile, Costa Rica, Bolivia, Uruguay, Peru, and Argentina. To illustrate the growing involvement of Venezuelan ophthalmologists it is worth noting that by April 2009, Cuban ophthalmologists in Venezuela had operated on 447,185 patients, while their Venezuelan counterparts had performed surgery on 221,659—for a total of 668,844 operations in Venezuela in less than four years.[13]

While there are now more than 60 ophthalmology clinics of differing sizes throughout Latin America and the Caribbean, both as stand-alone clinics and as part of an existing hospital, there are common aspects of the composition and mission of each. The nucleus of each center has the following personnel: a director, ophthalmology specialist, anesthesiologist, clinical specialist, nursing staff, specialist technicians in optometry and optical sciences, a pharmacist, a laboratory specialist, an epidemiologist, an engineer, and an accountant. Having visited three such centers I have been struck by the almost monastic living style employed. The medical personnel generally live together in a rather spartan fashion, working long hours at the clinic. They have few distractions, although e-mail contact with families and internet access, satellite television (to stay in touch with events in Cuba), and even dominoes are of paramount importance. They share domestic duties, have limited contact with locals, drink alcohol only on special occasions, and maintain a simple communal lifestyle.

The role of the director of the center is to keep up staff morale and deal with challenges that occur in a totally different culture, political system, and societal milieu. Many of the personnel understandably miss their families and home environment and are physically and mentally exhausted after hours of hard work at the clinic. It is no easy chore, demanding a variety of qualities, as one *internacionalista* has noted: "It implies for us the need to be revolutionaries, to assume a commitment to humanity, to feel love for our profession, to possess a spirit of sacrifice, and to meet all the requirements of medical ethics. These are the essential characteristics of people working in health, and of course the director has to provide an example for all to follow."[14]

The results of the first five years of Operación Milagro were remarkable, and 1,554,662 patients were operated on. Of these 267,267 were operated on in Cuba (the first phase of work undertaken) with the balance (1,113,602) receiving their surgery outside Cuba in any of the 61 ophthalmology centers set up by Cuba in some 20 countries. Since Venezuela paid for most of the expenses of the program, the greatest number of centers (23) were located there (although in total, ophthalmology operations have been carried out in 74 hospitals in Venezuela), and the single greatest number of patients were Venezuelan (635,401).[15] By contrast there were 173,793 Cubans operated on, as well as 668,532 from other Latin American countries. (The smaller number of Cuban patients reflects the decades of medical care which the population had traditionally received, whereas throughout the region many years of neglect and limited access to public health services, as well as the prohibitive cost for many, resulted in far greater needs for immediate medical attention elsewhere.) There were also 65,714 people from a number of Caribbean countries who were operated on, as well as 4,508 from Angola and 6,714 from Mali.[16] In terms of the distribution of the ophthalmology clinics, there were also 15 in Bolivia, 3 each in Ecuador, Guatemala, Honduras, and Nicaragua, 2 in Haiti, and 1 in Paraguay, Uruguay, Peru, Saint Lucia, Saint Vincent and the Grenadines, Suriname, and Angola.

The essence of the Cuban program is to provide ophthalmology services to the maximum number of patients who need these at no cost to them. It is a no-frills strategy, but one in which they follow a finely tuned approach based on years of experience. The principal components of the strategy employed have been defined as the following:

(1) Analysis of the major ophthalmology pathologies
(2) Determination of the necessary infrastructure
(3) Massive mobilization of patients to the location for examination
(4) Massive treatment of the identified pathologies
(5) Return to the home environment
(6) Follow-up care for all patients
(7) Training for professionals in the host country[17]

The adjective *masiva*, used several times, is in keeping with the Cuban socialist revolutionary objective and illustrates the Cuban determination to provide basic services to the greatest possible number of people. Of particular importance is the last point, since the fundamental nature of Cuban medical internationalism is to provide a sustainable system—one that is not dependent on foreign participation, but instead trains local talent to take over from the Cubans. That is the hallmark of the largest programs of Cuban medical internationalism, as in Venezuela, Bolivia, Timor-Leste, and Haiti.

The idea of setting up ophthalmology clinics in Latin America and the Caribbean, using Cuban medical talent and supported financially by Venezuela, is also a strategic option in terms of supporting the concept of Latin American integration—a goal of both Fidel Castro and Hugo Chávez. The advantages of treating the medical conditions of millions of poor citizens of Latin America and the Caribbean (previously ignored by multilateral agencies and banks of the industrialized nations) are clear. Combined with other initiatives related to this sweeping approach of medical internationalism, the strategy has exercised a major influence in winning the "hearts and minds" of many in the region. One patient at a Cuban ophthalmology clinic in Guatemala told me, "You have no idea how it feels to have the patch removed and to see—for the first time in many years—colors, members of my family. This is indeed a miracle."

In many ways the Cuban role in the José Martí Ophthalmology Clinic in Uruguay is typical of the approach employed throughout Latin America. It opened in 2007, and since then Cuban specialists have carried out more than 40,000 surgeries. Every week a team of Cuban and Uruguayan ophthalmologists set out to visit small rural towns in the interior of the country and hold clinics that been advertised several weeks in advance. They examine patients and then transport to Montevideo those who can be helped by surgery. According to Pilar González, director of the National Plan for Rural Health in Uruguay, this surgery would cost at least $5,000 in a private hospital, an amount which the majority of patients would never be able to pay.[18]

Another common denominator is the patients' gratitude for the respect with which they have been treated by Cubans, not common in their homeland where they are often considered with scorn because of their social standing, race, or lack of wealth. From my interviews with some 30 patients, it is clear that they are understandably appreciative of the medical treatment they have received, and the respect shown them. Typical in many ways is the attitude of Roberto Andrade, a Salvadoran bus driver who had cataract surgery on both eyes in Havana: "In my country, a surgery like that costs $8,000. . . . I make $12 a day. I would never, ever, be able to save that much. Now I am an ambassador. I go around El Salvador telling everyone how well I was treated."[19] Political support for the governments of Cuba or Venezuela is not a prerequisite, and patients are not asked about their ideological positions when they are screened for their medical history. This can be seen most clearly in the treatment afforded an old Bolivian, Mario Terán, the military officer who executed Ernesto "Che" Guevara in Bolivia on October 9, 1967. In August 2006, his cataracts were removed by Cuban physicians at a clinic recently inaugurated by President Evo Morales.

The Cuban approach seen in Operation Miracle has provided many benefits to the people of Latin America and the Caribbean. The establishment of a series of clinics throughout the region allows people to receive medical care in their own countries. The Cuban model has also resulted in the transfer of technology and the training of local personnel so that they can eventually replace the Cuban medical staff. Some of these clinics are situated in a central geographical location with the intention of treating patients from neighboring countries, in this way strengthening the concept of the need for Latin American and Caribbean unity. There are large clinics in Kingston, Jamaica, to which people from smaller Caribbean countries come, and several clinics in Latin American are located to facilitate treatment for patients from neighboring countries.

This is seen in Bolivia, where there are clinics designed to treat both local patients and those from neighboring countries. A report from September 2011 noted, for instance, that almost 600,000 patients had been treated at the Copacabana hospital. The clinic there, operated by Cuban medical staff, had been established in 2006. By late December 2007, it had operated on 196,000 patients, and by September 2011 this had increased to 600,000. The origin of patients is instructive: 492,231 Bolivians, 48,270 Brazilians, 35,265 Argentines, 22,285 Peruvians, 312 Paraguayans, and an undetermined number of Chileans and people from other nationalities.[20] The clear political message that results is that the initiatives of ALBA pay practical benefits to the population and that Latin American integration is a highly desirable goal. A Cuban ophthalmologist working in Bolivia, Yanet Valdéz, summed up the role of the program there: "In Bolivia, Operation Miracle is everywhere and we give medical attention for free, from the first consultation to giving out spectacles, to surgery and medicines. The idea is to fully incorporate the blind and almost-blind back into society. We want to give our patients the chance to see the world through their own eyes—to give them the miracle of light."[21]

The development of dozens of ophthalmology clinics in Latin America and the Caribbean has not been without problems or controversies, however. Understandably local ophthalmologists are displeased with what they see as unfair competition, since the medical services provided by the Cubans are free. Moreover, the local specialists are often made to look like medical mercenaries, charging high fees and ignoring the needs of people with curable conditions who simply cannot afford to pay them. In many ways, however, the idea that patients are being "stolen" by Cuban and Venezuelan ophthalmology specialists is a false argument, since the vast majority of the patients lack the means to pay for any local professional services. In interviews with representatives of medical associations in Latin America, I have also noticed a definite political bias on the part of local specialists, who are critical of all aspects of Cuban medical internationalism (and indeed, usually of the Cuban revolution itself). They are generally from privileged backgrounds and clearly feel uncomfortable with the nature of the training received by Cuban and Cuba-trained physicians. Many also disagree with the underlying philosophy held by the Cubans that access to healthcare is a fundamental human right and that it should be free to all. In terms of the provision of ophthalmology services offered (at no cost) by the Cubans, local doctors are understandably concerned by the impact on their own practice.

A useful synthesis of these complaints can be found in an article written by seven ophthalmologists based in the United States and several Latin American countries. They present several complaints about the Cuban approach employed in Operation Miracle: most of the reports on the Cuban and Venezuelan programs "tend to be nonscientific and strongly focused on political propaganda" and offer conflicting data; there is insufficient evidence that all of the patients treated were actually blind; and there is a lack of information on some aspects of the program (such as whether the "management of chronic diseases such as glaucoma and diabetic retinopathy are part of the program or not)." Perhaps the most serious criticism is that the system is not sustainable: "The best way to combat blindness worldwide is through development of integrated and self-sustainable eye-care services at the local and national levels, by improving the local ophthalmological services that will still be there to serve the people when the visitors go home. None of these things are being done by Misión Milagro."[22]

This article, one of the very few that is critical of the Cuban/Venezuelan ophthalmology initiative, does offer food for thought. However, it suffers from an overly simplistic approach (confusing Operación Milagro and Misión Milagro and not recognizing the existence of many professional medical journals in Cuba that do offer specific data). The concluding thought about the need for a sustainable system is patently incorrect. The training of skilled medical personnel in Cuban medical faculties has been a priority since the Escuela Latinoamericana de Medicina (ELAM) opened in 1999, and Cuba has done more than any country to train doctors from throughout the Third World. In July 2012, for instance, while 5,315 Cuban students graduated as physicians, 5,694 from 59 nations also graduated as doctors. The largest number of graduates (all trained at no cost to the student) was from Bolivia (2,400), followed by Nicaragua (429), Peru (453), Ecuador (308), Guatemala (170), and Colombia (175).[23] How can one accuse Cuba or Venezuela of developing an unsustainable system when they have made a commitment to train tens of thousands of physicians for the region and to reduce dependence on the services of Cuban doctors?

Perhaps the real reason behind the critique is the implicit support which the authors provide for local professional medical societies ("Cuban doctors are not usually well accepted by medical societies nor by local citizens"). The latter point is nonsense, and most of the 3 million patients who can now see would presumably disagree with the coauthors. From my own experiences talking with patients at three clinics run by Cuban ophthal mologists in Guatemala, it is clear that they were delighted to be able to see again, especially since the surgery was carried out at no charge.

Sadly, two conservative governments in the region have taken advantage of friction with Havana to interfere with the medical services offered in their country by Cuban medical professionals, thereby substantially reducing services offered to their own people. In 2009, for instance, the government of conservative president Alan García in Peru criticized Cuba's Operación Milagro program, noting that Peru's own government-sponsored ophthalmology program, "Ver para Creer," was soon to be launched and would provide up to 5,000 cataract operations each year.

This brought a blistering reply from Fidel Castro, who referred to Cuba's role in Peru in 1970 following a devastating earthquake. At that time the two countries did not have diplomatic relations, yet 100,000 Cubans donated blood for the victims. In terms of García's criticism, Castro noted in an article that "since 2006, Operation Miracle has restored the sight to, or improved the vision of, 19,496 Peruvians. Of these, 16,907 were treated at the Ophthalmology Center operated by Cuba in Bolivia and 2,589 in the Cuzco Clinic, which began its work on December 15, 2008. The Peruvian president has not mentioned Cuba's role in any of these clinics."[24] The Peruvian government initially stated that it would provide free surgery annually for 5,000 patients of limited means, yet in its first year of operation it only operated on 1,500, and by May 2010 only 5,000 people had been treated, although it is unclear if they had been operated on or merely examined.[25]

This politicization of criticisms against Cuban medical care also occurred in Panama, resulting in the withdrawal of the successful Cuban ophthalmology program there in 2010. Some 50 Cuban medical staff had been employed in the Omar Torrijos Herrera Ophthalmologic Center—named after the former president of Panama. Prior to this, in the first stage of Operation Miracle, the Cubans had operated on 5,229 Panamanians in Cuba, and in the second stage, on 44,486 patients in the state of Veraguas, where some Cuban medical staff worked. In 2009 the conservative Ricardo Martinelli, known for his anti-Chávez positions, was elected president, and he made it clear that the Cuban medical cooperation was not welcome.

On January 5, 2010, the Panamanian press reported on a speech given by the national minister of health in which it was mentioned that a new program, Visión 20–20, organized by Panamanian specialists, was to be launched, replacing the Cuban services, which were to close by April 30.[26] This had been done without any consultation with Cuban officials. As a result the Cuban government decided upon an immediate withdrawal of its services, while offering to operate at no charge in Havana on the 22 Panamanian patients who had received pre-op assessments and were awaiting surgery. Odalys González, head of the Cuban medical brigade in the country, was frustrated by the lack of attention that would now be provided in Panama for tens of thousands of patients who needed surgery: "Logically we all know that behind this there are the avaricious interests of Panamanian ophthalmologists who have been opposed to our program from the very beginning."[27]

The new program was supervised by a committee headed by Martinelli's wife and involved the active support of his sister-in-law, an ophthalmologist. The proposed surgery under Visión 20–20 was to be carried out in private clinics and paid for by the government. Panamanian media reports have been extremely critical of the subsequent project, which did not live up to claims by Martinelli's government. There have been resignations, a lack of equipment, long delays in initiating the program, reports of corruption and—most disturbing of all—a limited number of surgeries. The Kiwanis service organization has also become involved, and U.S. ophthalmologists have flown in for brief surgical visits in a clearly tokenistic program. Local politics and professional greed got in the way of the provision of medical care for those who needed it most. Even worse, according to the World Health Organization, in Panama there were "69,521 people who suffer from a lack of vision. Of these, 32,056 suffer from different kinds of cataract pathologies, and of these 15,351 have lost vision completely in both eyes."[28] So much could have been accomplished if the Cuban ophthalmology clinic had been allowed to continue. Instead, a limited program, politically motivated, has replaced it. The tone of the new approach can be seen in the support of the Kiwanis service club of Panama, which in February 2013 organized the ninth "Cataratón," using the volunteer services of two American doctors over a two-day period. They treated 100 Panamanians, bringing the number of patients treated to 900 since the program was initiated.[29] Without taking anything away from the intensive two-day program and the volunteer work of the two ophthalmologists, this approach is a rather superficial reply to the 50 Cuban specialists who had previously worked full-time in Panama.

Unfortunately, the governments of Peru and Panama rejected the approach used by the Cuba-Venezuela initiative in Operation Miracle and were suspicious of its goals. To no small degree this is because the two conservative governments are unaccustomed to the model of providing medical care at no cost to the patient. After all, why would Cuba and Venezuela do something like this? Typical of this attitude is an article written in November 2007 with the provocative headline "Cuba, in a Campaign against Blindness, Uses Doctors to Bolster Its Image." Emphasis is added, but the point remains the same: Cuba is not doing this for any humanitarian reason but rather as a "poignant advertisement for the benefits of Cuban socialism." It is also presented as "an ingenuous way to export one of the few things the Cuban state-run economy produces in abundance, doctors."

The argument about proselytizing is a major error. It is worth noting that Cuban medical personnel serving abroad are expressly forbidden by their own government from becoming involved in politics of the country where they are serving. In their pre-departure briefings this is emphasized at some length, and *internacionalistas* have confirmed this to me in dozens of interviews. In recent years where decidedly conservative governments have taken power (including through clearly illegal means), Cuban medical personnel have deliberately refrained from making political comments, instead focusing on their humanitarian work. Cuban medical personnel did not comment on the overthrow of the democratically elected Honduran government of Manuel Zelaya in 2009, for instance, or the "parliamentary coup" that resulted in the ouster of President Fernando Lugo in Paraguay. The 16-person ophthalmology clinic in Paraguay continues the work it has been doing since the end of 2007 (significantly during the time of a conservative government), and during this period 18,000 Paraguayans have improved or recovered their sight.[30] The same has been true in Honduras ever since Zelaya was overthrown in 2009. Recognizing this, in January 2014 outgoing president Porfirio Lobo, a man with particularly strong right-wing views who is a close ally of Washington, decorated the Cuban medical brigade with the José Cecilio del Valle order, thanking them for their support to the Honduran people since 1998.[31]

Cuban medical humanitarianism as a policy thus makes every effort to remain distant from any comments on political developments in the host country of its medical personnel. That said, it cannot help but influence the way in which grateful patients view this treatment, since it represents an example of political alternatives to established systems wherever Cuban doctors practice medicine.

Misión Milagro in Venezuela

Special attention is owed to Cuba's role in Venezuela, where it has its largest ophthalmology program outside the island and where it has made a commitment to the delivery of a sustainable public health system. The provision of medical care to the population of Venezuela under Hugo Chávez has been extensive. In 2005 the Cuban and Venezuelan governments decided to provide surgery in Venezuela, after several years of performing ophthalmology operations in Cuba, where some 204,000 people were operated on.[32] In October of that year Venezuela took over the direction of the program. Cuban medical personnel are still extremely active in Misión Milagro (having attended 691,479 patients of the over 1.5 million operated on since 2005, and are active in 18 states),[33] but Venezuela is now in charge of the huge program at home.

One of the objectives of Cuba's medical internationalism program is to ensure a sustainable system of healthcare. A fundamental aspect is therefore to train local medical personnel to assume greater responsibility until the Cuban presence is greatly reduced and eventually not necessary at all. That has happened with Misión Milagro, as the Cuban role has gradually decreased. Today ophthalmology surgery is carried out in 54 well-equipped hospitals, with an ever-increasing role of Venezuelan physicians. To put this in perspective, in that first year of the program some 5,000 patients were operated on by Cuban ophthalmologists in Havana—the same number of patients now undergoing surgery in Venezuela on a weekly basis. The data are quite startling: since 2004, some 21 million patients have been screened, 26 million pairs of glasses have been distributed, and by July 2012, a total of 1,553,458 ophthalmology surgeries had been carried out in Venezuela. Of these operations, 700,000 were for cases of pterygium, 205,000 for cataracts, and 15,000 for strabismus.[34]

Data on the trends in ophthalmology operations undertaken in both countries is revealing. From 2004 until June 2012, a total of 893,434 people had been operated on in Cuba through the program, while from June 2005 to June 2012, some 647,547 had undergone surgery in Venezuela. The growth in the number of ophthalmology surgeries carried out in Venezuela is remarkable: 6,947 in 2005, 39,464 (2006), 70,088 (2007), 83,191 (2008), 99,599 (2009), 134,232 (2010), 141,608 (2011), and 65,643 for 2012 until June 20 of that year. Many of the patients operated on were foreign. For example, from October 2005 to June 2012, some 33,375 foreigners and 606,568 Venezuelans had undergone eye surgery. Of the Latin American patients treated under Misión Milagro in Venezuela, the largest group were from Ecuador (6,767), followed by Salvadorans (5,792), Nicaraguans (3,406), Hondurans (2,832), and Guatemalans (2,588).[35]

In August 2013, further announcements were made by Gabriela Soler, the director of Misión Milagro in Venezuela. A new phase in the goals of the Misión had just started. High-tech workshops were established to create glasses and contact lenses, state-of-the-art equipment was to be installed in some of the surgical clinics, training had been ramped up to increase the number of Venezuelan ophthalmologists and optometrists, and a statistics center was to be inaugurated in order to keep track of the patients treated and those in need of treatment. In addition, 22 hospital clinics were to be set up as pilot programs in order to reach patients not normally targeted, including prisoners in penitentiaries, people with disabilities, and the indigenous.[36]

Operación Milagro at Work

A personal note might be pertinent here. In February 2010 I accompanied Cuban ophthalmology teams in their work in three clinics in Guatemala—in Escuintla, Nueva Jalapa and Guatemala City. I talked with patients from all walks of life (but mainly of indigenous origin), as well as the Guatemalan administrators of two hospitals in which the clinics were located, the mayor of Nueva Jalapa, and Cuban medical personnel. I also accompanied patients as they passed from each of the stages of the process until they were discharged following surgery. It was a moving and humbling experience.

What struck me about the three experiences was how uniform they were. The dedication of the Cuban medical personnel, and the professional respect of the Guatemalan hospital administrators and ophthalmologists for the level of dedication of their Cuban counterparts (who earned substantially less, and who did not have profitable private clinics which they left for every day) were very noticeable. Also fascinating was the attitude of the patients, the vast majority of whom were of modest means and, as several confided to me, could never have afforded to have this surgery if it were not for the Cuban program.

There are several key principles at play in the Cuban medical system, both on the island and abroad. Equitable treatment of all patients, with all social groups having the right to access medical care, is the keystone of the approach used. All services are free of charge to the patients. An underlying concept of humanitarian solidarity in the physician-patient relationship is essential in order to facilitate trust and communication. Accessibility is an absolute necessity in terms of material needs (distance, transportation, scheduling). Economic realities have to be minimized for patients (cost of travel to the hospital, affordability of medical treatment). In addition, social or cultural differences have to be respected (overcoming any barriers based on cultural or linguistic differences). Healthcare has to be available to all people, regardless of gender, age, race, ethnic group, or any other such distinctions. Finally, it is seen as a humanitarian duty by Cuban medical personnel to provide care for all patients, one which they are obliged to respect.[37]

Final Thoughts

The loss of vision inevitably causes tremendous suffering for the victims, their immediate family and friends, and ultimately society as a whole, since the person usually cannot contribute effectively to the economy and indeed comes to depend on others. Having our sight is an invaluable asset, of fundamental importance for the enjoyment of all other freedoms. Jamaican commentator Robert Buddan has commented on this ability, one which we take for granted: "Operation Miracle makes you wonder what good is freedom of movement if you can't see to move around; freedom of speech if you can't see to read and write; freedom of religion if you can't see to read your Bible; freedom of property if you can't see to run your business. If you are sight-dependent, how can you truly be free?"[38] Setting the context in this fashion is crucial.

By restoring the vision to millions, this Cuban-Venezuelan medical initiative contributes to the well-being of patients, their families, and their society. The cost of this program is relatively small, although its impact—socially as well as in economic terms—is significant. The key element in the Cuban approach, supported by Venezuela, is political will and the ability to employ a humanitarian philosophy to meet the essential needs of society. There is, however, a stark contrast between what Cuba and Venezuela seek to achieve through this medical internationalism program and what is offered by multinational organizations. As Buddan noted, "If anyone can find in the thousands of pages of the FTAA or the WTO any plan for bringing water to the poor, housing for squatters and slum dwellers, and making the blind see, I'd love to know of it. These are the very things that ALBA and Operation Miracle plan to do."[39]

The facts are simple: Cuban ophthalmology clinics are located in several countries of Latin America and the Caribbean and, supported by the Venezuelan government, have restored sight to over 3 million people (most of modest resources) from 34 countries, and hope to continue to cure millions more of blindness and vision problems. The expanded role of Venezuela in providing the medical care there has become increasingly important since 2005. And all of this has been accomplished since July 2004. The vast majority of beneficiaries of this ophthalmology surgery are Venezuelans, but the benefit of Cuban-Venezuelan cooperation has been extended to other countries in the region. Table 4.1 illustrates the evolution of this program.

A detailed report from July 2014, on the tenth anniversary of Operación Milagro, documented the gains made. The information, provided by Reinaldo Ríos, director of the Cuban Institute of Ophthalmology, noted that 55 clinics had been established. This had resulted in 3 million people, from 34 countries, receiving the gift of sight. Cubans had also benefited from this program, with the number of cataract operations increasing from 13,000 in 2004 to 35,000 in 2013. The number of ophthalmologists had increased from 700 in 2004 to 1,800, and many ophthalmologists had been trained at ELAM to provide a sustainable source of medical specialists for the countries of Latin America and the Caribbean.[40]

These numbers are worth reflecting on. Since 2004, over 3 million people of low and modest income around the world have been given their sight back, allowing them to earn a living, receive an education, support their families—and at absolutely no charge. Some 69 ophthalmology clinics are now providing medical care in 15 countries, and more than 2,000 Cuban specialists have worked in this program since 2004.[41] Operación Milagro also provides corrective lenses, a proactive approach to seeking out patients with ophthalmology needs, and education programs to help avoid eye diseases. Speaking in 2006, Cuba's ambassador to Bolivia, Rafael Daussá, summarized the approach: "Cuba does not weigh its collaboration in dollars, but in lives, in citizens who have recovered their sight and

Table 4.1. Surgical interventions, Operation Miracle, 2004 through May 10, 2013

Countries	2004	2005	2006	2007	2008	2009	2010	2011	2012	2013	Total
Venezuela	18,845	156,604	130,481	174,071	108,775	145,685	66,779	57,004	66,411	22,592	**947,247**
Latin America		5,743	85,331	234,283	236,916	291,475	143,842	96,331	81,088	23,248	**1,198,257**
Caribbean		10,649	13,917	16,533	16,158	26,309	9,306	6,620	6,488	2,545	**108,525**
Africa				5,021	6,847	4,707	5,582	4,950	3,044	2,163	**32,314**
Cuba		36,193	61,044	54,568	20,463	3,342	27,285	32,297	31,806	-	**266,994**
Total	**18,845**	**209,189**	**290,773**	**484,476**	**389,159**	**471,518**	**252,794**	**197,202**	**183,837**	**50,548**	**2,548,341**

Source: José de la Osa, "2.5 Million Patients Benefit: Miracle of Solidarity," *Granma*, June 13, 2013.

happiness."[42] In order to appreciate the impact, it is worth consulting the dozens of articles about this program found at http://www.oftalmologia.sld.cu/mas-sobre-operacion-milagro. Proud of the impact of this Cuban-Venezuelan program, President Nicolás Maduro met with Pope Francis in June 2013 and proposed an alliance between the Holy See and Venezuela to extend Misión Milagro to people of limited resources throughout the world. While this is unlikely, the fact that it should even be considered is noteworthy.

In a provocative article published in late 2008, José Manzaneda lamented the fact that so little is said in North America about the impact of Venezuelan-Cuban medical cooperation in poor countries. He referred in particular to the role that Operación Milagro has played in providing sight to hundreds of thousands of people from developing countries. He contrasted this with extremely limited missions carried out by institutions and clinics from the "developed" world that helped comparatively few patients. He concluded by noting that Operación Milagro represented a "huge challenge for the Latin American elites and for the large international communication media. It demonstrates that the ideology of solidarity can triumph over the ideology of money. And solidarity is incompatible with the business interests or huge fortunes. It is a profoundly subversive project."[43]

In a visit to ELAM in January 2014, UN secretary-general Ban Ki-moon recognized many aspects of Cuba's medical internationalism. He praised the role of ELAM, the ubiquitous Cuban medical presence which he frequently encountered in many countries of the developing world, and Cuba's long-standing role in Haiti. "You create doctors who are miracle workers," he noted. He also praised Cuba's role in Operation Miracle, noting that Cuba was the world leader in this approach to restoring vision. He added, "Besides returning the capacity to see, Operación Milagro has given us a new vision of the world—one of generosity and solidarity: we are all one, human beings who are all brothers and sisters. Healthcare has to cease being a privilege for a few, and should become the right of the majority."[44]

5

Cuba's International Disaster Responses

From 1960s Chile to the 2005 Henry Reeve Brigade

> Not once, throughout the selfless history of the Revolution, have our people failed to offer their supportive medical assistance to other nations in need of this aid at times when catastrophes have hit them, regardless of wide ideological and political differences, or the serious insults received from the government of any of these countries.
>
> Fidel Castro, at the graduation of the Henry Reeve International Contingent of Doctors Specialized in Disaster Situations and Serious Epidemics, and the National Graduation of Students of Medical Sciences, Ciudad Deportiva, September 19, 2005

The growing number of natural disasters resulting from climate change has produced a new term, "disaster tourism." This refers to the issue of those traveling to disaster areas specifically to have an "experience" rather than provide meaningful assistance to those affected. After the 2010 earthquake in Haiti, for example, an astonishing 10,000 NGOs from all over the world participated in the recovery operation and, despite the best of intentions, many only got in the way of the serious rescue attempts and made matters worse. Most stayed for just a few weeks—including the Canadian and U.S. naval presence, and their contribution garnered a tremendous amount of coverage in North American media. In many ways the role of international aid organizations appeared more as a public relations exercise than a humanitarian mission. The Cuban response could not have been more different. Their strategy in disaster response is one that is large-scale, long-lasting, and has developed over time to help millions of the most marginalized and underserved.

Cuban disaster response is characterized by the fact that their specialists help any country in need, regardless of the state of diplomatic relations that they have with Havana. They stay while they are needed, go to work in the areas worst affected, and are both well-trained and experienced in the realities and challenges of developing nations. They send medical staff, trained in complex emergency medicine procedures, and often their emergency assistance evolves into long-term medical support, as is the case in Honduras, Guatemala, and Haiti. All have extensive training for national disasters and significant experience in such situations. As a result Cuba is a world leader in disaster response, and in the last decade has responded on a government level to international natural disasters more than any industrialized country. This chapter will explore the phenomenon of Cuba's international disaster response, including its history and development, and in particular will focus on the activities of the Henry Reeve Contingent, formed in 2005 precisely for this purpose. Several thousand strong, obligated to participate regularly in specialized training to keep its skills sharp and permanently on standby, it has an exemplary record in disaster areas of the world. The second part of the chapter examines the evolution of the Cuban emergency missions in two specific cases, Guatemala and Honduras, where emergency assistance provided by hundreds of Cuban medical personnel was followed up by a commitment to provide a comprehensive medical program to the underserved communities and continues to this day.

As noted in the introductory chapter, the tradition of responding to natural disasters started in 1960 with Cuba's support in Chile after a major earthquake devastated the city of Valdivia, causing 5,000 deaths. Cuba responded with a medical team which set up and staffed six rural field hospitals. A decade later a massive earthquake hit Peru, causing 80,000 fatalities. In less than 72 hours, Cuba had arrived with a medical brigade of 40 emergency specialists and more than 10 tons of supplies.[1] Moreover, in Cuba (and within just nine days), 106,000 people donated their blood for the Peruvian victims, despite the fact that Cuba had strained diplomatic relations of both countries.[2] These disaster response missions have continued throughout the decades, as Cuban medical brigades, supplies, and medications were sent to several countries in Latin America, as well as Asia, the Middle East, and Africa in the wake of natural disasters. Table 5.1 provides details on these missions.

One of the most notable examples of Cuban disaster response came in the wake of the devastation of Hurricane Mitch, which hit Central America on October 22, 1998. Mitch was a category 5 storm on the Saffir-Simpson Hurricane Scale, with winds of 180 mph and gusts of over 200 mph, and it lasted 33 hours. Wave heights reached 44 feet, and total rainfall was 75 inches. The resulting mud slides and floods destroyed massive infrastructure in Honduras, devastated parts of Nicaragua and Guatemala, and caused significant damages in Belize and El Salvador. In total, the hurricane was responsible for the deaths of 30,000 people and resulted in 3 mil-

Table 5.1. Cuba's international disaster response

Year	Country effected	Disaster	Cuban disaster response
1960	Chile	Earthquake, 5,000 fatalities	Sent medical brigade and 6 rural field hospitals.
1970	Peru	Earthquake, 80,000 fatalities	Sent medical brigade of 40 and more than 10 tons of various supplies; in addition, in Cuba, within 9 days, 106,000 Cubans voluntarily gave their blood for the victims.
1971	Chile	Earthquake	Sent medical brigade.
1972	Nicaragua	Earthquake, 5,000 fatalities	Sent a medical brigade of 48 and 10 tons of various medical materials.
1974	Honduras	Hurricane	Sent a medical brigade of 61 and 12 tons of various medical materials.
1985	Mexico	Earthquake	Sent medical brigade of 40 and 13 tons of various medical materials.
1986	El Salvador	Earthquake	Sent a medical brigade.
1987	Ecuador	Earthquake	Sent medical brigade.
1988	Nicaragua	Hurricane	Sent a medical brigade of 39 and 12 tons of various medical materials.
1990	Soviet Union/ Ukraine	Chernobyl nuclear meltdown	Provided medical treatment in Cuba for some 25,000 of the people (mainly children) who were affected.
1990	Iran	Earthquake	Sent a medical brigade of 21 people and 50 tons of various medical materials.
1990	Brazil:	Radiation poisoning	Provided treatment in Cuba for 52 patients.
1991	Nicaragua	Flooding	Sent medical brigade.
1992	Nicaragua	Volcanic eruption	Sent medical brigade.
1998	Honduras, Guatemala and Nicaragua	Hurricane Mitch, 30,000 fatalities	Sent 2,000 personnel in medical brigades and began the Comprehensive Healthcare Programs.
1999	Colombia	Earthquake	Sent medical brigade.
1999	Honduras	Dengue epidemic	Sent medical brigade.
1999	Venezuela	Floods	Sent a medical brigade of 447.
2000–2003	El Salvador, Ecuador, Nicaragua, and Honduras	Dengue epidemic	Sent various medical brigades, including advisors and equipment; in El Salvador in particular, Cuban medics treated 10,000 cases in a 16-week period.
2003	Algeria	Earthquake	Sent a medical brigade of 31 and 4.8 tons of medical supplies.

Year	Country effected	Disaster	Cuban disaster response
2005	Sri-Lanka and Indonesia	Tsunami	Sent medical brigades of 24 and 25 respectively and over 12 tons of different medical materials to each country.
2005	Guyana	Flooding	Sent a medical brigade of 40 and 6 tons of various medical materials.
2005	United States	Hurricane Katrina	Offered the assistance of the Henry Reeve Contingent, including 1,600 medical professionals and 36 tons of medication and equipment.
2005	Pakistan	Earthquake	80,000 fatalities; 2,500 members of the newly formed Henry Reeve Contingent sent with 32 field hospitals (all donated to the Pakistani people); 1,000 medical scholarships provided to local students.
2005	China	Earthquake	70,000 fatalities; 36 members of the Henry Reeve worked at local hospital.
2005	Guatemala	Hurricane Stan	1,500 fatalities, 600 members of Henry Reeve worked with Cuban medical personnel already there.
2006	Bolivia	Flooding	Sent medical brigade.
2006	Indonesia	Earthquake	Sent medical brigade.
2007	Bolivia	Flooding	1,700 members of the Henry Reeve Brigade supported other Cuban medical personnel working in Bolivia.
2007	Peru	Earthquake	540 fatalities; Cuba sent 77 specialists and 2 field hospitals.
2007	Mexico	Flooding	47-person medical brigade sent to Tabasco area.
2009	El Salvador	Hurricane Ida	199 killed; Cuba sent 20 members of the Henry Reeve brigade and a field hospital.
2010	Haiti	Earthquake and dengue outbreak	Sent medical staff to support efforts of Cuban medical staff already on the ground, and Haitian graduates of Cuban medical training.
2010	Chile	Earthquake	500 fatalities; 62 members of the Henry Reeve brigade sent and set up two field hospitals.

Source: Data based in part on *CubaCoop*, "Antecedentes históricos de la asistencia de Cuba ante situaciones de desastre," supplemented by Cuban media accounts.

lion people—10 percent of the population of Central America—being left homeless.[3]

Honduras was the most affected, with 6,500 dead, 11,000 missing, and 1.5 million people displaced or homeless (20 percent of the country). Some 80 percent of the infrastructure was destroyed, as well as 70 percent of the crops.[4] Damages were estimated at around $1.7 billion. As Honduran president Carlos Flores stated, "We lost in 72 hours what we have taken 50 years to build, bit by bit."[5] International aid came largely in the form of loans. The IMF and World Bank, for example, released $201 million in emergency loans for Central America,[6] while Canada loaned Honduras $25.3 million, and the United States offered $96.2 million. The Cuban government took a different approach, immediately sending specialists in emergency medicine and supplies. On November 21, Fidel Castro announced that Cuba would provide up to 2,000 emergency medical personnel to the affected areas in Central America and offered to establish a Comprehensive Healthcare Program (PIS in the Spanish acronym) there. In his address, President Castro swore "revenge" on the hurricane and made a commitment to carry out this revenge by saving many more lives annually than the hurricane had taken.[7] He also announced that 14,800 of Cuba's 21,000 medical students had volunteered to help if they were needed.

In addition to the commitment of sending 2,000 medical staff, the government also stated that it would be offering medical scholarships in Cuba to students from Central America, allowing them to train to become doctors. The scholarship program (directed toward students from underserved rural areas) would span ten years, with 1,000 awards offered in 1999 and 500 in each subsequent year. As Castro also explained following Hurricane Mitch, "We need to do more than weep for those who have died. We need to concentrate on those who die silently every year."[8] This led to the inauguration in 1999 of ELAM.

Cuba immediately sent 14 health workers and six tons of medicines, as well as two field hospitals and other materials. Ten days later, seven more brigades arrived, totaling 119 Cuban medical staff, and all went to the areas that were most affected and underserved.[9] Scores more Cuban medical personnel soon followed and remained for several months, providing medical care. In September 1999, however, as a result of pressure from the Honduran Medical Association and the local school of medicine, the Cuban doctors were informed that their services were no longer required, since they lacked the legal Honduran qualifications to practice medicine there.

This situation soon changed. In the wake of a massive popular outcry from the Honduran public, which demanded that the Cuban doctors remain, the government relented. An agreement was reached which translated into several more collaboration projects in the field of health, as well as a larger number of Cuban professionals working within the country, mainly in rural communities where the Cuban physicians offer little competition for the Honduran private medical sector. The Honduran Medical Association disagreed with these arrangements, but the popular resistance to the idea of the Cuban doctors leaving was so great that the government was obliged to bow to public pressure, and the Cubans were allowed to remain. These agreements continue until today. Following the new agreement on collaboration, some 264 medical staff worked in the Cuban Medical Brigades (BMC), covering 33 percent of the Honduran population (working in 3,307 of the country's 9,943 municipalities).

Guatemala was the second most affected country by Hurricane Mitch. Some 268 Guatemalans were killed and 106,000 were displaced; 6,000 homes were destroyed. In addition, 20,000 homes, seven health care centers, and 48 rural health stations (which served some 50,000 people) were damaged. In total, losses were estimated at $750 million.[10] Within 72 hours of the end of Mitch, the first Cuban doctors arrived, working in the areas where the need was greatest—predominantly in the jungle and mountainous regions. These areas were among the poorest in the country, with an average life expectancy of between 35 and 40 years. Living conditions were very bad: there was often no electricity or schools, and the only means of transportation was by foot, donkey, or canoe.[11]

When examining the contributions of other countries and organizations in the wake of Hurricane Mitch, Cuba's support was significant in many ways. Not only did the country provide a large medical contingent and numerous scholarships, but Cuba also established the Comprehensive Healthcare Program (which continues today) for both Central American countries. In late 2013 the Guatemalan foreign minister, Fernando Carrera, and the president, Otto Pérez Molina, praised Cuba's contribution in improving the health of their people, particularly in underserved areas. Carrera maintained that at least 50 percent of the decline in the national infant mortality rate was due to the work of the Cuban medical brigade, which still numbers about 300. For his part the president praised the "extremely important contribution of the Cuban doctors, because they have gone to rural areas, where they were most needed, and where there was no hospital, clinic, or health post."[12] He refrained from saying that these were areas in which most Guatemalan doctors had remarkably little interest in working.

In terms of preparations for disaster relief, Hurricane Mitch marks a milestone in the Cuban response to natural disasters. This was because of the enormous size of the operation it developed in Central America and for the way this emergency response evolved into a program of sustainable support for several countries in the area. In addition it laid the foundation and provided the necessary apprenticeship for many members of what would become the Henry Reeve brigade, founded shortly after Hurricane Katrina devastated New Orleans seven years later.

Sadly, President George W. Bush refused to allow Cuban emergency medical specialists to set foot in the United States in the wake of Katrina, despite repeated offers of assistance. The hurricane arrived first in Florida on August 25, 2005. It soon reached the level of a Category 4 storm and with some vengeance hit the states of Louisiana, Mississippi, and Alabama on August 29. On the morning of August 30, President Fidel Castro contacted Washington to express his sympathy and offer medical assistance. Specifically, the Cuban government offered to send three field hospitals and the personnel to staff them. No reply ever came, and on September 1 the United States held a press conference where State Department spokesman Sean McCormack formally thanked 50 organizations and countries that had provided aid or offered to do so. Cuba was a significant omission from his list.[13]

As Castro explained in the September 2 graduation speech, Cuba was fully prepared to send 1,100 doctors by air within 36 hours of any official request for assistance. Of these, 100 specialists in comprehensive general medicine could arrive within just 12 hours, with two other groups of 500 to follow shortly afterwards. The Cuban medical staff would be transporting 26.4 tons of medication and diagnostic kits. Each doctor had two backpacks of 52.8 pounds containing vital medicines and diagnostic kits—the basic tools to address the normal forms of distress found in these situations such as dehydration, high blood pressure, diabetes mellitus, and a variety of infections. Each emergency medicine specialist also had medicine to suppress vomiting, as well as painkillers and drugs to lower fever and medication for the immediate treatment of heart conditions, for allergies of any kind, as well as for treating bronchial asthma and similar complications.[14]

By September 4, the quantity of medications and supplies that the Cuban medical staff would be bringing was increased to 36 tons, and in addition 86 recent graduates from the Latin American School of Medicine and an additional 400 doctors volunteered their services. The 1,586 volunteers were brought together and waited with their emergency backpacks, ready to leave at a moment's notice, in the Convention Center in Havana. While waiting for the United States to accept the offer, they participated in workshops to improve their English, as well as refreshing their skills in epidemiology. The call from Washington never came.

The group was made up of specialists in family medicine, cardiology, pediatrics, epidemiology, and other fields, and all were trained in disaster response and the health risks associated with them. Of the group 857 were women, 729 were men, and their average age was 32. In all, 699 had previously worked overseas, they had an average of 10 years of clinical experience, 1,097 were specialists in family medicine, and 72 had two or more medical specializations. Collectively they had worked in 43 countries.[15] In addition these doctors volunteered not just to work in the areas most affected but also to stay as long as they were needed, as they had done in other countries following natural disasters. Despite the fact that their offer was ignored by the Bush administration, the Cubans remained on standby, hoping for Washington to recognize their willingness to help. Given their extensive experience in several emergency missions, they seemed ideal candidates to assist the people of New Orleans.

Certainly that beleaguered city needed support, because the situation was disastrous. It is generally estimated that some 1,800 people died as a result of Katrina, including approximately 1,500 in Louisiana. Louisiana governor Kathleen Blanco was fully aware of the need for extra medical personnel. She outlined this in Executive Order No. KBB 2005-33, the "Declaration of Public Health Emergency and Suspension of In-State Licensure for Medical Professionals and Personnel Licensed Out-of-State," noting that "although scores of people have been rescued, there are many more persons waiting for rescue, evacuation, and medical assistance, and many citizens have suffered or will suffer injury and/or illness." The declaration explained that "the number of medical professionals and personnel currently available to the state to respond to this emergency are insufficient and there is a need to immediately supplement their number in order to serve those affected by this disaster." The state of Louisiana therefore declared that all pertinent laws were "hereby suspended for those medical professionals and personnel from other states or other countries offering medical services in Louisiana to those needing medical services as a result of this disaster."[16] Unfortunately, despite her plea for badly needed medical assistance, and despite Havana's offer to help, Cuban personnel were unable to provide any relief, since authorization from the federal authorities was never granted. Castro angrily noted, "It is a harsh lesson for those whose false pride and mistaken concepts led them to decide not to respond, even belatedly, to our offer, which isn't the first time in these circumstances."[17]

From this frustrating experience a new stage in Cuban disaster response emerged, with the group of approximately 1,500 doctors waiting to assist in the aftermath of Hurricane Katrina being officially named by the Cuban government on September 4, 2005, the Henry Reeve Contingent. When the graduation of students of medical sciences in the Ciudad Deportiva (Sports City installations) took place on September 19. Castro explained:

> On this day a so far unprecedented organization will be formed: the International Contingent of Doctors Specialized in Disaster Situations and Serious Epidemics. This will take the place of the Medical Force formed to help the people of the United States when Katrina hit the south of this country with all its brutal force. Its aim will not just be to help a certain nation, but to give immediate assistance, with its specially trained staff, to any country that suffers a catastrophe, particularly those that are hit by hurricane, floods or other natural phenomena of this severity.

The brigade was named after Henry Reeve, who was born on April 4, 1850, in Brooklyn, New York. He fought in both the U.S. Civil War and Cuba's First War of Independence from Spain. In Cuba he was renowned for his bravery, fighting in scores of battles over a seven-year period, being wounded on several occasions, and obtaining the title of brigadier general. On August 4, 1876, wounded and facing imminent arrest by Spanish forces, he shot himself.[18] Fidel Castro named the contingent after Henry Reeve because of his strength, bravery, and tenacity. The irony of his American heritage is also worth noting.

The brigade was originally made up of 2,000 health care workers, including 300 fifth-year medical students who were trained specifically to provide health care following natural emergencies. Members of the contingent are required to participate in a 315-hour training session in which they learn about each kind of disaster (including hurricanes, volcanic eruptions, sanitary disasters, chemical spills, and floods). Following the training session, and based on their specialty, the members are divided into three groups within the brigade: the Basic Brigade, the Specialized Brigade, and the Recuperation and Rehabilitation Brigade. Each section has its own responsibilities during the contingent's disaster response.

When the Henry Reeve makes plans to assist at a disaster site, the Basic Brigade is the first to arrive, and its principal function is to provide primary health care and, where needed, to perform minor surgeries. The Basic Brigades are individual units, each comprising 70 professionals, who represent 20 specialties. They generally include an administrator, two epidemiologists, four anesthesiologists, three hygiene specialists, eight nurses, one logistician, one pharmaceutical technician, and two internal medicine specialists. By contrast, the Specialized Brigade can work in two distinctive capacities, either immediately after a disaster (fulfilling similar duties to those of the Basic Brigade), or tending to the more complicated needs of people affected in disaster areas. They have the capacity to perform both primary and secondary health care functions. These brigades are made up of 120 personnel, with 41 specialties. Finally, the Recuperation and Rehabilitation Brigades arrive after the disaster is no longer categorized as an emergency, and the situation is stabilized. These brigades are each made up of 18 personnel with nine specialties and concentrate largely on restoring public health care structures in the community.

The basic philosophy behind the contingent is solidarity with the victims of natural disasters. As one contingent member has explained, "Many people ask why do Cubans do this? For me, the answer is simple. Health, education and internationalism are the heart of our system, and what we believe [is that] if you can help people who need help and you are able to—then why not?"[19] As has been the case with each of their missions abroad, they go to the areas that are most affected and stay for an indefinite length of time. The constitution of the Henry Reeve brigade sums this up well: "We offer professionals to fight against death. We show that there are answers to many tragedies of the world. We show that human beings can be better. We show the power of conscience and ethics. We offer lives saved."

It did not take long for the newly established Henry Reeve Contingent to be put to work. On October 9, 2005, the Kashmir area of Pakistan was hit by an earthquake that reached 7.6 on the Moment Magnitude Scale. There were 80,000 fatalities, 120,000 wounded, and 3.3 million left homeless. Moreover, 80 percent of the health centers in the areas affected by the earthquake were destroyed. To place this in context, the damage caused by the earthquake was five times greater than that caused by the tsunami, which had occurred the previous year and affected several Asian countries. Following the disaster, the international community came to assist the affected areas. The United States and European countries sent approximately one base camp each—though they only stayed for a month. The United States sent their last MASH field hospital to Pakistan—an old model that the government no longer employed. Sadly, while the international community pledged over $6.5 billion, the Pakistani government received only a little over $1 billion. The Cuban government sent their newly formed Henry Reeve brigade.[20]

Following the earthquake, and despite the fact that Cuba did not have diplomatic relations with Pakistan, Fidel Castro offered President Musharraf his condolences and followed up on October 12 with the proposal to send 200 doctors, 85 of whom arrived in forty-eight hours. On October 17, after the severity of the damage was better understood, Castro sent an additional 30 surgical teams and 30 field hospitals, with enough equipment to perform 20,000 surgical operations in 90 days and house 600 hospital beds. The field hospitals that the Cuban medical personnel set up were equipped with advanced technology to provide surgeries, ultrasounds, electrocardiograms, X-rays, and laboratory services.

By October 20, the number of Cuban medical staff was increased to 800, and within a week another 260 had arrived, along with 100 tons of medication and surgical instruments, as well as 150 tons of hospital equipment. Within a number of weeks, the figures of Cuban medical staff increased to 2,500, 51 percent of whom were women (a figure which increased from the original 44 percent since, due to local religious beliefs, male physicians could not attend to female victims). The Cuban medical staff lived in tents in the poor, mountainous communities among their patients, and in bitterly cold temperatures. By contrast, international aid organizations and workers mainly stayed in nearby hotels.

By November 19 (five weeks after the Cuban medical staff arrived), the brigade had assessed 60,000 patients, performed 2,000 surgeries, saved more than 200 lives, and introduced widespread preventive campaigns. All communities in the earthquake zone were declared free of the risk of epidemics. The Cuban medical staff then began a program of rehabilitation and prosthesis and orthopedic service to support those affected most severely by the earthquake. The most complicated amputee cases were flown to Havana for treatment. A survey was conducted to determine the number suffering from reversible ophthalmological problems who could then be treated through Cuba's Operation Miracle program. Moreover, the Cuban medical staff started a training program for fourth- and fifth-year Pakistani medical students to show them how to maintain the field hospitals after the Cubans left, and the Cuban government offered 1,000 scholarships to students in rural areas wishing to study medicine in Cuba.[21]

In 2007 the first cohort of students from the area started their education in Havana, and in February 2014 the first group of students, some 297, graduated as doctors in Cuba. One of the graduates, Muhammad Nabeel Shafqat, spoke on behalf of the Pakistani doctors, dedicating their graduation to the former Cuban president, adding, "We are young people from poor families who would never have been able to study medicine. As a result I cannot find words to thank Cuba for its solidarity."[22] The remaining 600 graduated in February 2015.

The Cuban field hospitals were well designed. All 32 had been purchased abroad (mainly from Russia) and were adapted to meet the needs of any emergency. While each is designed for extreme circumstances and equipped with enough space for an outpatient center, operating theatre, ICU, and diagnostic and recovery services, they are also altered and customized to comply with local conditions. The field hospitals, for example, were divided into separate areas for men and women (to accommodate religious customs). They had extra blood transfusion areas (frequently needed following earthquakes, due to the types of injuries and trauma sustained), as well as extra medicine and materials for burn victims (often the result of accidents in the overcrowded tents with open cooking areas). They also had running water in the operating room, increased X-ray developing areas (due to the high numbers of broken bones), and increased capacity for pre- and postnatal care (as 17,000 women in the area were pregnant when the earthquake hit).

The Cuban medics in Pakistan employed their own standard approach to delivering family medicine as a model for treating such large numbers of patients. A team of two doctors (male and female) would tend to a community of approximately 350 survivors (living in 80 tents) and evaluate their medical needs. This method worked to reduce the number of patients seeking medical treatment in the hospitals, as well as offering a preventive measure to resolve health problems before they became life-threatening. Between October 2005 and January 2006, Cuba's medical personnel of 2,378 worked in 44 locations of the Kashmir region and maintained 32 field hospitals. According to official data, they saved 1,315 lives, treated 601,396 people (276,491 of whom were women), performed 5,925 surgeries (2,819 of which were major), attended 125 births, and performed 24 caesarean sections.[23]

The Cuban medical staff of the Henry Reeve brigade stayed for seven months. In that time, they treated 1,743,000 patients, which represented 73 percent of the medically assisted cases in all of Pakistan following the earthquake.[24] They performed 14,506 surgeries and treated 166,000 people with rehabilitation and physiotherapy programs.[25] Cubans were responsible for

32 of the 44 field hospitals in the country, and—after training 450 Pakistani army doctors to operate the equipment—donated them when they left so that the areas affected could continue to receive medical care. Along with the hospitals, they also provided 234.5 tons of medicines and supplies, as well as 275.5 tons of equipment.[26] They charged nothing for the entire mission. Cuba's efforts can be summed up best by Pakistani author Tariq Ali, who noted that "the gesture of the Cuban doctors will go down in the history of internationalism. Many of my compatriots have learned a new word for love: Cuba."[27] Sadly, little international media attention was paid to their efforts.

The Henry Reeve brigade also proved its worth following the devastation of Hurricane Stan, which hit Central America on October 4, 2005.[28] Heavy rainfall led to massive flooding and mudslides, and Guatemala was greatly affected. The storm caused 1,482 deaths and destroyed 9,000 homes.[29] In total, 3.5 million people (31 percent of the Guatemalan population) and 40 percent of the Guatemalan surface area (15 of the 22 departments, and 133 of the 333 regions) were damaged by the storm.[30] Of those, 1.5 million were directly affected, including 500,000 children, and more than 107,000 people were forced to remain in temporary shelters.[31] By October 9, Guatemalan officials had abandoned the communities buried in mud and landslides, declaring the areas to be mass graves. The Guatemalan government immediately declared a state of emergency and requested international support.

Following the devastation, international aid began arriving. The United Nations World Food Program, for example, provided enough food for 87,000 Guatemalans for seven days.[32] The Inter-American Development Bank approved two grants of $200,000 each to Guatemala and El Salvador, as well as making $20 million available in emergency loans.[33] Doctors Without Borders also worked in two towns, providing 11,500 kilograms of relief materials.[34] The United States Agency for International Development (USAID) in partnership with Project Concern International (PCI) awarded a grant of $472,192 over a period of 14 months to help 37 communities with small-scale reconstruction projects.[35]

The Henry Reeve brigade also arrived—600 strong with medication and supplies. The first 300 medical personnel arrived October 8, followed by 300 in the following weeks. They worked alongside the other 233 permanent Cuban medical staff of the Comprehensive Healthcare Program already working in Guatemala since Hurricane Mitch in 1998. Unlike organizations that left within a few weeks, the Henry Reeve brigade stated that they would remain in the areas affected as long as they were required, in order to deal with the risks associated with the flooding and mudslides (including epidemic outbreaks and infections). The brigade stayed for two months, during which time they saved some 1,360 lives, treated 442,618 patients affected by the storm, and attended to almost half a million Guatemalans in 4,850 communities in 69 municipalities in 11 of the most affected departments (including Sololá, Suchitepéquez, Chimaltenango, and Retalhulei).[36]

The following year saw the brigade called into action, again following an earthquake, this time in Indonesia. On May 27, 2006, an earthquake in Indonesia caused the death of over 6,000 people. In addition, 100,000 homes were destroyed and some 650,000 people were displaced. The international community provided notable support and relief. The World Health Organization, for example, donated emergency health kits for 50,000 people for three months and surgical kits to support 600 operations. Doctors Without Borders sent a staff of 35 (including surgeons, doctors, nurses, psychologists, logisticians, and water and sanitation experts). Countries either pledged money (Canada, for example, committed $5.4 million, and international pledges amounted to $47.7 million) or sent emergency staff (including medical personnel from Japan, Italy, Australia, and Spain). However, pledges often do not translate into concrete funds for the government or area affected by the disaster, and emergency staff are often unable to remain in the affected areas for longer than a few weeks. The Cuban government, however, sent a 135-strong medical team from the Henry Reeve Contingent (96 of whom had worked in Pakistan following the earthquake of 2005), as well as two fully equipped field hospitals. They stayed for three months, until the crisis had abated.[37]

By August 20, a little more than two months after their arrival in Indonesia, the Cuban medical brigade had treated 89,550 patients—47,451 of whom received medical care on home visits. Moreover, in the two field hospitals that Cuba established in Prambanan and Gantiwarno, 1,865 surgeries were performed.[38] The medical staff also carried out thousands of lab tests, X-rays, and ultrasounds scans and vaccinated 10,000 against tetanus. An estimated 800 patients visited the hospitals daily, often from the neighboring province of Yogyakarta and from the remote surrounding villages. The Cubans were regarded with great respect, and as Khalida Ahmad of UNICEF noted, "They treat patients like people, not just cases. Everyone I spoke to from the affected areas was so grateful. They felt they could always go to the Cuban doctors to ask a question, despite language difficulties."[39]

In three months, the 135 members of Henry Reeve brigade treated

103,000 Indonesian patients in two field hospitals.[40] They performed 773 major surgeries and 1,436 minor surgeries and assisted in the delivery of 34 babies.[41] Moreover, as was the case in Pakistan, both field hospitals were left behind when the Cuban medical staff returned to Cuba, so that the local communities could continue to receive medical care. Dr. Oscar Putol, a Cuban doctor working in the intensive care unit and member of the Henry Reeve brigade, explained their approach to emergency medicine: "It is about humanity and saving lives. We are here to help. We are permanent members of the Henry Reeve Medical Brigade. Today a volcano, tomorrow an earthquake, the day after floods. Cuba is prepared to go to any country if the government requests us."[42]

Over the following years, the Henry Reeve Contingent would prove themselves on several occasions. They worked, for example, in China after an earthquake killed 70,000 in June 2005. The Cuban government sent 36 specialists in surgery, orthopedics, intensive medicine, and radiology to the disaster zones. This time, however, they were asked by the government to work in local hospitals. In 16 days and in two hospitals in Chengdu, the capital of the Sichuan province, they treated 1,000 victims.

Cuba was also involved in dealing with emergencies closer to home. In October 2007, for instance, massive floods occurred in the southeastern Mexican state of Tabasco. Some 70 percent of the state was under water, and the state's crops were destroyed. An estimated 20,000 sought refuge in emergency shelters, and 1 million were affected by the flooding. The international response was not overly generous. The United States gave $300,000 in emergency aid, while Canada gave $500,000, and even Wal-Mart donated $600,000. The UK government sent 10 inflatable dinghies. The Cuban government sent a 47-member medical brigade, and while their main focus was on minimizing risks of epidemics such as dengue and malaria, they also treated any injuries and medical conditions they encountered.[43]

Earlier that year a far larger response had been required to assist victims of flooding in Bolivia, with the Cuban government sending 1,700 medical workers from the Henry Reeve brigade.[44] In 2006, the brigade had also carried out a similar mission there when flooding affected 40,000 families. The medical personnel provided assistance as well as working to decrease the risk of yellow fever, malaria, dengue, diarrhea and respiratory infections. In total, the Cuban medical staff worked in 236 municipalities of the nine Bolivian departments, treated 3,617,434 patients, and saved 4,642 lives.[45] They were assisted by many of the almost 2,000 Cuban medical personnel already working in Bolivia, in the Operation Miracle, and Comprehensive Medical Programs there.

Cuban emergency medical staff also participated in relief efforts in Peru, following the August 2007 earthquake, which registered 7.9 on the Richter scale. The earthquake caused 540 deaths, destroyed 80 percent of the buildings in central Pisco, and left 16,000 people homeless. International support and emergency medical teams arrived from France, South Korca, Mexico, Venezuela, NGO groups, and the U.S. Air Force. Cuba again sent the Cuban Henry Reeve brigade. Seventy-two hours after the earthquake, 60 Cuban medical professionals arrived, followed by 17 within 24 hours. They included four orthopedic surgeons, two anesthetists, a gynecologist, a pediatrician, two epidemiologists, and 23 general practitioners, along with 10 nurses and 14 technical assistance staff. They brought two field hospitals—one in each of the areas most affected. The hospitals were fully equipped with operating theaters, diagnostic equipment, including electrocardiogram and X-ray, and a complete pathology laboratory. Within three weeks, they had treated more than 15,000 patients. They also performed 115 surgical procedures, including treatment of upper and lower limb fractures, amputations, and appendix removals. In total, 77 members of the Henry Reeve brigade participated, staying from 18 August 2007 to 25 March 2008 and treating 153,292 patients.[46]

In early 2010 the Henry Reeve brigade was called upon again, in both cases responding to earthquakes. The case of Haiti is dealt with in detail elsewhere. The response from Havana was immediate, given the magnitude of the event and the long-standing relationship with that beleaguered country—where Cuban medical personnel had been stationed since 1998. There was also a major earthquake in Chile in February 2010, which triggered a deadly tsunami in the south-central part of the country. Over 500 people lost their lives, and damage was assessed at $15 billion. Some 500,000 homes were deemed uninhabitable in the wake of the earthquake. The Cuban response was much the same as in the earlier cases. The Henry Reeve brigade responded immediately and a first group of 26 specialists flew out, installing a major field hospital in Rancagua and transporting 12 tons of equipment, instruments, and medicine. At the request of the Chilean government, a second contingent of 36 members was sent to install a second field hospital in Chillán, 319 kilometers to the south. More than 100 Chilean graduates from ELAM volunteered their support, coming to work on the weekends after finishing their regular work in local hospitals.[47]

While the Henry Reeve brigade has proved vital in immediate disaster response, it is also important to look at the broader context of the Cuban response to disasters in general. In other words, while the assistance provided by the Cubans was important, it was the combination of the work of the brigade and subsequent actions to support a sustainable public health program that was particularly valuable. In many cases, for example, the emergency assistance of the Henry Reeve brigade was subsequently supported by scholarships given to students from the affected areas to study medicine in Cuba. As noted above, in Pakistan this resulted in 1,000 students being able to train to become doctors for free in Cuba, and the offer of similar scholarships to study at ELAM has been extended to several of the countries where emergency medical assistance is provided. In other cases Cuba has followed up its emergency missions with the offer to provide a Comprehensive Healthcare Program, with the support of medical personnel in areas where there was no or very little health care, as is the case in Bolivia. As previously outlined, following the devastation of Hurricane Mitch, the Cuban government began such a program in the areas affected.

In Guatemala the Cuban program was staffed by 270 professionals including doctors (largely specialists in family medicine), epidemiologists, nurses, laboratory technicians, radiologists and anesthesiologists, statistic technicians, engineers who specialize in medical technology, secretaries, drivers, and entomologists. They worked in 17 of Guatemala's 22 departments in the rural, underserved, and predominantly Maya areas. The financial responsibility for the doctors was divided between the two governments. The Cuban government was responsible for providing transportation and staff, while the Guatemalan government provided a monthly stipend of up to $250 to each professional.[48] The medical personnel worked where the Guatemala government sent them—-usually in poor areas where Guatemalan physicians preferred not to work.

The Cubans did not take over any existing local health care support or seek to change any traditional medical techniques or remedies. Rather, they worked within the local customs, creating a hybrid of the two approaches. In particular, Cuban doctors worked with local religious leaders or *curanderos*.[49] As Yoandra Muro, a leader of the BMC in Guatemala stated, "Our mission is to help the Guatemalan people and to do everything we can for the health of children, the elderly, and the general public."[50] In my own interviews with Cuban physicians in rural areas of Guatemala I was informed that this approach continued and was essential among the indigenous communities. Childbirth, for instance, was usually carried out with the patient delivering the baby while in a squatting position (as was the local custom) rather than lying on a bed. In addition, many herbal remedies used by local faith healers were used together with drugs imported from Cuba, as well as surgery, to provide a holistic form of medical care.

By 2004, 1,700 Cuban medical personnel had worked in Guatemala.[51] Their impact has been extremely positive. For instance, child mortality rates in the areas in which Cuban doctors were working decreased from 40.2 per 1,000 to 13.8 per 1,000 live births, and according to official reports, some 157,226 lives had been saved. That same year, Alfonso Portillo, Guatemalan president at the time, in his last official presidential address, praised Cuban medical staff:

> As my last state duty, I didn't want to miss out on presenting our highest order of state (the Order of the Quetzal) to the heroic brigade of Cuban doctors who, often enough, risked their lives in order to save those of Guatemalans. . . . The doctors, nurses, and health care assistants have done everything imaginable during their stay here. They were doctors, mechanics, patient transporters, and repairers of kitchen equipment. They have survived threats, misunderstandings, being ignored, and loneliness. But they stayed and put into practice what friendship between peoples really means and demonstrated Cuba's international solidarity.[52]

Cuban physicians were soon assisted by newly graduated Guatemalan students trained at ELAM. In 2005, the first 187 Guatemalan students graduated from the Latin American School of Medicine—150 of whom returned to Guatemala to do their internships alongside Cuban physicians.[53] By 2006, 2,500 Cubans had worked in the Cuban health program in Guatemala[54] and had carried out over 20 million consultations, 56,458 surgeries, and health care to 2.5 million people.[55] In 2007, the Cuban medical mission was also presented with the Father Manolo Maquieira Human Rights Award. The ceremony was presided over by former president Oscar Berger, former vice president Eduardo Stein, President Álvaro Colom, and Vice President Rafael Espada. The ceremony also presented the 340 Cuban medical brigadiers in attendance awards "for their solidarity with the people of Guatemala, in favor of the right to life, good health, and a better living standard."[56]

As of 2009—11 years after the Comprehensive Medical Program was instituted—there were 297 Cubans still working in Guatemala.[57]

These professionals worked in 89 of the country's 363 municipalities (26.8 percent), 17 of the 22 departments (77.3 percent), 48 of 278 health centers (17.3 percent), 13 of the 43 hospitals (30.2 percent), and were responsible for providing health care to over 2.6 million of some of Guatemala's poorest.[58]

The Impact of the Combined Cuban Health Program (1998–2009)

Cuba's role in improving the health profile in the areas in Guatemala where they work has been important. Table 5.2 illustrates the impact of a decade of medical cooperation. Significantly, given the focus on prevention and community health care, infant and maternal mortality rates have greatly decreased. In particular, by 2008, in the areas in which the Cuban doctors were working (where they attend 90 percent of births), infant mortality rates had decreased from 40.2 per 1,000 live births, to 8.9. Similarly, maternal mortality rates decreased from 491 per 100,000 live births, to 113.8. According to official records, between 1998 and 2008 they were directly responsible for saving the lives of more than 255,292 Guatemalans.[59] This calculation is based on an analysis of historical data, detailing the number of people who traditionally had died of particular pathologies before the Cubans had arrived, and extrapolating conclusions from the health profile since their arrival. The most recent data, from February 2014, show that the Cuban presence remained strong in underserved regions of the country, particularly among the indigenous population. There were 472 Cuban medical personnel, working in 16 of Guatemala's departments. The most significant statistic, however, was the total of lives saved, now noted as 287,658.[60]

The Cuban role in Guatemala is not unique. Cuba's Comprehensive Healthcare Program (or PIS in the widely-used Spanish acronym) has also greatly contributed to the health care of Honduras, which instituted the program after Hurricane Mitch. A collaborative arrangement was then established between the two governments, and 264 Cuban staff arrived to introduce this program. Following a new agreement, the Cuban government increased the number of medical staff to 305. Since its inception, Cubans have continued to provide health care to 33 percent of the Honduran population and have worked in 3,307 of the 9,943 communities in the country. By 2006, a total of 1,400 Cuban health care personnel had worked in Honduras. Approximately 58 percent were women, 23 medical specialties were provided, and the average age of the Cuban participants was 43. Also by 2006 they had provided 3.3 million medical consultations, attended 61,930

Table 5.2. Impact of the combined Cuban healthcare program in Guatemala, 1998–2009

Population treated	2,199,146
Doctor/patient ratio in areas served by Cuban specialists	1 × 8145
No. of medical consultations	25,004,914
No. of surgeries	40,677
No. of births attended	74,237

Source: Conner Gorry, "Cuba-Guatemala Cooperation: Building Viable Models for Health," *MEDICC Review* 11, no. 3 (Summer 2009).

births, performed 289,845 operations, rebuilt or maintained 135,300 pieces of medical equipment, and saved 219,960 lives.[61]

One of the most notable projects that came out of the Cuban program in Honduras was in the community of Ciriboya, an isolated community in the eastern La Mosquitia region. In particular, a project called "Luagu Hatuadi Waduheñu" (for the health of our people) was started in 1999 by local students who were studying at ELAM.[62] They began expanding the medical services at a local hospital in which the Cuban doctors were working. The hospital soon became one of the most important medical facilities in the area. Moreover, following the graduation of the ELAM students, the hospital continued to expand as they returned to work there. The hospital maintains a family residency program and since 1999 has been responsible for providing health care to over 12,000 patients.[63]

By 2009, the Cuban doctors had given more than 22 million consultations in Honduras, performed more than 350,000 operations (including 108,000 major surgeries), presented 18,500 educational activities, and saved the lives of some 237,000 Hondurans.[64] Furthermore, they developed cooperation projects regarding mental health, HIV/AIDS, and programs to decrease dengue rates. They also introduced new services and areas of specialization in hospitals and medical centers (including biomedicine as a career in universities), as well as repairing and maintaining 18,635 pieces of medical equipment (with the latter contribution being valued at $8,438,000.)[65]

Perhaps most telling is that, as is the case in Guatemala, in the areas where the Cuban doctors are working, infant and maternal mortality rates have drastically decreased (By 2006, Cuban doctors had attended 61,930 births.)[66] Prior to the arrival of the Cuban medical brigade, the infant mortality rate had been 37 deaths per 1,000 live births, but by 2006 it had dropped to 10.8. Maternal mortality rates also fell by 80 percent.[67] In total, more than 1,600 Cuban professionals have worked in the most rural and underserved areas of Honduras. The coverage of these traditionally underserved areas continues to grow, through the efforts of the Cuban medical personnel and the arrival of newly minted graduates from ELAM.

In Summary

Cuba has a tradition of responding to natural emergencies that stretches back to their support for the Chilean people after a 1960 earthquake. Since 2005 this role has been formalized in the Henry Reeve brigade and has responded to disasters around the globe. Their contribution in the fight against Ebola in 2014–15 in West Africa is the latest example of this tradition. The Cuban approach is different from that found elsewhere. What is most striking about their contribution is that, unlike the proponents of "disaster tourism" noted earlier, the Cubans have specialized training and experience. They draw upon a body of several thousand medical personnel specialized in dealing with natural disasters, the vast majority of whom have extensive experience working in developing countries. In addition they stay for much longer than many of the other organizations that respond to natural disasters. Most important of all, they seek to contribute to a post-emergency sustainable solution to the problems of the areas affected.

In many ways their role in emergency medical response comes down to a combination of political will, humanitarian commitment, and long-term planning. As a result of Cuba's Henry Reeve missions, thousands of lives have been saved, and a standard has been set in the international context for emergency response. Of particular note is the underlying humanitarian concept, the lowest common denominator of Cuba's medical internationalism program. Indeed in many ways it can be traced back to the maxim of nineteenth-century Cuban revolutionary José Martí that "Patria es humanidad"—all of humanity is the homeland.

6

South-South Cooperation in Biotechnology

Medicine for the Masses

> It gives me great pride to inaugurate this Center, right in the middle of the Special Period. It represents a promise of health and well-being for our people, as well as the potential for our economy since it has a great production capacity. It also constitutes the possibility of coordinating with all the other research centers here. That is why we have created these scientific complexes in the *polo científico*. The idea is for every center in science research to work together in close coordination, and not act independently, ignoring the others.
>
> Fidel Castro at the inauguration of the Center for Molecular Immunology, December 5, 1994

International interest in Cuba's biotechnology potential was aroused in May 2002 when U.S. undersecretary of state John Bolton condemned what he alleged to be Cuba's offensive biological warfare program. This claim was strongly rejected, including by former president Jimmy Carter, since Bolton's objective was clearly political. Nevertheless, the incident caused many to examine Cuba's increasing role in biotechnology. It soon became clear to Western media that Cuba had in fact developed a sprawling complex of biotechnology research and development facilities in the west of Havana known as the *polo científico*. This consisted of dozens of well-designed new buildings, equipped with modern technology, in which thousands of engineers, technicians, and doctors were producing a wide array of medicines, vaccines, and related products, primarily for the Cuban population, but also increasingly for foreign markets. It was obvious, too, that Fidel Castro was the prime mover behind this initiative, a fact confirmed through several interviews with leading scientists in 2013 and 2014.

This poses many questions. Why and how did applied interdisciplinary research in biotechnology evolve so early and so readily in Cuba in the 1990s? Why were preventive medications and vaccines prioritized? How could a small country like Cuba produce such an array of medications and vaccines and indeed most of the medications consumed domestically? Why was it being praised by international bodies such as the World Health Organization (WHO) and the Pan American Health Organization (PAHO) for its exportation of massive amounts of low-cost drugs to the developing world? Apart from the occasional flurry of reporting on events such as Bolton's claims, and infrequent articles in professional journals, remarkably little has been reported in mainstream media.

In recent years Cuban medicines have been increasingly used throughout the developing world and sold at a fraction of the cost of drugs produced by multinational pharmaceutical companies in the industrialized world. A 2009 editorial in *Nature* emphasized its leading position in the Global South, as well as its distinctive model, calling it "the developing world's most established biotechnology industry which has grown rapidly even though it eschewed the venture-capital funding model that rich countries consider a requisite."[1] This recognition came belatedly, however, since Cuba had started this research initiative several decades earlier, and the origins of Cuba's impressive biotechnology growth may well be traced back to the statement in January 1960 by Fidel Castro that "the future of Cuba has to be of necessity a future made by people of science, of thought."[2]

This chapter offers some observations to show how South-South cooperation in biotechnology constitutes a significant support to Cuba's medical internationalism program. At first glance it might appear odd that a book examining MI, which in essence revolves around the contribution of doctors, nurses, and medical technicians in developing countries, would explore the role of biotechnology. Yet this is an important complement to the work being done by medical personnel in the field. In sub-Saharan Africa, for example, the role of Cuban physicians working in the most distant rural communities to treat patients suffering from malaria and dengue is clearly strengthened by the application of Cuban biolarvicides to kill mosquito larvae. Likewise, in Venezuela the use by Cuban physicians of Heberprot P, which has reduced drastically the need for amputations among diabetics, also assists doctors treating diabetes.[3] In the state of Mérida, for example, of 1,091 diabetic patients who received this treatment, only 5 went on to need an amputation.[4] Recent Cuban data show that since 2007 more than 29,000 Cubans with diabetes have received this treatment and that the risk of amputation has been reduced 80 percent.[5] This integrated approach to the care of public health, both at home and abroad, is a fundamental characteristic of the Cuban healthcare model, and biotechnology is an invaluable support.

In essence the Cuban approach to healthcare focuses on attending to the greatest healthcare needs of the population. In terms of biotechnology this translates into the development of products that will best assist and protect that population, preferably (but not exclusively) in a preventive mode. Since the early 1980s Cuba has built up the human capital capacity and physical infrastructure to attend to these needs, first for the Cuban population and increasingly for developing countries. And as noted, people's needs, and not profit, have traditionally been the driving philosophy behind the approach to biotechnology. As Simon Reid-Henry has noted, "Cuba's policy of putting biotechnology to work within a public health framework, focused on preventive medicine, and often tied to a mission orientation, might seem rather incongruous, but it has worked. . . . Despite the difficulties of the Special Period, the country has maintained a relatively high level of public health and has continued to export some of its most basic life-enhancing technologies to other countries in need."[6] Given the small size of domestic demand, in order to be financially viable Cuba's biotechnology industry had to look abroad.

The use of Cuban biotechnology also helps to illustrate the Cuban approach to public health in general, with the use of preventive medicine being of paramount importance, and not solely on the island. In 2000 the WHO recognized the potential of Cuba's role in this area, approving their hepatitis B vaccine in UN vaccination programs, mainly in developing countries. Since that time Cuba has been involved in scores of cooperation agreements throughout the world. Thus, in addition to being a profitable export product for Cuba, Cuban biotechnology products have saved countless lives at a more affordable cost—and are therefore important in Cuba's medical internationalism program around the globe.[7]

Cuba: The Evolution and Nature of Biotechnology

In the early 1980s, and with the strong backing of Fidel Castro, Cuba embarked on a journey to develop its nascent biotechnology program, based around the large science cluster west of Havana. According to UNESCO, approximately $1 billion was invested within the first two decades, resulting in the establishment of a science node of 52 institutions, in which over 20,000 scientists, engineers, and technicians are employed.[8] Cuba produces almost 70 percent of its own medications, which are provided at extremely low prices domestically and at affordable prices abroad. One of the principal drivers in the Cuban approach to developing its biotechnology industry was the need to become self-sufficient in the production of medications and vaccines for its own use—and in order to accomplish this, collaboration across disciplines and extensive teamwork among those researchers was an absolute requirement. The export of biotechnology products has become lucrative for Cuba, generating some $800 million in export earnings, second only to nickel in terms of income from products sold abroad. It has been estimated that it will generate $1.04 billion in 2016.[9] When the U.S. embargo against Cuba is lifted and American consumers can use these significantly less expensive medicines, it will prove one of the most lucrative industries in Cuba.

The integrated nature of the Cuban approach to biotechnology is very different from anything found in industrialized countries. Collaboration and not competition across several disciplines is the major philosophical factor behind its approach. Also important are the connections in the entire process of products, from initial research to the final stages of marketing. This "loop" combining various facets of the development and production process can probably be most effective in a socialist society with decades of cooperation in scientific research, supported by the government, and with an education system that from childhood has encouraged a collaborative approach to problem-solving.

Agustín Lage, probably the most significant figure in Cuban biotechnology and the director of the Center for Molecular Immunology (CIM), has explained the origins of the prestigious center, at first a small laboratory on the fourth floor of a Havana hospital. In September 1989 Fidel Castro entered the CIM and spoke of his ambitious vision for biotechnology in Cuba: "He talked about building a new Center; we just wanted to improve the small laboratory that we had. Fidel spoke about developing an industry; we had not thought of that for the immediate future."[10] From this humble origin a biotechnology industry grew.

Biotechnology research and production have increased steadily since the first building was constructed. By late 2012, according to Lage, "products from the Cuban biotechnology industry were either being used, were in clinical trials, or had been registered in 50 countries. In terms of cancer treatment, Cuban products were being used in more than 25 countries, with clinical trials being carried out in 12."[11] Cuba's reputation as a producer of quality medical goods has increased dramatically in recent years, and Cuba is the only country in the world that has developed an effective vaccine against type-B bacterial meningitis.

There are many quality pharmaceutical products from Cuba being used both domestically and abroad. These include the world's first synthetic vaccine against Haemophilus influenza type B (Hib), the bacteria responsible for almost 50 percent of infections. Nimotuzumab, an anti-cancer epidermal growth factor receptor, is currently in clinical trials in several developing and developed countries, while a second vaccine against advanced lung cancer, Racotumomab, is now being used following the success of CimavaxEGF.[12] In 2013 clinical tests were initiated for Itolizumab, for patients with severe psoriasis. Particularly successful among the hundreds of products is Heberprot-P, a treatment for diabetic ulcers, which has generated support worldwide, even among influential U.S. politicians, and may eventually be allowed in the United States, an exception to the U.S. embargo of Cuba.[13]

Heberprot-P has been registered in 25 other countries (ranging from several in Latin America to others in Asia), and patents have been taken out in 14 countries, including the United States. To date, more than 60,000 patients in Cuba and abroad had benefited from this innovative treatment, which has reduced the need for amputation by some 90 percent. In the case of Venezuela, by late 2011 almost 34,000 patients with diabetes had avoided having their feet amputated as a result of this treatment.[14] It is significant that, instead of simply exporting the drug to target markets, Cuba also provides training on the use of Heberprot-P. In June 2012, for instance, the Ministry of Health in Ecuador bought 1,012 doses, worth $3,275,000, in an arrangement that included training for Ecuadoran specialists.[15]

One of the major research institutions in the science cluster is the Center for Genetic Engineering and Biotechnology (CIGB), with over 1,400 researchers involved in more than 50 major projects. This modern building with cutting-edge technology would not be out of place in any science complex in Western Europe or North America. According to a catalog advertising their current research, over 60 medical inventions have been accorded to the CIGB, which has also been granted 406 patents worldwide.[16] The research program undertaken by the CIGB is ambitious, including the production of vaccines against Hepatitis C, cancer, dengue, and Human Papillomavirus 16m and treatments for rheumatoid arthritis and multiple sclerosis. There are also dozens of research projects being undertaken on agricultural biotechnology projects at the CIGB. As is the case with the other institutions mentioned, the medical products made here are also used throughout the developing world—at a fraction of the cost charged by multinational pharmaceutical companies.

Agustín Lage's Center for Molecular Immunology has also produced a series of vaccines against meningitis B, hepatitis B, and dengue which are used around the globe, especially in the developing world. For many years the CIM has also been working on a vaccine for HIV/AIDS. By 2007 the center was already producing two recombinant proteins, seven monoclonal antibodies, and five cancer vaccines. It was also operating factories in China and India, with stringent quality control standards, where its products were being manufactured for use in the domestic and export markets, mainly in Asia.[17] In recent years another major research center, LABIOFAM, has produced encouraging results with its anti-cancer drug Vidatox, made from the poison of blue scorpions. (This has been registered in 15 countries, and by late 2012 it was being used by 55,000 patients including 40,000 outside Cuba. It has an analgesic, anti-inflammatory effect, and has been used to treat cancer of the prostate, uterus, and pancreas.) Other well-known research centers in this biotechnology cluster are the National Center for Bioproducts, the Finlay Institute, the Pedro Kourí Tropical Medicine Institute, the Immunoassay Center, the National Center for Neurosciences, and the National Center for Scientific Research.[18]

In terms of Latin American countries' investment in research and development (R&D) in biotechnology, Cuba ranks third, just below Chile and Brazil. Cuba spends 0.6 percent of GDP on R&D, compared with 2.7 percent in the United States.[19] However, Cuba's approach to biotechnology research has provided far better results for its population in terms of ensuring accessibility of (free) products for its citizens, and has resulted in enhanced health outcomes. Despite spending four times the GDP rate on R&D, the U.S. approach has not led to the same wide access to needed products for its citizens. In poorer countries the development of new biotechnology products is extremely difficult, and the cost is prohibitive, even when there is a clear need for drugs to combat widespread diseases. In industrialized countries potential profit, and not need, is the major driver for new product area research. As a result, lifestyle drugs such as Viagra or cures for baldness are favored because of their high profit margins over the development of new antibiotics with more limited market potential, despite the greater need. The Cuban case shows that this state-supported approach, focused on the needs of the people and not exclusively on profits, drives research and production in a different direction—towards the most needed products that support better health outcomes. In essence Cuba is "developing a paradigmatically capitalist form of science in a developing socialist country."[20] This strategy does not preclude innovations, however, as the production of the drugs and vaccines mentioned above illustrates. It is also the result of a decades-long strategy of the state supporting this sector. The unusual nature of this strategy is also found in the Cuban approach to South-South cooperation in biotechnology.

There are significant differences between the Cuban approach to biotechnology research and that found in industrialized nations. For example, while private biotech companies seek to maximize profits for their shareholders, this does not apply in the Cuban case, where the state pays for all research and development activities and so has no obligation to produce profits for the shareholders. The state is thus less driven by market considerations and the need to focus on producing the most lucrative products.[21] By contrast, the Cuban approach concentrates on the greatest need, primarily for the Cuban people, but also for the population of countries in the world, especially those who cannot afford medical care. The director of the Finlay Institute, Concepción Campa, explained the differences in philosophy:

> We have spoken with several foreign companies, but from the outset they inform us "we are a for-profit company, and our principal objective is to make profits. We of course also work to improve people's health." That principle puts us at a disadvantage. More than anything else we work to improve human health—not to make profits. And we don't have the financial resources for marketing.[22]

Put simply, for a multinational corporation, the production of drugs to be used to save lives in impoverished sub-Saharan countries is not a profitable venture and therefore will never be a priority. By comparison, the development of medications for middle-class North Americans suffering from impotency or hair loss will generate significant profits.[23] As a result, developing profitable products for that target population will be their main goal. The Cuban approach therefore places it squarely in opposition to the dominant capitalist paradigm.

Moreover, many of the pathologies encountered in developing nations, such as dengue or malaria, are not common in the developed world. As a result, U.S. and European pharmaceutical companies have relatively little interest in such research, since market potential for these products is limited in developed countries. By contrast, while the need for drugs to combat these diseases in developing countries is great indeed, the comparative financial reward is small—and so research and production in these areas are limited. The way in which Ebola was ignored by transnational pharmaceutical companies for many years, despite the need in Africa, illustrates clearly this reality: it was simply not a profitable enough business venture. The Cuban philosophy is thus very different from that of multinational drug producers in the developed world and is based upon the belief that products of biotechnology are not primarily intended to generate profits but rather to help people, both in Cuba and abroad. If the human need is great, then so must be the research interest. The question of producing medicines primarily on the basis of the financial bottom line is thus an alien concept in the Cuban approach.

This does not mean that profit is not welcome in terms of Cuban exports of pharmaceutical products, and this has clearly come to the fore since Raúl Castro became president in 2008. Yet commercial returns on biotechnology of necessity must be fair and not exorbitant. In addition, wherever possible the Cuban approach limits the price of medicines by producing generic drugs which are far less expensive than those produced in the developed world. Cuba's focus also differs in its emphasis on prevention. It seeks to develop vaccines to avoid diseases in the first place, thereby reducing the costs of medication to the patient rather than heavily focusing research on developing treatments and cures once disease has occurred. Many result in technological cooperation with other developing countries—as is seen most clearly in the case of cooperation with Brazil.

Another significant difference is that pharmaceutical products, the result of state-funded research, are provided free or at very low cost to Cubans and are part of an integrated approach to accessible, public healthcare, available to all on the island without charge. Indeed from the Cuban perspective, access to public healthcare is seen as perhaps the most important human right for people. Moreover, in this cluster of scientific research facilities, the integrated process of working closely with local hospitals and sharing production and distribution tasks, eschewing competition and secrecy in favor of collaboration and support, provides an exceptional base for solid, cost-effective R&D. Cooperation among these institutes, rather than competition, is pursued diligently.

Based on a half-dozen visits to several of these research institutes over the past decade, several points can be made about this distinctive Cuban approach. Andrés Cárdenas summarizes his analysis of some key components, of which strategic control is perhaps the most important.[24] By this he refers to the integrated planning process involving the stakeholders of all of the major research centers and government ministries, setting out goals for the entire (shared) direction of the biotechnology industry in the monthly meetings attended by representatives from the various centers. Research priorities are established, scientists are tasked to work with colleagues from other centers on a particular project, and support is provided by the state.

Cárdenas also refers to the long-term commitment of the state to the industry, in good times and bad. Even in the worst moments of the Special Period following the implosion of the Soviet Union and the loss of its major trading partner, government support for research in biotechnology remained firm, as did the commitment to public healthcare, guaranteed in the national constitution. The government strategy also shows the close relationship between R&D in biotechnology and the delivery of healthcare to the population. Another difference can be seen in the manner in which intellectual property is handled, since all patents are owned by the Cuban state and are used to support the interests of the Cuban population, instead of generating profits for an individual corporation. Since Cuba's scientists, researchers, and doctors have all been trained at no charge to the individuals, the official position is that the fruits of their research belong to the people and the state which had provided them with that education.

An important development in the industry occurred in November 2012 when the Cuban government formally established the Group of Biotechnology and Pharmaceutical Industries, better known as BioCubaFarma. The objective was to centralize the many diverse institutes, research centers, and biotechnology groups into one central body, with the ultimate goal of making the organization more efficient and ultimately generating more income for the state. Research, production, equipment-manufacturing, and marketing have now been brought together formally, involving more than 21,000 people. The 60 organizations that had previously existed were now reduced to 38, with a centralized management group in charge of them all.

In addition, these groups are no longer to be financed totally by the state. Instead, they are seen increasingly as business enterprises, capable of making profits for their research center—but significantly not for themselves. Their fundamental goals remained the same, namely, to produce high-tech medicines, equipment, and services focused on improving the health of the Cuban people, while also providing goods and services for the export market, principally focused on developing countries. The incoming leadership of this new organization claimed that income would double within the next five years with all profits generated to be reinvested in the centers. As was the case with other aspects of medical internationalism, from training doctors from wealthy countries to establishing hospitals in Qatar and Saudi Arabia, under Raúl Castro financial matters have become increasingly important, although in all cases profits revert to the state.

Under this government it was clear that one of their principal goals was still people's health, both in Cuba and abroad. It was also obvious that the use of all forms of healthcare—from the exportation of medical services to biotechnology production—were to be used to generate economic gains for the good of the nation. In many ways this runs parallel to the general belief under Raúl Castro that, while medical cooperation would still remain a priority of the government, this had to be at least cost-neutral with, where possible, a fair return for Cuba's support to be expected. In both cases profits would be directed back into the state coffers, where they would be used to support the Cuban public healthcare system.

South-South Collaboration in Biotechnology

Cuba's reputation as a major biotechnology power in the developing world was established by the new millennium as it strove to develop cheaper, more accessible pharmaceutical products for markets there. The discovery of the first synthetic vaccine for the prevention of meningitis and pneumonia, for example, meant a significant decrease in the cost of the vaccine traditionally manufactured by pharmaceutical companies in the industrialized world. This has resulted in millions of children being immunized. Many would otherwise not have received the vaccine, and they could have died.

Cuba has also developed the commercial side of its approach to cooperation in biotechnology. The country has been keen to share its knowledge with the developing world, and countries from Asia were among the first to receive this transfer of technology. In 2003, for instance, Biocon India Ltd. signed an agreement to establish a production plant, with Cuba providing support to its Indian partner in "the production of recombinant monoclonal antibodies for use in cancer treatment designed to target tumors."[25] (The term *recombinant* refers to the process of bringing together artificially, such as in a laboratory setting, genetic material from multiple sources.) This followed a 2002 agreement with China to produce treatments for head and neck cancers, and several joint ventures with Beijing have followed. By 2008 Cuba had signed science and technology agreements with 32 developing countries (13 in Latin America and the Caribbean, 12 in Asia, and 7 in Africa). Particularly well developed were biotechnology agreements with

Brazil, India, Malaysia, Iran, and China.[26] Within Latin America there are also comprehensive bilateral agreements with Argentina, Brazil, Colombia, Mexico, and Venezuela.

The Cuba-China collaboration is a model that is both lucrative and mutually beneficial in terms of biotechnology production. Cuba is currently involved in two joint ventures in China. The larger (Heber Biotech) is in Beijing (where 260 workers are involved in the development and marketing of monoclonal antibodies for cancer treatment), while the other (ChangHeber) is in the northeast and focuses on the production and marketing of interferon (both for the Chinese market and to export elsewhere in Asia). Another significant line of research in this process is the production of glucose biosensors for diabetics, a project on which the Cubans have been working for several years.

In February 2012 Biotech announced that it was increasing its investment, since it hoped to triple production of the monoclonal antibody Nimotuzumab, to be used for the treatment of head and neck cancer. By that time more than 10,000 Chinese patients had benefited from the Cuban treatment.[27] Its sales in 2011 were reported as $46 million,[28] and since then sales have continued to increase at an average annual rate of 30 percent. More significant was the increase in research results, with two new drugs now in the clinical trial stage, one of which was a therapeutic vaccine used for patients with lung cancer. Biotech was also awaiting approval to start clinical trials for another product, a monoclonal antibody already being used in Cuba to treat autoimmune conditions such as rheumatoid arthritis, severe psoriasis, and multiple sclerosis.[29] The new research and production center at ChangHeber, inaugurated in June 2013 by Vice President Miguel Díaz-Canel, is especially important as its focus will be increasingly on the production of a Hib vaccine against Haemophilus, a major gap in China's universal immunization program for children.

The Cuban biotechnology presence in China is held in great esteem. In 2009, for example, President Hu Jintao presented Dr. Agustín Lage, director of the Center for Molecular Immunology, with the Prize for Collaboration in Science and Technology in the treatment of cancer patients. As a further sign of the importance given to this collaboration in biotechnology, in August 2013 the Chinese and Cuban ministers of Science and Technology inaugurated the Sino-Cuban Center of Molecular Immunology there. Commenting on the value of the Cuban role, Chinese specialists noted that "the development of these cooperative projects help the development of biotechnology, serve the Chinese people, and improve the research and development level of biopharmaceuticals with marked social and economic effects in China."[30]

In many ways this cooperation with the Chinese projects resembles the relationship which the Cuban Center for Molecular Immunology has with the Indian company Biocon. There, Cuban scientists have been working for a decade, focusing on the development of recombinant proteins. The objective is to develop therapeutic products based on biotechnology that can be used to treat chronic ailments. As a result of this joint research and development program they have already marketed in India and other countries a monoclonal antibody used in cancer treatment as well as medication used to control anemia in patients with chronic kidney conditions.

An offshoot of this successful and profitable Sino-Cuban partnership through Heber Biotech also resulted in the establishment of a commercial alliance with the Vietnamese pharmaceutical group AMV. In December 2011 a $5 million agreement was signed for the transfer of technology and sale of Cuban products. Earlier that year Hapharco, a unit of AMV, had agreed to purchase Cuban vaccines against Hepatitis B, as well as the Pentavalente vaccine which immunizes babies against five common childhood diseases. AMV also agreed to sell a dozen Cuban biotechnology products, with the value increasing from $100,000 to $3 million.[31]

A final example of South-South collaboration of this kind can be seen in Cuba's relationship with the Algerian company Saidal. This partnership was established in 2009, when the Center for Genetic Engineering and Biotechnology (CIGB) transferred the appropriate technology to its Algerian partner in order to produce a Hepatitis B vaccine. In 2010, a similar agreement was signed, with the express understanding of forming a strategic alliance in the production of generic medicines and advanced biotechnology. The objective was to reduce the high cost of importing drugs while increasing the variety of biotechnology products available for the local market. There was also an interest in exporting these products to other countries in the region. Once again, while Cuba benefited from the technology transfer process in terms of licensing and royalty benefits, also important was the availability of cheaper pharmaceuticals in North Africa.

One of the most important research centers in the Havana science cluster is LABIOFAM (Laboratorios Biológicos Farmacéuticos), which makes a wide variety of chemical and biopharmaceutical products for the domestic and international markets. Originally focused on the domestic farming market (to which it still supplies 98 percent of the veterinarian drugs used in Cuba), it now also exports many products. Its main research focus, however, remains on agricultural biotechnology. One of its first exports to support Cuban medical cooperation was in 1994, when an outbreak of the bubonic plague in Peru resulted in Cuban specialists using the biological rodenticide BioRat (particularly important since it is biodegradable). Since then its products have been used in many countries—from Central America to Guinea, from the Mongolian steppes to the jungles of Benin.[32] In October 2010 some 52 tons of the rodenticide were donated to Nicaragua after 353 cases of leptospirosis were detected throughout the country, and BioRat was distributed within a week to over 323,000 Nicaraguans.[33] In early 2011, some 960 tons of BioRat were applied in Angola following a rodent plague, with a 95 percent success rate.[34]

LABIOFAM's fundamental goals are to prevent the transmission of diseases to humans—such as leptospirosis or hemorrhagic fever—as well as to protect crops. The twin goals of protecting health while generating profit can be seen in their investment in Vietnam, where a BioRat production plant of LABIOFAM was built with the support of both governments. LABIOFAM did not seek just to export the rodenticide to Vietnam, even though this would have been in its best commercial interests. Instead it sought to contribute to a long-term approach for the country by transferring Cuban technology, establishing training programs, and building a factory.

The president of LABIOFAM, José Antonio Fraga Castro, has explained the approach employed in such circumstances: "When we identify a market niche in a specific—usually developing—country, we diagnose the problem and suggest the appropriate technology. After a contract is signed our specialists travel to work on the project. They then train personnel from the client country so that, when they leave, the program is sustainable."[35] As a result, BioVietnam was established, producing the rodenticide for both domestic use and exportation. In addition to the clear medical benefits, it also has economic value, since in Vietnam the rodents eat 17 percent of the rice harvest (approximately $500 per hectare), whereas it costs only $15 per hectare to implement coverage with BioRat.[36]

Together with the Pedro Kourí Institute, LABIOFAM has also been involved for years in the production of bioplagicides, to be used as an alternative to chemical insecticides in controlling vectors, which cause many diseases in the developing world. It has also produced biolarvicides as a means of reducing malaria, and these products have been applied in 60 countries. (The biolarvicides prevent mosquitoes from laying their eggs in stagnant water and thereby spreading malaria. These biological products do not have the environmental contamination problems of DDT and other chemical pesticides.) In the case of Africa, seven countries—Angola, Ghana, Burkina Faso, Nigeria, Equatorial Guinea, Tanzania, and Zambia—have successfully applied the Cuban products, and several other sub-Saharan countries have expressed an interest in doing so.

Again, the objective is not just to sell the product but rather to transfer the appropriate technology and skills in order to develop a sustainable approach to eradicate malaria through the application of the biolarvicide, substantially decreasing the mosquito population. This understandably has a significantly positive impact upon the local population. As a result, factories to manufacture this product have been built in Tanzania and Ghana, while others will be built in Angola, the Ivory Coast, and Nigeria. Other facilities in China and Argentina have also been established to produce larvicides in order to support pest control and thereby address local health needs.

The role of Cuban biotechnology in the struggle against malaria is particularly well developed. For example, between January 2009 and August 2010 a group of 174 Cuban technicians using LABIOFAM products covered 91 percent of Angolan territory, working in 44 of the country's 164 municipalities. Educational campaigns to advise people about insanitary practices, as well as the application of larvicide and the training of 1,400 Angolans and hundreds more volunteers to implement the program, were key components of the campaign. The strategy was successful: the rate of morbidity caused by malaria was reduced by 53 percent in the capital, Luanda, and 52 percent in the rest of the country.[37] Figures provided by the Angolan Ministry of Health showed that between January and October 2010, 6,770 people died from malaria, compared with 10,249 the previous year.[38] By 2012 the biolarvicides Bactivec and Griselesf, produced by LABIOFAM, were being used widely in Angola, Tanzania, Ghana, Zambia, Nigeria, Burkina Faso, and Equatorial Guinea.[39]

In April 2012 a significant step was taken in an agreement between LABIOFAM and the Economic Community of West African States, held in Nigeria. The objective was to move ahead with Cuba's role in a program to eliminate malaria in the member states. Malaria is a major health problem, and in Ghana alone it is the cause of 13 percent of deaths each year. Pilot programs were initiated in Ghana, Nigeria, and Burkina Faso, since they were the countries where the greatest concentration of attention was to be focused. Following the completion of this first stage, production of the larvicide using Cuban materials was to be established in Ghana and Nigeria by late 2014 and the Ivory Coast by 2016. In addition to setting up production facilities in West Africa, Cuba also committed to a program of training local personnel to ensure the sustainability of the program. This was to be done in two phases, with the first focusing on the training of members of the military and the second of civil society members. In April 2014 Cuban experts from LABIOFAM also participated in the campaign, organized by Roll Back Malaria, in a traveling caravan that visited Tanzania, Malawi, Zambia, the Democratic Republic of Congo, Mozambique, Zimbabwe, Swaziland, South Africa, Angola, and Namibia.

A smaller program against dengue took place in Ecuador in 2013, and again it was led by Cuban specialists from LABIOFAM, who built a plant to produce bioplagicides and biofertilizers for local use. This resulted in a decrease in the costs of the chemicals previously used in a campaign against the *aedes aegypti* mosquito. By September 2013 there were 80 Cubans working in four provinces of the country in this campaign to end dengue. Within the first six months of their campaign they had been able to reduce the rate of dengue by more than 90 percent.[40]

In sum, Cuban biotechnology centers have also provided cost-cutting equipment to medical and research centers in many developing countries, again to promote public health. Profits are made, but not at the exorbitant rates of return expected by multinational pharmaceutical companies. The transfer of Cuban technology, to ensure the sustainability of the project, is also common.

Cuban research centers also produce a wide array of diagnostic equipment. The Immunoassay Center, for instance, has for years pioneered an ultramicroanalytic system, or SUMA, capable of carrying out a number of diagnostic tests used to detect and monitor several health conditions. In 2008 they produced the SUMAsensor, "a glucometer designed specifically for tropical climates."[41] This diagnostic tool, available at a modest price, is being used in 496 laboratories in half a dozen countries, including Brazil, Argentina, China, and Mexico. The same research center, together with the International Center for Neurological Restoration (CIREN) provided the Alejandro Posadas hospital in Argentina with Estereoflex, an automated system designed by both Cuban research institutes and used to detect neurophysiological responses in neurosurgery.

Two other centers in Havana's biotechnology complex, the Cuban Neuroscience Center (CNC) and the Central Institute for Digital Research (ICID), have produced sophisticated medical equipment, to be used both in national hospitals as well as by Cuban medical brigades working in developing countries. They are also exported to developing countries, where they are sold for significantly less than similar equipment manufactured in industrialized countries. Among this equipment are portable electrocardiograms, the CARDIOCID BB (used to monitor and analyze heart rhythms), the CARDIODEF 2, a defibrillator monitor, and the HIPERMAX, an ambulatory monitor to record blood pressure and heartbeat. Other monitoring equipment includes the TERAPLUS (a therapeutic electro-stimulator) and the DOCTUS VI (used in intensive care units to monitor physiological reactions such as blood pressure, heart rate, and respiration rate). At the CNC, created in 1990, the MEDICID (a digital electro-encephalograph) and the AUDIX (which records electrical brain activity) are exported to China, Venezuela, Colombia, Mexico, Spain, and Italy.[42] As is the case with the exportation of pharmaceuticals, the commercialization of these products is largely focused on developing countries, which often do not have the funds to buy similar equipment manufactured in the industrialized world. The Cuban equipment is sold by a local company with offices in Venezuela and Algeria. By contrast, in developed countries the major market share remains in the hands of large multinational companies, where brand recognition is an important factor and where Cuban equipment would have obvious difficulties penetrating.

South-South Collaboration: Cuba and Brazil

Perhaps one of the best illustrations of the application of Cuba's approach to collaboration with other partners from the South in terms of biotechnology and public health can be seen in the production of meningitis vaccines, in this case with the economic powerhouse of Latin America, Brazil. Bacterial meningitis is a severe infection of the fluid and coverings surrounding the brain and spine that can often prove fatal. In some 20 sub-Saharan countries, bacterial meningitis, due to Meningococcal serogroup A, comes in epidemic waves. It can be prevented with a vaccination, but pharmaceutical companies have not been keen to ramp up production, since this type of meningococcal strain is rare in industrialized countries—and is therefore not overly lucrative. The lack of priorities for multinational pharmaceutical companies was seen clearly in 2006 when there was an outbreak of the disease in Africa. At that time the only producer of the vaccine was Sanofi Pasteur, which was cutting back on this particular line, since it was not considered to be particularly profitable.[43] Given the pressing need for the drug and the lack of interest shown by Sanofi Pasteur, in 2007 the WHO requested the support of Cuba and Brazil to provide large quantities of vaccine at inexpensive prices for the at-risk populations of sub-Saharan Africa.

Cuba and Brazil responded to the clear need for the vaccine by combining their efforts through the Finlay Institute in Havana and Brazil's Bio-Manguinhos Immunobiological Institute. Both developing nations face common difficulties of launching new products in a world dominated by wealthy multinational drug companies. Both also had to prove their capabilities, given the skepticism from the pharmaceutical industry in the Global North. Yet in light of the need for their products and the reluctance of multinationals to manufacture them, their role in the Third World was crucial in reaching populations with limited means. The price difference between the combined Cuba/Brazil product and that charged by multinational drug companies, for instance, was enormous: 95 cents compared to $15–20 per dose.[44] (The more expensive vaccine does last longer and has greater coverage than the Cuba/Brazil product, but the cost remains prohibitive.) By the end of 2012, some 19 million doses had been prepared and distributed throughout the region, with the largest shipments going to Mali, Ethiopia, Burkina Faso, Nigeria, Niger, and Chad. These vaccines were purchased by international organizations such as the WHO, UNICEF, the International Red Cross, and Médecins sans Frontières, who then administered them.[45]

Cuba and Brazil have been working together on a series of biotechnology projects since the 1990s. The initial focus was on a transfer of technology agreement, allowing Cuba to produce in particular two products for the Brazilian market: Interferon alpha 2b ("a recombinant protein used extensively as an antiviral or anti-neoplasic agent, particularly against hepatitis C") and recombinant human erythropoietin (rHuEPO), used for treating anemia in patients with chronic kidney conditions.[46] In this agreement Cuba trained Brazilian researchers to produce these drugs at an affordable price. As Halla Thornsteinsdóttir and Tirso Sáenz have illustrated, both "had an applied focus—to increase the availability of affordable health products that serve local health needs."[47] This goes to the heart of Cuba's exportation of biotechnology collaboration. Rather than maintain control over the development of drugs made in Cuba, the objective is to ensure a technology transfer process in order that people can obtain pharmaceutical products at a fraction of the cost charged by multinational drug companies.

To put this in context, 2,000 units of EPO would cost $50 in the international market, yet in Brazil—as a result of bilateral research and production—the cost would be $3.[48]

The agreement between the two countries illustrates the approach undertaken in several developing nations by Cuba. As a socialist country with a decades-old commitment to a comprehensive public healthcare system, Cuba follows a radically different approach than would be employed by a multinational drug company. This can be seen in its dealings with Brazil, where the "basic objective was to implement a gradual process of technology transfer that would first solve the immediate Brazilian need for these products and, over time, would build Brazil's capacity to produce them."[49] The transfer was clearly not done with the sole objective of gaining market share and extensive profit for Cuba, an alien concept in the capitalist business model. In short, the Cuban-Brazilian collaboration on biotechnology illustrates meaningful South-South cooperation. Cuba was able to receive compensation for its advanced biotechnology experience, while Brazil succeeded in meeting the need for a basic pharmaceutical product and providing its people with medical products that would have been otherwise unavailable because of their prohibitive cost on the world market. Moreover, the technology transfer ensured that Brazilian scientists would be able to produce the pharmaceuticals in the future.

In September 2011 Brazilian Health Minister Alexandre Rocha Santos Padilha and Roberto Morales, his Cuban counterpart, signed a memorandum of understanding to expand this relationship by making and distributing the diabetes treatment Heberprot-P, as well as 11 anti-cancer products and others for kidney disease. These would be produced in Brazil, using Cuban technology, both for the local market and for export. In all, 58 projects were agreed to, involving Cuban research institutes as well as Brazilian centers and private companies working in the health sector. Significantly, Padilha echoed the Cuban approach to the development of these biotechnology products, for the benefit of others as well as for both countries: "We expect to take concrete steps regarding cooperation, not only between our peoples but for the rest of the world, which hopes to be closer to access to medicine as a basic right to health."[50] It was announced the following month that joint research projects, using the monoclonal antibody Nimotuzamab, were being used to treat cancer of the cervix, esophagus, nervous system, head, and neck.[51]

Biotechnology for the Developing World

Cuba's biotechnology industry has become successful in recent years, both because of its impressive research into cutting-edge pharmaceutical products and its mass production of far cheaper generic drugs. Cuban researchers have been granted over 500 patents, including 26 in the United States, and Cuba is now the "largest medicine exporter in Latin America and has more than 50 nations on its client list."[52] This, it should be remembered, occurs in a country of 11.2 million, with an average monthly salary of $25.

In a recent study on South-South collaboration in biotechnology, it was shown how Cuba plays a leading role in sharing its knowledge through joint research projects. In a comparison of countries such as Brazil, China, India, South Africa, Egypt, and Cuba, for example, Cuba and South Africa were the most active in terms of seeking ties with other countries of the South, slightly more than even China. Cuba also has the most active clinical trial collaboration of the countries studied, and illustrative of this interest in expanding scientific ties with developing countries, a third of its internationally co-authored papers from 1996 to 2009 were with researchers from other low/middle-income countries.[53]

Furthermore, this interest in biotechnology has been profitable. The exportation of biopharmaceutical products increased dramatically—by a factor of five between 1995 and 2010—making it one of the most significant sources of hard currency for the cash-strapped country.[54] One of the largest markets, not surprisingly, is Venezuela, where the purchase of Cuban pharmaceutical products between 2006 and 2012 increased 2,905 percent—from just $10 million to $323 million in 2012. In June 2014 it was announced that Cuba and Venezuela had inaugurated a state-of-the-art factory in Venezuela (the Empresa de Producción de Medicamentos Biológicos) to mass-produce vaccines in order to "favor the development and independence in terms of pharmaceutical products" in Venezuela, another example of Cuba's commitment to South-South collaboration.[55] Larger markets await, however. Indeed, if Washington succeeds in normalizing relations with Havana and dropping the trade embargo, Cuba may well prove to be the first country that overturns the traditional North-South paradigm, with developed pharmaceutical products then heading from the south to the north. To a certain extent the success of Heberprot-P in Europe has already brought about a significant shift in acceptance of Cuba's high standing in terms of biotechnology. There are many other drugs, already successfully applied in Europe as well as in developing countries, that could be beneficial to the U.S. population—and profitable for Cuba.

It is also clear that Cuba has used its considerable experience in biotechnology to support its long-standing tradition of medical internationalism. At times this has been seen in the donation of medicines when health crises arose abroad. In February 2008, for instance, Cuba flew yellow fever vaccine to Paraguay following an outbreak there. The following month Paraguay received 50,000 doses of medicine after malaria was detected. In August 2010 Nicaragua received 600,000 vaccines against Hepatitis B. From the exportation of the cancer treatment Vidatox-30Ch to Laos and Mongolia to the use of the diabetes treatment Heberprot-P in dozens of countries, from the use of biolarvicides to fight malaria in the Ivory Coast to the transfer of Cuban technology in Algeria, Brazil, and China, from courses in Guinea Bissau training people to prevent dengue and malaria to donations of vaccines against H1N1 and hepatitis B in several Latin American countries, Cuba's role in the use of biotechnology to complement its policy of medical internationalism has been successful.

Particularly successful is its cooperation with developing countries, as the example of its partnership with Brazil shows. South-South collaboration has resulted in countless lives being saved in developing countries, as was seen in their shared production of the meningitis A vaccine for Africa, a process which clearly "reflects solidarity with other developing countries. It demonstrates how such collaboration can be harnessed to address a health threat spurred by demand and funding from an international organization."[56] The role of Cuba in biotechnology projects in sub-Saharan Africa has also grown steadily in recent years and will continue to increase because of its cost-effective, environmentally friendly campaigns against malaria and dengue.

Equally noteworthy is the South-South model of collaboration in which Cuban experience and advances in biotechnology are paired with local companies in joint venture projects. In these cases—as seen in India, China, Algeria, and particularly Brazil—the objectives are to transfer technology to the host countries, so that they can develop a sustainable industry producing an array of generic drugs for local consumption, while collaborating in the production of goods to be exported. In all cases reasonable profits will be accrued, but this is not necessarily the primary goal. Indeed it is significant that in countries where Cuba is providing extensive medical support, the host countries are not obliged to purchase Cuban-made medicines. Even in Venezuela, where there are some 30,000 Cuban medical personnel, the government buys medical supplies from all over the globe. Members of the medical brigades from several countries in Latin America and Africa have commented in personal correspondence that most of the pharmaceutical products used are from major drug companies in the United States and Europe. The concept of "tied aid" (a common process among industrialized countries which insists that developing nations purchase goods from the same country that is providing "aid") is not applied by Cuba.

In the case of Brazil, the increasingly close political ties between Brasilia and Havana offer greater potential, both as a market for Cuban products (given the 195 million population of the South American country) and as a source of bilateral research and production. Under the governments of Lula da Silva and Dilma Rousseff, Brazilian investment in Cuba has also increased dramatically—most clearly seen in the massive port development of Mariel outside Havana, but also in manufacturing and even sugar processing. To put this in perspective, bilateral trade increased sevenfold between 2003 and 2012.[57] These closer commercial ties have also resulted in greater interest in cooperation in biotechnology.

Joint ventures in this field have increased, and their combined efforts in several regions have illustrated the potential for growth. The fact that Brazil is taking a significant role in supporting Cuba's campaign to improve Haiti's public healthcare system which Cuba is leading also helps to strengthen shared interests in biotechnology. The United Nations is well aware of the value of using the technical capabilities of both countries to produce cost-effective drug campaigns for the developing world, as was noted earlier. The 58 cooperation projects in this field agreed to by both countries in September 2011 continue to provide mutually beneficial results, and this bilateral approach to biotechnology also offers great potential for Cuba. A sign of these increasingly close medical ties can be seen in the employment of 11,400 Cuban physicians in 2013–14 to work in underserved areas of Brazil.

In terms of future development, an important consideration will be the role of ALBAmed, a regulatory institution, in terms of medical care for the member countries of ALBA (the Bolivarian Alliance for the Peoples of Our America), which was consolidated in 2013.[58] The objective is to unite member countries in order to centralize the production of drugs and medical goods and to determine the needs of each member country. This represents a potential market of 70 million people, with a GDP of $636 billion. As the largest producer of these materials in the ALBA membership (and of course provided that ALBA remains functioning), Cuba will naturally benefit from this association, while this participation will result in a reduction of costs for ALBA member states.[59] The aim is to provide enhanced "concerted regional planning for sustainable pharmaceutical production and to save the participating governments between 20 percent and 50 percent in medical purchases."[60]

The same report notes the vast array of generic drugs made in Cuba, including antibiotics, antiretrovirals, drugs for infectious diseases, and anti-inflammatory drugs, as well as many kinds of vaccines. Medications to treat many chronic diseases are also manufactured in Cuba, ranging from treatments for diabetes to cancer. The next major related project will be ALBAfarma, a centralized agency responsible for the purchasing, storage, and distribution of drugs for ALBA members, and it is likely that this will be located in Cuba. Despite obstacles from opponents of the left-wing governments in ALBA countries, it is clear that the potential for the expansion of Cuban exports in biotechnology is great indeed.

In his study of Cuban biotechnology, *The Cuban Cure: Reason and Resistance in Global Science*, Simon Reid-Henry analyzes in some depth the evolution of the Cuban approach to science. In the Global North, economic conditions have traditionally held sway over social utility in the field of biotechnology—yet the Cuban model went totally against the grain. At a time when biological sciences were becoming focused on producing profits, "Cuba's biotechnology project—along with not dissimilar experiences in countries such as India and Brazil—*was* an alternative, and one that has pointed up some of the contradictions inherent in Western science more broadly."[61] To a large degree this was due to the political will of the Cuban leadership, which was determined from the outset to use biotechnology both for the benefit of the Cuban people and for the developing world.

Over a decade ago Agustín Lage Dávila talked about the gains made by biotechnology in an essay entitled "Socialism and the Knowledge Economy." He waxed eloquent about the Cuban experience ("successful by any indicator one chooses to measure it by: the generation of products, biopharmaceuticals, and vaccines, the impact on public health, patents, exports, cash flow, profit margins, or return on investment").[62] He outlined the basic elements of the Cuban experience, the socialist alternative, noting in particular the integrated approach (research-production-marketing between dozens of research and production centers), the export orientation of the industry (used to finance the goods and services of the Cuban healthcare system), and the need to view scientific research—the result of the formation of "massive, highly qualified human capital with motivation and commitment"—as investment for Cuba's development. He concluded by emphasizing the essence of the Cuban approach: "Ours is a new and creative path. There is no one to imitate. There is much to be done, but we can do it, and the people of Cuba, socialist owners of our economy, demand that we do it right."

7

The Cuba-Venezuela Medical Partnership

The Castro-Chávez Dream Lives On

> We have a mutually beneficial, generous, and humanistic integrating system that is not based on competitive mechanisms. We are assisting each other to give the best to our peoples. . . . We are proving that we can achieve big goals with few resources but with a lot of willingness and love.
>
> Hugo Chávez, November 8, 2010

Fidel Castro and Hugo Chávez are widely recognized as two larger than life figures that strode the world stage for many years. Yet remarkably few people are aware of the impact of their partnership in terms of public health, both in Venezuela and indeed throughout Latin America and the Caribbean. This chapter seeks to shed some light on the large medical cooperation program in which both countries engaged and in particular to analyze developments concerning the Cuban role in Venezuela since 1999. As is seen throughout this book, the benefits of Cuba-Venezuelan cooperation for developing countries (largely using Cuban medical personnel and Venezuelan financial resources) go far beyond the limits of this bilateral approach. For example, financial support for the delivery of Operation Miracle programs in many countries, for the reconstruction of the Haitian public healthcare system following the devastating 2010 earthquake, and for many medical support missions throughout Latin America and the Caribbean (and indeed Africa), could only have been possible with the committed support of these two crucial components.[1]

This chapter narrows the focus, examining how Cuban medical cooperation was applied in the case of Venezuela, a program that started following Cuba's offer of assistance in December 1999 in the wake of massive flooding and landslides in Vargas state. Given the size of Cuba's medical cooperation in Venezuela (where some 30,000 medical personnel were working in 2014), an analysis of the nature and evolution of the program employed there is a necessity. In particular three areas of Cuban participation will be assessed—its role in the Barrio Adentro (Inside the Barrio) program, its contribution to Misión Milagro (Mission Miracle), and finally its participation in the Medicina Integral Comunitaria (Comprehensive Community Medicine, with MIC being the Spanish acronym) training of medical students.

To a large extent the Cuba-Venezuela alliance as well as its cooperative missions throughout the region, have been responsible for laying the foundations of a reinvigorated sense of regional unity and pride in Latin America. For many years the Cuban revolution had been the only major challenge to U.S. hegemony in the region, a situation that changed dramatically with the election of Hugo Chávez in 1998. The resulting alliance culminated in the political map of Latin America being irrevocably changed. In bilateral terms too, both Cuba and Venezuela benefited significantly from closer ties. On a pragmatic level Cuba badly needed the subsidized oil that Venezuela, with its massive reservoirs, could provide at reduced rates, while Chávez following his election in 1998 also needed to show Venezuelans that he could provide them with significantly enhanced public health services—an area in which Cuba had ample experience and a large supply of doctors.

The relationship between the two countries went far beyond that, however, since scores of bilateral agreements (from fishing to oil exploration, shipbuilding to agriculture) have been implemented over the years. Indeed in April 2013 a further 51 collaboration projects were signed in Havana between the two governments, and a work plan from 2013 to 2019 was laid out. In many ways Chávez saw himself as the heir apparent to the Cuban president, often referring in emotional terms and with tremendous respect to the influence of Fidel Castro, whom he saw as a mentor and father figure in terms of ideology and understanding of development issues. For his part Castro consistently praised the grasp of international politics of his younger Venezuelan counterpart, whom he regarded with great personal affection. In many ways Chávez was the political apprentice of Fidel Castro—and he quickly came to appreciate the enormous importance that public health constituted for Castro. The death of Chávez in March 2013 and the election of Nicolás Maduro have resulted in a continuation of the strong bilateral relationship, with a lesser dependency on the two leaders (Maduro and Raúl Castro) and greater emphasis on pragmatic bilateral relations. The charismatic presidents may have left power, but the mutually beneficial relations have continued.

In terms of images, while there is a general (and simplistic) view of the Venezuela-Cuba relationship as one based on an "oil for doctors" arrangement, the basis for this strong bilateral partnership is far more deeply rooted. It goes beyond this one-dimensional presentation, and in fact has drawn both countries together in a way never before seen, especially in medical cooperation. The large Cuban presence today can be traced back to the original support provided following the December 1999 flooding and landslides in Vargas. An estimated 15,000–30,000 people died or disappeared (presumed dead) in this natural disaster, and the hospital and transportation networks were largely destroyed. Cuba responded immediately by sending some 450 medical personnel (including 250 doctors, as well as nurses, epidemiologists, and emergency medicine specialists). The first contingent arrived two days after tragedy struck, and the rest within a week, and the Cuban government committed to them staying as long as they were needed by the Venezuelan government. They in fact remained in Vargas until 2002, but also extended their medical services to several neighboring states. This was roundly condemned by the Venezuelan Medical Federation (FMV in the Spanish acronym), concerned with the "Cubanization" of medical services to people. For their part, however, the local population was generally pleased with the medical attention provided by the Cuban medical brigade, since for many their healthcare needs had been ignored by the medical establishment for decades.

This basic tension between the FMV and the government, between traditionally educated Venezuelan doctors and those trained in the Cuban medical philosophy, would continue for many years later. Sadly, it remains to this day, with the same phenomenon also found in other Latin American countries where there are large numbers of Cuban physicians and graduates of Cuban medical programs. Most recently this situation has been seen in Brazil, where the Rousseff government is paying for the services of 11,400 Cuban physicians, after Brazilian physicians failed to respond to a program (Mais Médicos) for physicians to work in sparsely populated, rural communities largely in the impoverished North East of the country. Once again the local medical federations are opposed to the Cubans' services, while there is overwhelming support from the population, most of whom live in traditionally underserved regions, mainly poor and rural.

The current tensions between Cuban-trained physicians in Venezuela (proponents of Comprehensive Community Medicine, or MIC as it is referred to locally) and the traditional approach to medicine supported by the FMV can be traced back to December 1999 with the arrival of the emergency response medical support from Cuba and subsequent assistance to local communities in Vargas. The FMV position rested on two principles: the Venezuelan Federation of Medicine accused the Cuban doctors of spreading left-wing ideology among their patients and also stated that, since they did not have a license to practice medicine in Venezuela, they were working there illegally and should be expelled. For their part the Cuban medical brigade countered that it was providing badly needed medical care in the coastal area, where 90 percent of the sewage system had been destroyed and where there was a grave danger of an epidemic of water-borne diseases. There were clearly insufficient medical resources in these areas, and Venezuelan doctors were loath to transfer there. Moreover, the Cuban physicians were not working to provide competition to Venezuelan doctors and their private clinics—because the people whom they treated could not afford to see local specialists. Cuba also made clear that it would help in any way that the people needed, that it would serve only as long as the Venezuelan government wanted its doctors to remain—and at no charge. Hugo Chávez, elected the previous year and a great admirer of the Cuban revolution, was impressed by the commitment of the Cuban medical contingent.

There are several key dates to bear in mind when assessing the evolution of Cuban medical cooperation in Venezuela, mainly revolving around a series of bilateral agreements, each building on the other as progress in the impact of public health services was noted, and each being more ambitious than the previous one. The election of Hugo Chávez in 1998 obviously signaled the beginning of a different era in both domestic politics and bilateral relations. Another important step to formalize ties came on October 30, 2000, when he and Fidel Castro signed the first broad Cuba-Venezuela Cooperation Agreement. Among other areas of cooperation, one major objective was to improve the healthcare system of Venezuela with the support of Cuban medical personnel. The agreement was quite specific in terms of the services that Cuba would provide. Its key significance was that the Venezuelan government now legalized the medical services being provided by Cuba at that time and opened the door for further avenues of cooperation. The FMV strenuously opposed this agreement.

There were four main areas of the planned medical cooperation. The first allowed for the transfer of Cuban medical personnel to areas where there were insufficient Venezuelan doctors, as well as the possibility of the Cubans training local people in basic public health education matters. The location of Cuban medical personnel was to be decided solely by the Venezuelan government, which insisted that the doctors would be sent where they were needed. The second component supported the training of Venezuelan doctors and nurses in Cuba (both in specialized areas and in general medicine). Medical technicians and nurses were also to be trained for missions in isolated areas where there were again insufficient medical services.

A broad area of medical treatment in Cuba was offered to Venezuelans as the third component. This ranged from check-ups and treatment for members of the Venezuelan oil industry to care for the Venezuelan population at large for a variety of medical conditions—addictions, orthopedic surgery, treatment for neurological conditions, skin disease, and transplant surgeries. This was significant in several areas: first, because it provided the services of Cuban specialists and allowed patients with insufficient funds to obtain medical care free of charge in Cuba; and second, because it fostered broader people-to-people contacts with Cuba, a process in which it helped to demystify the overwhelmingly negative portrayal of Cuba found in large sectors of the Venezuelan media. Eventually tens of thousands of Venezuelans, mainly from disadvantaged socioeconomic backgrounds, took advantage of this opportunity. In March 2014 the tenth flight of the year headed for Havana, taking patients with serious health conditions (ranging from heart disease to neurological conditions) to be treated there, and it was stated that some 60,000 Venezuelans had benefited from this bilateral agreement in Cuban hospitals to date.[2] The fourth area of the bilateral agreement allowed for the sale of Cuban medical products and equipment, ranging from diagnostic tools to vaccines. The agreement was signed for a five-year period and was renewed in 2005. It remains in effect to this day and has benefited millions of Venezuelans.

Another key development in this evolving medical accord came in 2004, when Operation Miracle was initiated, a process which resulted in tens of thousands of Venezuelans being flown to Cuba for ophthalmology surgery—again at no charge to the patients. In August 2005 the Sandino Commitment was signed (in the town of that name in western Cuba) by Chávez and Castro to broaden the original agreement, with the key promise of providing Cuba's widely recognized ophthalmology program to Venezuelans. This program revolved around a clear need for eye surgery to be provided for people of limited resources. Initially these services were for Venezuelans, but the program was soon increased to include patients from Latin America and the Caribbean. They involved mainly straightforward operations, but were still too costly for millions of people in Latin America and the Caribbean. The commitment made was to provide basic eye surgery to 6 million people throughout Latin America and the Caribbean within a decade, and as of early 2015 over 3 million have been operated on. In Venezuela this program was named Misión Milagro.

Finally, what is called the New Program of Training Latin American Doctors (later crystallizing in the Medicina Integral Comunitaria or MIC training program) also resulted from that agreement. Both countries committed themselves to the ambitious goal of pooling resources (largely Cuban human medical personnel and Venezuelan petrodollars) to train 60,000 physicians for the region in a program of practical medical care, also at no cost to the medical students. The training was to take place in Venezuela, with the teaching to be carried out mainly by Cuban medical professors and doctors. To date, more than 20,000 physicians have graduated from this innovative approach. Any one of these programs would have been a major breakthrough in terms of assisting the Venezuelan population—let alone the people of Latin America and the Caribbean. Together, though, they represented a major challenge for the Cuba-Venezuela partnership, two countries of just 11.2 and 22.9 million people, respectively. It also offered the possibility of improving the lives of millions throughout the region.

In the case of Venezuela, all of these programs were badly needed in a country with a 20,000 physician deficit in 2004, according to Héctor Navarro, the former minister of higher education.[3] Until Chávez was elected, however, none of these initiatives would have been possible. Indeed just the opposite had happened under previous governments. During the decade when policies of neoliberalism were applied by the predecessors of Chávez, resources had been reduced from public health facilities and programs, while private clinics had flourished. That changed dramatically under Chávez, most notably with the arrival of the Barrio Adentro program.

The major breakthrough in Cuban medical cooperation in Venezuela came in January 2003, when Freddy Bernal, the mayor of the Libertadores municipality in Caracas, sought to deliver a reform program of badly needed medical services to people living in marginalized and underserviced areas of the capital. It was to be called the Barrio Adentro Integral Plan for Caracas. He explained the pressing needs and appealed to Venezuelan doctors to participate. The idea was to have small consulting rooms in the *barrios* in which medical care would be provided for the local population, as well as a series of educational programs designed to promote healthy living and disease prevention. The response from the medical profession, however, was poor: only 50 doctors agreed to brave the poor living conditions of the slums and provide basic medical services. Some 30 left soon afterwards, refusing to live in the *barrio*, and the 20 who remained were assigned areas of medical specialization.[4] Transportation difficulties, personal safety, and a lack of understanding of conditions in the *barrio* were the principal causes for the doctors' reluctance to become involved. Frustrated by the Venezuelan doctors' lack of solidarity, the mayor of Caracas then approached Cuba. Would Havana be interested in sending family doctors to live in these underserved districts and provide assistance for people who had been overlooked by Venezuelan doctors? Their supportive role after the flooding in Vargas state was already well known, and with Hugo Chávez as the newly elected president, the time for extended cooperation seemed to have arrived.

In April 2003, 53 Cuban medical personnel, specializing in comprehensive family medicine, arrived in Caracas to help in a pilot project, and they were distributed in 10 of the districts of Libertador municipality. Each was responsible for the medical care of 222 families, and all lived in the community, in a spare room offered by one of the locals in the region where they were working. The arrangement was highly informal, and the only requirement of the family that took in the Cuban doctor was to provide a bed, wardrobe, fan, and access to a bathroom. In this initial stage there was no budget for food or rent, and the host family—supported by the community—agreed to provide food, accommodations, and protection for the Cuban doctor.

The small contingent of Cuban medical personnel proved to be extremely popular with the barrio inhabitants. For the first time people now had medical care close to their homes—and without any charge to them. Plans were soon made to formalize the program and to increase its size. Between April and June 2003, a further 303 Cuban medical personnel arrived, to be followed by another 686, who were sent to the state of Miranda in July and August. This process of adaptation went well, and between October and December a further 9,179 Cuban physicians were deployed throughout Venezuela. By the end of the year there were 10,169 Cuban medical personnel installed in Venezuela, of whom 52 percent were women.[5] The original group of just 53 medical personnel had thus been replaced by an army of thousands of Cuban doctors, nurses, and technicians. It would be further strengthened by the support of Venezuelan doctors trained in the Comprehensive Community Health program by Cuban physicians/tutors. In turn, this increasing Cuban presence in the *barrios* led to a major development of public health services (initially primary care assistance and ultimately in specialized hospitals).

The Impact of Barrio Adentro in 2003

Prior to the establishment of Barrio Adentro in underserved urban areas, Venezuelans faced a stark choice. When there was medical care available, they could pay exorbitant fees for private service, or wait long hours in a poorly staffed public hospital, often far from their homes. For many, particularly in impoverished rural areas, these options were simply not possible. Most doctors preferred to remain in comfortable and lucrative middle-class practices and were not interested in working in the *barrios*, where they were concerned about the lack of security and the difficult living conditions. Douglas León Natera, president of the Venezuelan Medical Federation (FMV), supported their position: "The government says that it cannot guarantee our safety. How are we then going to go into the hills where there are all kinds of marginalized people?"[6] The doctors were largely from upper-class backgrounds (and therefore with the funds to pay for their medical education) and had little understanding of difficult socioeconomic conditions found in the *barrios*. Attending to the needs of "all kinds of marginalized people" was generally not an attractive option to the doctors from middle- to upper-class backgrounds, keen for higher salaries and employment in private clinics. To a large extent this attitude was responsible for the Chávez government's decision to train a new breed of doctor—one who would come from a poorer socioeconomic background, would understand the needs of those traditionally underserved, and would make a commitment to change the delivery of healthcare, particularly for the marginalized.

In 2003 the dean of the medical school at the prestigious Central University of Venezuela in Caracas explained the mind-set of graduates of his faculty. His own students were not interested in following the Cubans into the *barrios* or the underserved rural areas. "Almost all of the new doctors," he noted, "want to live in Caracas and other big cities and engage in lucrative specialties, such as plastic surgery." The breakdown of what medical graduates did, and where they went after graduation, is worth noting. Between 1,200 and 1,500 doctors qualified annually in Venezuela. Of that number just over half went into private practice, and some 10 percent left to work abroad. In terms of the number of physicians working in the primary care or family medicine sectors—where the need was greatest—sadly there were only about 4,000 (approximately 10 percent of doctors in Venezuela). And this occurred at a time when 17 million people, out of a population of 24 million, did not have regular access to medical care.[7]

By contrast the Cuban medical personnel were generally from working-class origins and of various ethnic backgrounds. They were more pragmatic, having weathered back home the worst of the "Special Period" following the collapse of the Soviet Union. Many had also worked in other developing countries and were aware of the challenges of dealing with patients in poor living conditions, often unable to pay for medical services. Cuban physicians had also been socialized from daycare to believe in access to medical care (and at no cost to the patient) as a basic human right, and the need to cooperate with all, regardless of social position or race. Moreover, their hands-on training was extremely different from that received in Venezuela, relying less on complex technological equipment and spending more time with their patients to give an exhaustive physical examination, to visit them in their homes, and prepare a thorough clinical history. Unlike their counterparts, Cuban doctors often also live in the communities that they serve and have daily interactions with community members. They are full-time neighbors rather than professionals who parachute into the barrio for a few hours. Cuban training is based largely upon a preventive medical philosophy, uses popular education strategies to inform the population and involve them in order to improve their health, and is typified by a pragmatic, proactive approach.

After some initial skepticism (since Venezuelans in the underserved areas where the Cuban doctors were sent were not used to the idea of free medical care, much less having doctors visit them in their homes or live in the same communities), the population came to respect the role of the Cuban doctors. Two quotations from a 2006 report by the Pan American Health Organization illustrate the dramatic developments in the *barrios*. Prior to the arrival of the Cubans, people living there generally "distrusted the doctors who took care of them in the emergency rooms of the Caracas hospitals. Many others in the neighborhoods had never known a doctor who would go to someone's home." The views now commonly held were summed up by the comment of a nursing auxiliary from the same report: "How things have turned upside-down in this country! It used to be that those who had a bedside doctor were the rich people. The rich! Now we are the ones who have the good doctors, and they are not in it for the money.

We have dedicated doctors who are with us day in and day out, who feel with us, who live with us in poverty. That's what means so much to us."[8]

By 2005 some of the teething problems of the Barrio Adentro program had been resolved. There were then 8,573 medical stations (*consultorios populares*) established in which 14,345 Cuban doctors worked alongside 1,104 Venezuelan physicians. There were also 293 Cuban and 3,193 Venezuelan nurses. Each doctor was responsible for 250 families (approximately 1,500 people), which amounted to 70 percent of the local population. That year the government had also built 600 small consulting clinics, formalizing the rather loose organization that had existed until then with medical care being provided from people's living rooms. There were also 1,415 dental clinics that had been set up, in which 3,071 Cuban and 1,320 Venezuelan dentists operated. In addition 1,440 Cuban optometrists worked in 457 clinics. A large number of Cuban sports technicians (approximately 5,000) worked with their medical counterparts, promoting sports activities through the clinics and through various associations and clubs for young people, seniors, and pregnant women, as well as support groups for people with varying pathologies such as diabetes or heart conditions.[9] For the Cubans, keeping physically active was an integral part of maintaining good health—hence the involvement of the sports trainers to support the many community health initiatives.

Within just a year the arrival of some 11,000 Cuban family doctors (referred to in the Venezuelan media as "un ejército de batas blancas," or an army of white coats) changed the situation in underserved areas in a manner that was unimaginable for many. Poor Venezuelans could now receive healthcare service, in their own community, and at no charge. Moreover, the doctors lived in their communities, saw them on a frequent basis, and made house calls every day. Patients interviewed refer with surprise to this radical departure from the old system. By 2010 approximately 14,000 Cuban physicians, supported by 15,000 nurses, dentists, physical therapists, optometrists, and technicians, were providing medical care to Venezuelans at almost 7,000 doctors' offices and 500 larger diagnostic clinics.[10] In the early stages of Barrio Adentro, many of the doctors' offices were rather primitive—often just a spare room in somebody's house—while the physician usually slept in another room that nobody was using. The term *consultorio* was thus a rather grandiose term. Yet this army of white-coated Cubans living in spartan conditions provided free healthcare, as well as free medicines and respect. They lived in the barrio alongside the locals, ate the same food, went to the same stores, engaged socially with their neighbors, and were available for consultation on a 24-hour basis. Not surprisingly, after overcoming initial concerns about "communist doctors" coming to brainwash them, Venezuelan residents in the barrios were soon welcoming them warmly.

By 2006 it was obvious that the Barrio Adentro system (a phrase allegedly coined by Chávez) had been extremely successful. In fact, in many ways it was too successful, requiring Cuban and Venezuelan community health planners to revise the approach being used and decide how to support the vastly increased numbers of patients who now sought medical care. As noted, the first stage of this program consisted of a series of community health clinics manned by Cuban family doctors who specialized in basic primary healthcare. While successful, the system was rapidly being overwhelmed by patients whose more complex pathologies could not be treated adequately by family doctors. The end result was the formation of Barrio Adentro II, which included the construction of hundreds of more specialized institutions—Comprehensive Diagnostic Centers (Centros de Diagnóstico Integral, or CDI), Comprehensive Rehabilitation Centers (Salas de Rehabilitación Integral, or SRI), and Advanced Technology Centers (Centros de Alta Tecnología, or CAT), in which Cuban and Venezuelan doctors worked side by side.[11] The objective was to provide more specialized care, as well as to use more sophisticated technology, to assist primary healthcare physicians in their diagnosis.

While most medical conditions can be diagnosed by a detailed physical examination in a doctor's office, it is also important to use technology to support findings, employing equipment such as X-ray, ECGs, and laboratories. Until Barrio Adentro II, that had been extremely difficult, since the one-room *consultorios* in people's homes were clearly not equipped for that purpose, and those services were available mainly at private facilities. Given the need for such services, the Venezuelan government now built the CDIs, where a variety of diagnostic tools were located, in many ways based on the role of polyclinics found in Cuba. They provided 24-hour emergency and diagnostic services, clinical laboratories, intensive therapy, endoscopy, ultrasound, electrocardiogram facilities, an ophthalmology clinic, and even a section for making plaster casts. Patients now came to the CDIs in an emergency or following a referral from their family physician. There were also a small number of emergency beds for intensive care patients, as well as offices for doctors.

Comprehensive Rehabilitation Centers were instituted to assist with a variety of therapies for patients following medical treatment. "Rehabilitation" was provided in a number of modalities. The most common pathologies were treated—through occupational therapy, electrotherapy, physiotherapy, and hydrotherapy—and treatment for stroke and accidents, fractures, and herniated discs was provided. But the SRIs expanded the term to include rehabilitation in speech and hearing therapy, optometry, podology, bursitis, treatment for burns, and also a clinic for natural medicine.[12] Barrio Adentro I was maintained (albeit in increasingly improved, stand-alone clinics), but it was now increasingly supported by more sophisticated equipment in the CDIs and SRIs. For their part, the CATs provided treatment for specialized conditions needing extremely sophisticated diagnostic equipment such as nuclear magnetic resonance, computerized axial tomography, noninvasive tridimensional ultrasound, mammography, electrocardiography, and the like. These were reference hospitals for patients who needed more specialized treatment than the CDIs could provide.

The increase in medical facilities was rapid. In 2013 the Pan American Health Organization released a report to document the evolution of healthcare from 2006 to 2010, and their data coincided largely with those provided by the government. Among their findings were data on the number of primary care clinics that had increased by 153 percent (from 1,433 in 2006 to 3,630 in 2009). Similarly the number of outpatient care centers in the neighborhood clinics (Misión Barrio Adentro II) had increased 90 percent (from 529 to 1,006). Moreover, "477 new centers were built and equipped, bringing the number of comprehensive diagnostic centers to 466, comprehensive rehabilitation centers to 509, and advanced technology centers to 31."[13] In addition, 5,916 locations had joined the National Vaccination Program, providing free vaccinations to Venezuelans as the drive to emphasize a preventive medicine approach developed. Primary healthcare was increasingly delivered by Venezuelan physicians, either trained by Cuban medical school professors in Venezuela or at ELAM, and it is the Cubans who run the academic program in Comprehensive Community Medicine program. To date, some 20,000 doctors trained in Venezuela have graduated from this program.

Perhaps one of the most important pieces of information to gauge how successful the Chávez approach to public healthcare services was came in the 2008 Household Survey. When asked about the medical services provided by Barrio Adentro, 93.5 percent expressed their satisfaction. This was not at all surprising in light of the extent of the growth in accessibility of healthcare services for the marginalized sectors. The arrival of the Cubans participating in this program in 2003 had an immediate impact on the population, many of whom had never seen a doctor before—much less had one visit them at home. A summary of the work of the Cubans during just one week in 2005 is helpful in appreciating this new reality for many.

Between April 10 and 16 Cuban medical personnel performed 1,513,475 medical consults. Of these, 556,616 were home visits. There were 382,785 nursing consults, and 18 births were attended. Since a large part of the Cuban mandate was to promote health education, a total of 915,641 Venezuelans attended educational activities. This analysis of a week's work of the Cuban medical mission provides a window into their activities. This microcosm of the work carried out on a weekly basis is reflected in the data for the entire year: 20,760,019 medical consults, as well as 7,743,539 nursing consults and 278 births.[14]

* * *

Clearly Barrio Adentro is the major structure on which the national healthcare policy of Venezuela is based. It is the focal point of primary healthcare for the majority of Venezuelans, accessible to all. While there are still many private clinics, mainly in larger cities, the vast majority of the population receives medical care from the Barrio Adentro system, including many people opposed to the ideas of the socialist government. The initial primary care facilities still exist, and while they are mainly manned by Cuban physicians, increasingly they are supported by Venezuelan graduates trained by Cuban medical professors. (From the first year of their training, medical students in Venezuela engage in practicums held at the clinics with patients, preparing them for the days when they will be in charge. The students are supervised by Cuban physicians, who often double as professors.) And, just as the first stage of Barrio Adentro evolved into one in which hundreds of rehabilitation centers and polyclinics (the comprehensive diagnostic centers) were established, so too stages III and IV have also developed within the national system of hospitals and specialized treatment centers.

Barrio Adentro III seeks to modernize and integrate some 300 hospitals in Venezuela, to improve the quality of the equipment, and to introduce advanced training for the staff, while Barrio Adentro IV has concentrated on building new specialized reference hospitals, each focusing on areas such as cardiology, ophthalmology, neuropsychiatry, gastroenterology, infectious diseases, nephrology, urology, endocrinology, and plastic surgery.

This process has evolved rapidly since the first contingent of Cuban family doctors arrived in Libertadores municipality in 2003, and Cuban medical personnel are heavily involved in each of these facets of the program.

A common complaint heard by those opposed to Chávez and his healthcare policies is that he is "turning the country over to the Cubans," and that Venezuelan doctors have little say in the direction of public health. It is argued that he (and his successor, Nicolás Maduro) paid too much for Cuban medical support, blinded by their personal respect for the historic Cuban leadership and fundamental political convictions. In addition, Venezuelan medical associations criticize the nature of instruction given to students under the Medicina Integral Comunitaria curriculum. The tens of thousands of doctors being trained by Cuban medical professors, opponents note, are poorly equipped for work in Venezuela (although they are being trained in the *barrios*, in a rigorous hands-on approach, and being taught in an extremely practical fashion how to provide badly needed primary healthcare). The same opponents from traditional medical associations claim that the Cubans are taking employment away from Venezuelan doctors, forgetting that most of the underemployed doctors refused to work in Barrio Adentro or in the impoverished rural areas where their salaries would be significantly lower.

Typical in many ways are the opinions expressed by Douglas León Natera, president of the FMV and an outspoken opponent of the Venezuelan government. In a 2009 interview with the BBC he condemned the situation of public health there: "What they have done in the past ten years is to destroy the hospitals, abuse doctors, and leave hospitals half-empty. . . . They now have a health system with some Cubans who are not really doctors and are here practicing medicine with the support of Chávez."[15] In such a polarized situation between those who support the Chávez government model and its opponents, and specifically the official medical establishment, there was little middle ground. Four years later, Dr. Pedro Martínez Latuff maintained a similar position, although his claims were more extreme. He claimed that the healthcare situation was the worst that it had been in decades. ("Before the election of Hugo Chávez, Venezuela had a healthcare system that worked. . . . But now all of that has disappeared. Malaria, yellow fever and enteritis have all increased. It is as if they had obliterated with the stroke of a pen all the medical advances developed over several decades.") He criticized the quality of the Cuban doctors ("I have to say that the Cuban doctors work with a great lack of professionalism and with antiquated methods. They are also responsible for bringing cholera to

Venezuela.") The Cuban influence in the Venezuelan health system was "a complete disaster and the start of all our problems in Venezuela. Many of them are not real professionals and have not been properly trained."[16] The same article also mentioned that 7,000 doctors had emigrated in the past decade, when they could have found work in Venezuela.

What has been forgotten in their criticisms is that Venezuelan doctors, nurses, and technicians are increasingly assuming the roles previously held by Cubans. By 2010, for instance, many Venezuelans worked alongside their Cuban counterparts in this program: 1,426 physicians, 2,095 dentists, and 2,495 nurses.[17] There has indeed been a notable increase in the participation of Venezuelan medical personnel since the early days when Cuban doctors were the backbone of Barrio Adentro I. In 2004, for instance, there were 81 Venezuelan doctors involved in the program, compared with 10,867 Cuban physicians and 675 dentists.[18] A comparison between 2004 and 2010, with data above, shows how quickly the Venezuelan participation has grown and continues to grow. The former head of the Cuban medical mission, Dr. Joaquín García, has emphasized that Cuban medical personnel work in Venezuela at the pleasure of the government ("until President Chávez decides otherwise"). He expected the numbers of Cuban staff to decrease as Venezuelans took a leading role. This was, he concluded "a genuine Venezuelan project, where the Cubans participate, and not the reverse."[19] With the large graduation classes in the MIC program, the process of Venezuelans assuming control of the system appears assured. Moreover, as the potential for employment and the need for medical care grew in Brazil under the Rousseff government, Cuban personnel began to transfer from Venezuela to Brazil. From personal correspondence with Cuban physicians who had been working in Venezuela, it is clear that many have left to return home or have undertaken similar work in the "Mais Médicos" program in Brazil.

Misión Milagro

There is a great deal of misunderstanding about the role of Cuban medical cooperation, often compounded by self-interest and clouded by ideology. Typical in many ways is an article written by several ophthalmologists who condemned the Cuban-Venezuelan approach to eye surgery. They quote Venezuelan specialists and raise several queries: "Visiting Cuban doctors are usually not well accepted by medical societies nor by local citizens. In Venezuela, where a general health program began under the name Misión

Barrio Adentro, with the declared purpose of providing primary healthcare to the poorest Venezuelans, doctors report that the entry of Cuban doctors weakened their health system and created tension between foreign and local physicians." This is a frustrating experience, they continue, "leaving the local population at risk, but with no possibility of holding the visitors accountable, and perhaps fueling a perceived high level of postoperative complications that must usually be handled by local ophthalmologists."[20]

This is a rather shallow interpretation since, while local medical societies do indeed not welcome the Cuban specialists (who do not charge for their services, thereby representing serious competition), popular acceptance of Cuban personnel has been extremely high. Likewise it is disingenuous to claim that the healthcare system has been "weakened" when the large increase in facilities, new doctors, and accessibility of medical services is clear and when data on an improved health profile prove the opposite. The Cuban doctors live in the community, and any post-operative difficulties can be handled by Cuban ophthalmologists. The doctors quoted above end by calling for the Cubans to assist local ophthalmologists: "The best way to combat blindness is through development of integrated and self-sustainable eye care services at the local and national levels, by improving the local ophthalmological services that will still be there to serve the people when the visitors go home. None of these things are being done by *Misión Milagro.*" But that is exactly what the Cuban approach is doing, training Venezuelan specialists to replace them, and this is indeed happening, with the graduation of 60,000 physicians (mainly trained by Cuban medical professors) expected by 2019. They will be running the medical system "when the visitors go home."

One of the key elements of the Cuban medical role in Venezuela is the commitment to the sustainable nature of the public healthcare system there. This is seen most clearly in the successful section on training thousands of doctors in Venezuela in the Medicina Integral Comunitaria program, but it can also be seen in the approach to ophthalmology surgery, originally called Operación Milagro in Cuba and subsequently Misión Milagro in Venezuela. The Venezuelan program began in 2004 when patients were selected for surgery and flown to Cuba. According to the Venezuelan embassy in the United Kingdom, 204,000 Venezuelans received surgery there.[21] They, and a close family member to accompany them, were flown to Cuba where they underwent medical tests to ensure their suitability for surgery. They usually remained about a week in Cuba, staying at a hotel following surgery and received close follow-up care. There was no charge to them or their accompanying family member for any aspect of the week, with transportation, accommodation, meals, medical treatment, and drugs provided in Cuba.

The first stage of the program involved all surgery for Venezuelan patients—including ophthalmology cases—being carried out in Cuba, and the most complex cases are still referred there. Yet Venezuela has come into its own as a center for ophthalmology surgery and as of October 2005 started to treat its patients at home. By May 2010 Misión Milagro had already carried out 1,119,215 operations in Venezuela (using Cuban and Venezuelan medical personnel). Of these patients, 85 percent were Venezuelan, with the remainder coming from various countries in Latin America and the Caribbean.[22] Soon 5,000 patients were being operated on every week—in some 30 hospitals in 15 states in Venezuela. To put this in the proper context, this weekly average was roughly the same number of patients operated on in Venezuela on an annual basis before the program was initiated, according to Manuel Pacheco, the national coordinator.[23] This gives some idea of the rapid development of this program and the significance of its outreach. As is the case with Operación Milagro clinics throughout Latin America (Cuba currently has 69 ophthalmology clinics in 15 countries), the most common conditions treated were cataracts, pterygium, and strabismus.[24]

A fundamental goal of this program—as practiced both in Venezuela and Cuba and in the many countries where Cuban medical staff work—is to provide surgery for people of the Americas as a whole, especially those who cannot afford it. As a result, while approximately 90 percent of cases treated in Venezuela are national citizens, 10 percent are from other countries in Latin America. Pacheco noted that, between 2005 and 2012, more than 33,000 patients from Latin America had been treated at no charge in Venezuela, with the largest contingents coming from El Salvador, Nicaragua, Honduras, Guatemala, Costa Rica, Paraguay, Colombia, Brazil, Peru, and Argentina. By May 31, 2013, it was estimated that combined Cuban and Venezuelan efforts had restored sight to 2.5 million people in Latin America, the Caribbean, and Africa—people from 34 countries.[25] By early 2015, this had increased to over 3 million. In reviewing Latin American newspapers and media websites, it is fascinating to see the number of articles written about locals heading to Cuba or Venezuela for treatment or being treated by Cuban physicians in their own country.[26] Participants arriving in Venezuela for eye surgery often were handed T-shirts and caps that indicated they were participants in Misión Milagro. Fittingly, the slogan embroidered on the caps summed up the goal of the operation: "a people leaving darkness behind."

Misión Milagro has been an extremely successful program. Undoubtedly it will continue to be a government priority, and in May 2013, Nicolás Maduro announced that out of respect for the recently deceased Hugo Chávez, his eldest daughter, Rosa Virginia, would assume the presidency of the Misión Milagro Foundation. The following month, shortly after his election as president, Maduro met with Pope Francis in the Vatican. The president sees it as an important tool to help marginalized people throughout the world who lack in dignity because of a simple medical condition—one that can often be repaired within 15 minutes. In his audience with the pope he extolled the virtues of Misión Milagro, noting that over 2 million Latin Americans had benefited from this program since its inception. A modernization of Misión Milagro (updated equipment, fresh education programs on the prevention of eye injuries, workshops to produce glasses and lenses, and specialized training for ophthalmologists) was launched in May 2013 in order to make it even more effective.

Training Doctors: A Radically New Approach

Arguably the most important contribution by Cuba to the development of a sustainable healthcare system in Venezuela is their role in developing a new type of physician there—a revolutionary doctor. In 2005 Cuban physicians started to train Venezuelan students. For the Chávez government, the need to train a new breed of doctors who would go where they were needed, rather than remain working in middle-class suburbs of Caracas, was essential. Hundreds of Venezuelan doctors were being trained at ELAM in Havana, but far more were needed. It was time to develop a new approach to medical training. Speaking in 2008, Dr. Yiliam Jiménez, then deputy minister of foreign affairs and in charge of Cuba's medical cooperation programs, explained the new model to be used in both Venezuela and some parts of Cuba. The objective was to train more doctors than ever and to do so using a new approach: "Traditional models of medical training cannot resolve the terrible lack of health professionals and the urgent need for access to healthcare in today's world. . . . We are returning to the tutorial method supplemented by information technologies and other teaching aids, so that students from low-income families can be educated in classrooms and clinics in their own communities, where their services are sorely needed."[27]

The Venezuelan Medical Federation and its outspoken leadership have consistently criticized the Cuban medical personnel working there. They point to the thousands of unemployed or underemployed Venezuelan doctors and demand that the government find them positions and pay them better. In September 2013, the president of the FMV condemned a 75 percent increase in the salaries for doctors as being "insufficient."[28] The FMV reserves its worst criticisms, though, for the new generation of medical doctors being trained in Medicina Integral Comunitaria.

This Comprehensive Community Medicine program is an innovative six-year course in medicine unlike anything found elsewhere, other than Cuba, Gambia, Guinea Bissau, and Timor-Leste, where it is taught by Cuban professors.[29] It was founded in 2005 through an agreement between Hugo Chávez and Fidel Castro to train physicians in Venezuela, using the services of Cuban doctors and medical professors. Initially it was designed so that Cuban doctors working in the Barrio Adentro program could train young Venezuelans who otherwise could not afford to attend the traditional medical schools in the country. It was hoped that the new graduates would be able to participate actively in the new national public healthcare system that Chávez had initiated, eventually replacing the Cuban doctors. Students in the MIC program are largely from poorer socioeconomic backgrounds and are of a variety of ethnic origins, and ages.

The government's hope is that they will bring a totally new approach to community medicine, working where they are needed rather than where they would be paid the most. While it maintains much of the rigorous approach found in Havana's Latin American School of Medicine (ELAM) studied elsewhere, the MIC program has distinctly Venezuelan components. It is a pragmatic, hands-on approach that obliges students to see patients from the first year of the program, accompanying Cuban doctors of Barrio Adentro for part of the day, while during the rest they meet with MIC professors (mainly, but not exclusively, Cuban) in classes. (Premedical students are also involved in meeting with patients, as a way of preparing them for the actual medical degree program.) The daily practical sessions are particularly important, since they allow the students to understand better the challenges of life in the *barrio*, while observing and cooperating with the Cuban physicians. This teaching model took over from the education provided to Venezuelan medical students in Havana and is designed to train enough medical staff so that their Cuban counterparts can eventually leave. The goal of MIC is simple: "to integrate the training of family practitioners into the fabric of communities in a holistic effort that meets the medical needs of all citizens, making use of local resources, and promotes preventive healthcare and healthy living."[30]

It is important to emphasize the role and the character of the Cuban *internacionalistas*. From my own experience shadowing them in the field, and following interviews with medical personnel who have served abroad, it is clear that the Cuban physicians *are* different. The manner in which they treat their patients, taking the time to prepare a full clinical history, as well as the austere conditions in which they live, their humility, their human warmth and respect for patients from all walks of life, the way in which they speak with patients, their energetic and compassionate approach to medicine, the rigors of their training are all very different from those of their counterparts in other countries. As role models to people from non-traditional backgrounds who are studying medicine, they are a natural fit, and their influence as tutors for the first four years of the MIC program is enormously significant. In their third year students have two courses, Clínica III and Clínica IV, with two and three days of hospital practice per week, respectively, and in the last two years of their program they start hospital rotations. Moreover, as the Cuban mentors' own experience shows, the Venezuelan students have to be doctors for humanity and to go where the need is greatest.

The MIC model closely resembles the teaching curriculum in Cuban medical faculties. Much emphasis is placed on the need for a preventive approach to public health, and while curative skills are also taught, it is shown that these are to be subordinated to the need to prevent medical pathologies in the first place. This is, of course, a far more economical approach to public health, since it does not rely on expensive drugs made by multinational drug companies. Also important is the need for public education and for participation by all who live in the *barrio*. Campaigns are led in the communities by medical personnel to illustrate healthy living styles and to point out common health hazards. The essentially pragmatic approach of the MIC curriculum is also of great importance, since from the first year medical students are in direct contact with patients—in the *barrio*. They see their living conditions and are made aware of the need for hands-on solutions to the challenges faced by their patients. One recent graduate of the MIC program explained the significance of this, since it emphasizes the differences between them and graduates of the traditional programs: "The humanist element is what differentiates us most. We are in direct contact with the community from the first year of our degree, which doesn't happen in the traditional universities. It is during the fifth or final year of their degree when they do their three-month rural residency that they have contact with a community. . . . We do the house-to-house visits, the neighborhood surveys, and we are directly connected to the life of the patient and their family because we see the patient as a holistic being. Thus we don't only focus on the person's state of health but also their lifestyle, in such a way as to improve their standard of living and that of their family too."[31]

The Cuban doctors/professors emphasize the need for a holistic approach to the study of medicine and seek to overcome the traditional silo approach in which subjects are taught in isolation. By contrast, in the MIC an interdisciplinary strategy is followed, allowing students to see the connected nature of pathologies and socioeconomic conditions. Perhaps the most important aspect of the medical training, though, is the development of *conciencia* and commitment to their patients. The students see the approach of the Cuban preceptors in dealing with their patients, observe their living conditions, and learn from their value system. The objective is "to create doctors with values different from those of the market-driven model of healthcare prevalent in the United States and the wealthier echelons of Venezuelan society. Community doctors are expected to be both rigorously trained and socially conscious; committed to public healthcare and focused on the needs of their patients and communities rather than seeking lucrative careers in private clinics."[32]

This approach has been largely successful. Under Cuban guidance (and very much reflecting the value system found in Cuba), the traditional view of the medical profession has changed dramatically. No longer do physicians trained under MIC view their profession as a means of making money. Rather, they are socialized to see themselves as people fulfilling a duty to their nation and to their patients. This sense of duty, of fulfilling a social need, of not forgetting either their roots or their obligations to people just like themselves, is extremely important. Since they are trained—again following the Cuban model—to see their patients as bio-psycho-social human beings (and not as fee-paying clients), and since they understand the environment in which these patients live, they are far better equipped to assist them. For them the pathologies of their patients are the result of a far larger picture, involving their psychological well-being, their socioeconomic background, their surrounding environment, and the resulting medical condition that has brought them to the *consultorio* in the first place. This new breed of doctor, imbued with *conciencia* and willing to work day and night in the *barrio*, represents a major challenge for the traditional model of medical training, as well as the standard role of doctors. They are fully aware of the traditional difficulties faced in underserved communities, and they have been trained to ensure that public health has to be accessible to all. They constitute a dangerous example of a new breed of Cuban-trained doctor, now found in dozens of developing countries, and it is no surprise that the traditional medical federations are fearful of this model of healthcare.

The public healthcare system in Venezuela, greatly supported by Cuba, has changed dramatically since the first agreement signed by the two presidents. The traditional doctors, members of an élite who had controlled the medical system, have seen their authority gradually decrease as Cuban specialists have assumed a greater role and—more important—as Venezuelan students have increasingly become key members in the system. No longer on the social periphery because of their lack of resources, there is a large new group of doctors pressing ahead with a different agenda. A recent graduate has explained this shift well: "It also has to do with how medicine works in Venezuela, and how it used to work when it was completely commercialized. That is, every medical exam, laboratory exam, X-rays, everything, absolutely everything, had to be paid for. And with the arrival of the new revolutionary socialist government . . . this changed. It can be said that medicine in Venezuela changed completely. It spun 360 degrees."[33] Needless to say, the FMV and political opposition are displeased.[34]

The reaction of the FMV to both the role of Cuban physicians and to the MIC approach is similar to that of medical associations throughout Latin America where these approaches are used. In Honduras, Bolivia, and most recently Brazil, there have been demonstrations against what the head of the FMV called a revolutionary approach that was merely "dispensing ideology."[35] Daniel Sánchez, president of the Medical Society of Vargas Hospital, likewise condemned the Cuban medical presence: "The health policy implemented by this government has resulted in failure, because it consists of the creation of a parallel system with foreign personnel of doubtful reputation."[36] The National Academy of Medicine joined the fray, claiming (falsely) that doctors were only trained for three years, and casting aspersions on their ability to practice as doctors. In fact, the medical training is for six years, with the MIC program demanding significantly more class and practicum hours (14,084 vs. 8,500) than those found in the traditional medical school system. The difference between the two approaches was summarized by Antonio Torres, national coordinator of the MIC: "In traditional medicine . . . what is important is specialization, managing to get one's own private clinic . . . whereas the humanist and community vision of medicine prioritizes primary attention. . . . That isn't a small thing. It's at the first level where 85 percent of health problems are intercepted."[37]

In Venezuela, the traditional approach to medicine is gradually being overtaken by the MIC and ELAM-trained physicians. An American doctor who lived in western Venezuela in 2007 and 2008 has put this in perspective in the Venezuelan case. He quotes Chávez, noting that the current enrollment in the medical training program was almost 25,000, and concludes: "With more students enrolled in 2009 and 2010, it appeared that even with some attrition among the newcomers, there would be 30,000 students graduating with MIC degrees between 2012 and 2017."[38] This was almost as many doctors practicing medicine when Chávez was elected president in 1998. In April 2013 President Nicolás Maduro committed to his government training a total of 60,000 community doctors by 2019. In March 2014 he noted that 18,000 Venezuelans had graduated as doctors, with a further 20,000 pursuing medical studies, while the goal of graduating 60,000 graduates remained their target.[39] As in other facets of the sweeping reform in public health programs, Cuban medical personnel have played a crucial role, particularly since they are training a new cadre of tens of thousands of doctors who will gradually replace them.

While the leaders of the Venezuelan Medical Federation disapprove, the fact is that the delivery of medical care in the country has been irretrievably changed, in terms of numbers of MIC doctors and with regard to the kind of medicine being practiced. (Hugo Chávez once emphasized that he wanted community doctors to be "doctors of socialism," a request that must have infuriated the traditionalists among the Venezuelan Federation of Medicine leadership.) In December 2011 the first cohort of MIC physicians graduated (8,160), and 6,200 graduated in December 2012. They are now working in a two-year mandatory residency program in public hospitals and clinics. This wave of MIC-trained doctors has changed the delivery of medical care in Venezuela and will do so while Maduro remains in power. This is unsettling for the élite in the Venezuelan Federation of Medicine who have maintained control of healthcare delivery and now see their influence threatened: "To Venezuela's traditional medical sector, the influx of thousands of Cuban-trained doctors from low-income backgrounds, who are now working in public hospitals directly alongside doctors from the traditional sector, is at once a political and class affront."[40]

Cuba has made a major and lasting contribution in training tens of thousands of Venezuelan doctors, both in Cuba and in Venezuela. These new medical graduates are taking up roles in community medicine throughout the country, mainly where there are underserved communities. In addition, as of 2014 a new three-year postgraduate program, mainly taught by Cuban medical professors, was introduced to train specialists in Comprehensive General Medicine, and eventually between 6,000 and 7,000 of the MIC graduates will become specialists. The objective is to strengthen the public healthcare system with a large number of medical consultants, imbued with the values resulting from their MIC training. Indeed, as one Cuban physician noted, a very different approach to public healthcare is becoming firmly established in Venezuela: "What is even more satisfying for us to see is the creation of moral and ethical values that allow them to really influence their communities."[41]

Looking Back on Bilateral Medical Cooperation

So what has been the impact of this medical cooperation agreement signed by the two former presidents in October 2000? Speaking in April 2013 in Havana, in an emotional ceremony in which the shadow of the recently deceased Hugo Chávez loomed large, incoming president Nicolás Maduro thanked Cuba for its ongoing support in community sports activities (Barrio Adentro Deportivo), a literacy program (Misión Robinson I, in which 1,756,271 people had learned to read and write), and ongoing medical support—both in providing medical professionals and in helping to train 14,000 Venezuelan physicians. The goal of training 60,000 doctors by 2019, again with support of Cuban medical professors, remained on track. He also mentioned the reforms in medical facilities, largely staffed by Cuban medical personnel, although increasingly being joined by Venezuelan medical graduates. In all 6,712 local doctors' offices had been established through Barrio Adentro, as well as 651 Integral Diagnostic Centers (or CDIs), 583 Rehabilitation and Physiotherapy Centers (SRI), and 35 specialized High Technology Centers (CAT).[42] The number of doctors who had graduated in the MIC program was staggering: 8,160 in December 2011 and 6,200 a year later. Significantly there is a high proportion of women graduates—77 percent of graduates in 2012.[43] In November 2013 Vice President Jorge Arreaza emphasized the enormous medical support of Cuba: 1.9 million Venezuelans had received eye surgery at the hands of Cuban ophthalmologists, and almost 337,000 with disabilities had also benefited from Cuba's support. More than 700,000 lives had been saved as a result of Cuban medical cooperation.[44]

In March 2014 Maduro provided data on the number of patients treated by Cuban medical personnel, noting how 80 percent of the 647 million medical consultations that had taken place in the previous 11 years had been carried out by Cubans. He emphasized the "incalculable support that Cuba provides to Venezuela in the care of the population's health."[45] In addition 204,736 Venezuelan patients had received eye surgery in Cuba, at no charge to the patient. The future for accessible healthcare looked promising, since the ratio of doctors to patients had increased from 20 per 100,000 persons in 1999 to 80 in 2014.[46] None of this would have been possible without the strategic vision of Chávez and Fidel Castro, the profits from Venezuela's vast petroleum and gas resources, and Cuban experience in public health.

There is no doubt that Venezuelans have benefited extensively from Cuban medical support. Cuban medical personnel in Venezuela—as in any other country where they are employed—go where they are needed and where the local government instructs them. They do not choose the locations to practice medicine, nor do they impose their approach upon local physicians or members of the community. At all times they are the servants of the government and of the local population, as Venezuelan vice president Elías Jaua has made clear: "The dignified Cuban doctor can be found in the most distant locations, in the poorest districts. They take with them the medical attention, free medical attention, to people who were always excluded from receiving any healthcare."[47]

In October 2012 Venezuelan minister of health Eugenia Sader noted that 53,407 Venezuelan patients with chronic, complex health problems had been treated in Cuba.[48] These people, mainly of limited financial resources, would otherwise never have received medical care. In terms of the national health scene, the results of these bilateral health initiatives are also very clear. The infant mortality rate, for instance, decreased from 25 per 1,000 live births (1990) to 13 (2010). Misión Milagro has also been extremely beneficial, with tens of thousands of Venezuelans having been treated in Cuba and over a million back in their homeland at the hands of Cuban and Venezuelan specialists. The almost 40,000 fellow Latin Americans who have also received the gift of their sight back also bear eloquent witness to this success.

In Venezuela the population is still divided between those who supported Chávez passionately and those who hated him viscerally. One common theme in the opposition press is that the government in Caracas has been exploited by Cuba and that Chávez had fallen prey to that wily fox, Fidel Castro. Speaking in April 2010 Chávez responded with conviction to those charges: "What Cuba has given us is priceless. . . . If we start to add up, cent by cent, Cuba's contribution, it is clear that this is worth ten times the value of the petroleum that we have sold to Cuba." He continued, setting the scene to illustrate Cuba's massive medical support and posing a rhetorical question: "If a country has to contract the services of 30,000 medics from the United States or Europe to work in the *barrios* and the poorest towns, and live with the native population. . . . And in addition build the medical facilities, bring the equipment for the medical laboratories and operating theaters, and provide the medicines. . . . How much would a capitalist country charge us to bring that size of an army of doctors and that sea of medicines for our people, and be on call 24 hours a day?"[49]

In October 2013 I interviewed Dr. Jorge Delgado, deputy director of the Unidad Central de Cooperación Cubana, or UCCM, the large center in Havana which administers the functions and duties of all of Cuba's *internacionalistas*. This is where Cuban medical personnel undergo orientation and general preparation before setting out on a medical mission abroad. In the building there is a large room with a huge mural on which the data for various missions are kept. On the day that I visited, one of the functionaries was adding new data on the table to bring it up to date, a process which occurs with some frequency. One of the groupings—the only one devoted to a specific country—is for the "Special Program in Venezuela." The numbers provided illustrate clearly why there is so much attention paid to Venezuela at the UCCM. In total, as of mid-October 2013, there were 32,514 Cuban medical personnel working in the country, and 11,416 were doctors. Since Cuban physicians had first arrived in Venezuela in 1999, the number of patients who had benefited was 863,501,538 (presumably the number of patient visits). In addition there had been 1,720,734 surgeries performed and 73,800 births attended by Cuban medical staff. A total of 1,746,417 lives had been saved, a figure which refers to the number of patients, based on previous data, who would normally have died if medical care had not been provided.[50] Speaking in 2010 President Chávez summed up the significance of Cuba's medical role in Venezuela: "There is no such humanitarian operation of this size that has ever been recorded."[51]

It is worth emphasizing the shared vision of Cuban-Venezuelan medical cooperation that Hugo Chávez and Fidel Castro had when they first thought about pooling resources. The beneficiaries of their cooperation were to be the poor of the region, those who could not afford to go to see a family doctor, much less afford expensive surgery. In a moving article, Spanish journalist Pascual Serrano recounts his visit aboard a plane from Caracas to Havana that was full of Misión Milagro patients heading to Cuba for surgery. The passengers were almost entirely peasants, unable to pay the amounts needed for surgery in a private hospital in Venezuela, and the flight was unlike any he had taken before: "This is different from your normal international flight. . . . Here there are no ties, no briefcases or cell phones, no bags of goods purchased at airport stores. The only passengers are people who never left their provinces, much less flew on a plane. Nobody ever took any interest in their basic health problems—much less chartered a plane to restore their sight."[52] The two former leaders would undoubtedly be pleased to see who was sitting in those plane seats.[53]

8

Cuba's Role in Haiti

Hurricanes, an Earthquake, and Cholera

First [in importance] is God, and then the Cuban doctors.

Haitian president René Préval

It is often mistakenly thought that Cuba first provided medical support for Haiti at the time of the massive earthquake of January 12, 2010, which leveled the capital, killing 230,000 people. In fact, Cuba has been providing medical support to the Haitian people for many years. Large-scale Cuban assistance began in 1998, and more than 6,000 Cuban medical personnel have worked in Haiti while over 1,000 Haitians from poor backgrounds have been trained as physicians in Cuba at no charge to the students.[1] This chapter examines the evolving role of Cuban medical cooperation in Haiti, both in terms of emergency medical assistance—most clearly seen in natural disasters and in the 2011 cholera outbreak—and its contributions to sustainable public health in the poorest country in the Western Hemisphere.

1998: The Origins of Cuba's Medical Cooperation

Haiti has been plagued by natural disasters. In 1946 a tsunami killed 1,790 people, and hurricanes struck in 1954, 1963, 1994, and 1998. Floods killed 2,600 in 2004, and tropical storm Jeanne killed 1,900 more that same year. Tropical storm Noel triggered major mudslides and floods in 2007, and three hurricanes and a major tropical storm killed 800 Haitians in 2008. In September 1998, Hurricane Georges roared through the country, killing 230 people and destroying 80 percent of crops. More than 167,000 people were left homeless, and massive flooding resulted in unsanitary conditions throughout the country. In November of that year, an agreement was signed during the visit of Haitian president René Préval to Havana, the first accord since the breaking of diplomatic relations 36 years earlier. While the broad agreement called for Cuban support in education, agriculture, tourism, and sports, the most important component was for the provision of medical cooperation. This involved 200 doctors being sent to work in Haiti and for 100 Haitian medical graduates to obtain specialized training in Cuba.[2] On December 4, Cuba sent an emergency brigade to help the victims of Hurricane Georges, and in the following weeks 388 more emergency specialists arrived. Cuba adopted a dual approach to the disastrous public health situation in Haiti. First, they maintained a medical presence of between 300 and 500 personnel in the country for as long as they were needed, and second, they agreed to train hundreds of Haitians in Cuba as doctors, so that they could help their own people. The concept was to gradually withdraw Cuban medical staff as they were replaced by Haitians. That process has continued since 1998, and indeed at the time of the January 2010 earthquake there were 344 Cuban medical staff in Haiti as well as several hundred Haitian physicians trained in Cuba.

The training of Haitians sought to develop a sustainable public health system. Cuba made the same offer for young Hondurans and Guatemalans, whose countries saw catastrophic loss of life caused by Hurricane Mitch during the same hurricane season, and since 2005 hundreds of young doctors from each of these countries have graduated from the Latin American School of Medicine in Havana, the world's largest medical faculty. The first group of Haitian students was therefore selected, and they started at the Latin American Medical School in Havana in May 1999. The presence of Cuban medical personnel on the ground and the training of Haitian doctors continue to this day.

Even major political developments in Haiti had little effect on the Cuban medical cooperation role. In late February 2004, for example, President Jean-Bertrand Aristide, who had been elected in 2000, was ousted in a violent rebellion and spirited out of the country, eventually being sent in exile to South Africa.[3] Political turmoil had been swirling around the presidency of the former priest, who commanded popularity among the Haitian poor but had been accused of human rights abuses and corruption. Growing lawlessness, widespread instability, and spiraling violence (much of it politically motivated) became commonplace, particularly in the capital, Port-au-Prince. In February 2004, armed gangs took control of Gonaïves (Haiti's third largest city), and groups opposed to Aristide carried out attacks in several cities. These ongoing political disturbances and the climate of uncertainty and fear that prevailed had a major impact on the health situation in the country.

In a stormy UN press conference on the dire humanitarian situation of Haiti, held in March 2004 and sponsored by the Permanent Mission of Canada to the United Nations, concern was expressed about the crisis faced by the country. Representatives presented views on the crisis that in many ways were similar to those expressed after the January 2010 earthquake. Military intervention, for example, was criticized as being excessive and often unhelpful. Many suggested that an immediate and massive humanitarian intervention from abroad was desperately needed if a truly sustainable development model were to take root. There was also a widely expressed criticism of the fickle interest of the industrialized nations: as the crisis in Haiti disappeared from media attention, so had supplies of food aid. A representative of the World Council of Churches to the United Nations made a telling comment that "humanitarian aid could not be human if it was only publicized for 15 days."[4] Cuba's extensive support was largely ignored. In terms of recognizing the efforts of other nations that had come to help Haiti, there were only two lines about Cuba's cooperation in Haiti in a report by the Office for the Coordination of Humanitarian Affairs—and this despite the significant medical support provided by Cuba since 1998. In fact, there was a medical brigade of 525 members (of whom 332 were doctors) working in Haiti at that time. During those preceding five years Cuban medical personnel had treated nearly 5 million patients and saved the lives of nearly 86,000 Haitians. In the midst of the political crisis surrounding the departure of Aristide, Cuban medics had treated 406 patients, many with gunshot wounds, and Cuba had sent 12.2 tons of medical supplies. All of this was ignored in official United Nations documents and western media reports—much as was the case with the 2010 earthquake.

Political instability was replaced by further tragedy in September 2004, when the port city of Gonaïves suffered massive flooding, resulting in the death of over 2,800 people. At that time there were 18 Cuban medical personnel working in the city of 260,000. Shortly after disaster struck, Cuba sent an additional 64-person medical brigade, along with two tons of medical equipment and supplies to provide extra support. An abandoned hospital became the nerve center for both a surgical unit and a major intensive care unit, complete with ultrasound, laboratories, birthing room, sterilization chamber, and the normal consulting areas. Three mobile clinics were set up, and an NGO office and two churches were taken over by Cuban medical personnel as temporary hospitals. Eventually a network of six clinics was organized as the Cubans increased their medical presence. They used the local radio stations to share information about how to prevent epidemics. Gradually the crisis abated, but only after major damage and extensive loss of life had resulted.

The situation that Cuban medical personnel encountered when they arrived in late 1998 was exceptionally bad. Despite Haiti being only 90 miles from eastern Cuba, the two countries could not have had more different health profiles. The analysis provided by the Pan American Health Organization paints a bleak picture indeed. Infant mortality, for instance, had actually increased from 73.8 per 1,000 live births in 1996 to 80.3 in 2000, over 10 times the rate of Cuba. The principal health problem in infants was (and is) acute diarrheal disease, with the major cause of death in 1999 being intestinal infectious diseases (12.1 percent), closely followed by perinatal infections (10.2 percent), malnutrition (9.1 percent), and acute respiratory infections (6.9 percent)—all of which are preventable with proper living conditions and an adequate diet. Among adults the leading cause of death was AIDS (21.6 percent), while the maternal mortality rate in 2000 was a shocking 523 per 100,000 live births. Malnutrition in 1995 reportedly affected 67.3 percent of the population.[5] In 2005–2006 a useful study by Cuban physicians working in Haiti was undertaken through a survey of children under the age of five who attended one of the Cuban-run health centers during the course of the year. They examined 1,712 children and found that 33 percent were below the normal weight for their age and at risk of malnutrition, with a further 22 percent being malnourished. Among the patients, 72.5 percent suffered from anemia, while 34.0 percent had intestinal parasites.[6] These data, it must be remembered, came from a study of Haitians who actually sought medical assistance, and it would therefore be fair to assume that in areas where people were sick but did not seek medical treatment, the situation would probably be significantly worse. Clearly Cuban medical *internacionalistas* faced an enormous challenge.

The Value of the Cuban Contribution since 1998

Haiti has approximately 2,000 doctors, about 90 percent of whom are located in the capital city. Many depend on fee for service as the source of their livelihood, since the Haitian government has traditionally invested little in the public health system. UNICEF estimates that, in terms of public spending as a percentage of GDP between 2007 and 2010, the government only allocated 1 percent of its funding.[7] As a result, many physicians, including some of those trained in Cuba, are obliged to earn their living in the private sector. This has also led to a major scarcity of medical staff in rural areas, and when the Cubans arrived in 1998 to assist following Hurricane Georges, many were immediately sent outside the capital by the Haitian government. For many Haitians, Cuban doctors were the first that they had ever encountered, a sad reflection on the national public health system. They were also amazed to see that the Cuban medical personnel provided their services at no charge.

The long-term solution for Haiti's enormous health needs lies in the training of local students to become doctors—and for them to remain in their homeland and be employed. Graduates from the Cuban medical programs know that they are expected to work in poor, underserved communities, either their own or somewhere else in the developing world where their services are needed. It is worth noting that ELAM graduates from a variety of nationalities, including the United States, flew to work alongside Cuban doctors in Haiti after the 2010 earthquake. By April 1, 2010, in addition to the 783 Cuban medical staff, there were also 481 Haitians and 278 doctors from 28 countries—all graduates of the Latin American School of Medicine—working to help the people of Haiti.[8] When ELAM was inaugurated in 1999, Haitian medical students first studied in Havana. However, as the number of students grew, the decision was taken to train Francophone students at the Facultad de Ciencias Médicas No. 2 in Santiago de Cuba in the east of the island. A new stage of the medical training was then implemented as students from French West Africa joined their Haitian counterparts.

Cuban doctors worked in extremely challenging circumstances back in Haiti. The public health system was a disaster, particularly in rural areas.[9] This is where the Cubans mainly worked because, unlike foreign NGOs and others with medical projects in developing countries that set up private operations where they followed their own agenda, the Cubans worked for the established state. They followed guidelines set down by the Haitian government, working where they were needed, which meant in the slums of the cities and in marginalized rural areas. According to the agreements signed with Havana, the Cuban medical personnel are employees of the state in which they work, and therefore they set up their practice where they are told by the local government: they are provided with a small stipend and their living expenses are paid, and they usually work on two-year contracts—at which time they are replaced by colleagues. A detailed bilateral agreement was reached between the Cuban and Haitian governments to formalize this arrangement, according to which Cuba came to institutionalize the Comprehensive Health Program. This has remained in place since 1998, with a gradual reduction of Cuban medical personnel—as Haitian graduates from ELAM have steadily arrived since the first graduation in 2005 to replace them. By early 2011, 625 Haitians had graduated from ELAM, of whom 430 were working in Haiti, mostly in the public healthcare system or with the Cuban medical contingent.[10]

The Cuban medical personnel worked throughout the country in extremely poor living conditions among the impoverished communities there. This was an important factor in their being so widely accepted by the Haitian population, who were amazed to see the Cuban medical personnel sharing the same living conditions and not just visiting occasionally from air-conditioned hotel rooms in Port-au-Prince. Interviews with scores of patients have also shown that Cuban medical personnel were appreciated for their humanitarian spirit, the manner in which they treated their desperately poor patients with dignity and respect, and the fact that they took the time to listen to them. As a result the Cubans—many of whom were black—were highly regarded by the population. An article in a Mexican newspaper cites the director of La Paz University Hospital in Port-au-Prince as saying, "At times I feel ashamed because the patients only want to see the Cuban doctors."[11]

By 2004 there were 705 Cubans working in Haiti in veterinary medicine, the sugar and fishing industries, and a literacy program. The vast majority, however, were in public health—579, according to the Cuban ambassador at the time. They were responsible for the health of an estimated 75 percent of Haitians.[12] The following year they were joined by the first graduating class of 128 Haitian medical students from ELAM.

Cuban medical personnel are expressly ordered by Havana to refrain from political activities, regardless of the country in which they are working. Their role is to serve their patients and provide care. In a report in the *Dallas Morning News* at the time of the removal of President Aristide, and with violence breaking out all over Port-au-Prince, an American journalist noted that all the hospitals and the clinics in the capital closed but one—an emergency room operated by Cuban doctors. He quoted the head of the Cuban medical mission as saying, "We're here to help the people. . . . We don't take sides. We don't get mixed up in politics."[13] Whether it be in Somoza's Nicaragua in the early 1970s (at the time the greatest enemy of revolutionary Cuba in Latin America), or Guatemala and Honduras in the 1990s (when they did not even have diplomatic relations), the Cuban doctors came to provide badly needed medical care. This was the case in Haiti, since they have stayed regardless of the political stripe of the government of the day.[14] In April 2004 the Cuban ambassador to Haiti, Rolando A. Gómez González, articulated the Cuban philosophy: "We can't offer financial assistance . . . but we can give our human resources. . . . The cooperation isn't motivated by ideology or politics. We're helping the Haitian people who've suffered so much in the last 200 years."[15]

They are assisted in this mission by their training and upbringing and also by the society in they have been raised. They have been brought up in a socialist society and have been socialized to see everybody as their equal, in essence being blind to significant class differences. The concept of the need to work for the collective (as opposed to working for themselves) has also been a key factor in their education, even from preschool times, where an emphasis is placed on team-building exercises and games. Moreover, unlike their medical colleagues in the private sector, when they work as *internacionalistas*, the Cubans look after those patients who are marginalized, who usually cannot afford to pay for medical care, and who live in areas where doctors rarely go. Paul Farmer, Harvard Medical School professor and former deputy UN special envoy for Haiti, has noted the differences between Cuban and U.S. medical training: "Cuban physicians are trained differently. They're trained to understand the communities they're serving [making] home visits, for example, knowing their neighbors, who are also their patients. . . . In Cuba it's the rule. . . . Cuba was way ahead of the pack with their focus on prevention and health promotion. Prevention and promotion are highly regarded and are also worked very much into the curriculum from the beginning of medical school and throughout training."[16] They are renowned for treating their patients, whatever their social class, with respect and dignity. As one journalist noted: "I have seen the Cuban doctors in Haiti and they are like fish in water. There is a very good rapport with the masses, which is not the rapport of someone giving charity, but it is the rapport of fraternal solidarity."[17]

The Cuban role in Haiti was clearly beneficial, despite the horrible socioeconomic conditions in which the majority of the population live (and which constitute a breeding ground for many preventable diseases). Haiti is the poorest country in the Western Hemisphere, with a depressing litany of statistics: 62 percent of the population is below the international poverty line of earning $1.25 per day, only 50 percent attend primary school, only 49 percent of adults are literate, and life expectancy is 62.[18] These data, the most recent of UNICEF, are from 2011.

Yet despite the depressing picture of daily life presented here, from 1999 to the time of the earthquake in January 2010, health conditions had been steadily improving for Haitians, as the UNICEF website "At a Glance: Haiti" illustrates. For example, the under-five mortality rank (position 152) in 1990 had improved to 76 in 2007 and 40 in 2011; the infant mortality rank fell from 105 to 53, while life expectancy during the same period increased from 54 to 62 years. An analysis by the Pan American Health Organization of the role of Cuban medical personnel in Haiti between 1998 and 2003 reveals a significant improvement in the health of Haitians. In the areas where Cuban medical personnel worked, for example, infant mortality was reduced from 80 per 1,000 live births to 33, and mortality for children under five was reduced from 135 to 59.4. Maternal mortality rates had fallen by almost half, from 523 per 100,000 births to 285.[19] By April 2007, the two ophthalmology centers installed by Cuba had operated on 5,000 people, restoring their sight, and a million doses of vaccines had been administered.[20] In sum, while the health data for Haiti appeared disastrous compared with those of industrialized nations (and even many countries of Latin America), there is no doubt that the large number of resident Cuban doctors and the steady stream of Haitian graduates from medical school in Cuba had made a significant improvement in the lives of people there. This in many ways is the saddest point to be made about the devastating impact of the events of 2010, since Cuban medical cooperation had been making a major difference in improving access to public health. Then, however, came the earthquake and the subsequent cholera outbreak.

The Cuban medical brigade undertook its own detailed survey of the health profile of the Haitians in 2008, and their report shows an awareness of areas in which there were clear needs and problems, but also others in which progress had been made. Among the ongoing medical problems were the growth in AIDS (up 3 percent) and in pulmonary tuberculosis (up 2.1 percent). By contrast, infectious diseases (which constituted 34.9 percent of cases seen by Cuban medical staff) decreased by 19.2 percent between 2007 and 2008. Acute diarrhea-related diseases fell by 25.3 percent, typhoid fever was down 41 percent, malaria fell 41.8 percent, and cases of intestinal parasites were down 8.8 percent. Acute diarrhea-related diseases and typhoid fever (which represented 7.2 percent of all cases seen) are related to poor hygienic conditions, poor water quality, and inadequate nutrition.[21] Cuban officials themselves gathered some basic data, shown in table 8.1, to illustrate the significance of this extensive medical cooperation.

The same group produced a more detailed report for February 2008. In that month Cuban medical personnel treated 182,712 patients (an increase

Table 8.1. Selected statistics on the impact of Cuban medical cooperation in Haiti, December 1998–May 2007

Visits to the doctor	10,682,124
Doctor visit to patients	4,150,631
Attended births	86,633
Major and minor surgeries	160,283
Vaccinations	899,829
Lives saved (emergency)	210,852

Source: *Ministry of Foreign Relations (MINREX), International Cooperation, May 2007.* Published in Anna Kovac, "Cuba Trains Hundreds of Haitian Doctors to Make a Difference." Courtesy *MEDICC Review,* August 6, 2007.

of 17,544 over the previous month). Their report was critical of the high rates of diseases that were transmitted by vectors and made worse by poor hygiene and inadequate waste removal. Cuban medical personnel were thus encouraged to redouble their efforts to make Haitians aware of appropriate sanitary conditions. That said, there were noticeable improvements in comparison with the same period in 2007, as can be seen in table 8.2.

We have already seen how desperate the poverty was in Haiti—and this was before the 2010 earthquake. Yet Cuba too was facing major economic challenges. Economic growth dropped dramatically in the wake of Hurricanes Gustav and Ike in late 2008, which caused $8–10 billion in dam-

Table 8.2. Selected infectious diseases in Haiti, February 2007 and February 2008

Disease	February 2007 No. of cases	February 2008 No. of cases
Typhoid fever	6,889	3,654
Acute diarrhea-related diseases	14,446	8,818
Tuberculosis	482	293
Meningitis	21	50
Sexually transmitted diseases	4,997	4,616
HIV/AIDS	391	371
Dengue	752	82
Malaria	7,897	4,214
Intestinal parasites	15,517	11,046
Acute respiratory infections	22,589	20,957
Other infections and parasite-related diseases	11,186	7,490
Total	**85,167**	**61,591**

Source: Brigada Médica Cubana en Haití, Coordinación General, "Comportamiento de enfermedades transmisibles, Haití. Febrero 2008," mimeo.

age. (To put this in context, that loss amounts to over three years of gross income from the tourist industry for the entire country.) Prices for nickel, one of the principal sources of hard currency, fell to a third of its previous value. Government inefficiency, excessive control, and a lack of incentives, poor administration, and centralized control also accentuated the difficulties, as did five decades of U.S. animosity. As a result, Cuba's planned economic growth rate was reduced and then reduced again. Cuba, in short, was facing major challenges at this time and could be excused for decreasing its medical support to its impoverished neighbor.

Yet as Mexican journalist José Steinsleger has pointed out, Cuba's solidarity with its fellow members of the developing and underdeveloped world was maintained. At a time when Cuba's economy was suffering, it still managed to provide significant medical cooperation abroad, especially to the poorest of the poor. Using very conservative estimates, Steinsleger computes the cost of these medical services in Haiti: 14 million medical consultations at $10 each, more than 225 surgical operations at $100, more than 100,000 birth deliveries at $50, over 47,000 eye operations at $25, and the training of 570 Haitian medical graduates with 541 still being trained in Cuba at $5,000 each. At these remarkably low costs, he estimates that Cuba—itself a very poor country in terms of standard economic measures—had spent at the very least $215 million in helping Haiti.[22] Much of these 11 years of human solidarity were lost in just a few minutes on January 12, 2010, as an earthquake of 7.3 magnitude leveled the capital city and surrounding areas. In terms of Cuban medical cooperation in Haiti, this date is significant. It allows for a badly needed analysis both of the contribution of Cuban medical staff at the time of the hurricane and their contribution to the post-hurricane development of the Haitian people's health.

The Cuban Response to the Haitian Earthquake of 2010

> We send doctors, not soldiers.
>
> Fidel Castro, January 23, 2010

"The worst catastrophe that has occurred in Haiti in two centuries" is how Haitian prime minister Jean-Max Bellerive described the earthquake that destroyed Port-au-Prince.[23] Estimates of the casualties varied, but most agreed that at least 200,000 people had died, many being buried in mass graves. Most were the result of Haitians being crushed by collapsing buildings. Several thousand also needed amputations, a major burden in a developing country, where employment opportunities were already severely limited. Some 3 million people—one-third of the population—suffered the direct effects of the earthquake. In the capital, the scene was one of total chaos. More than 200,000 homes were destroyed or so badly damaged that they needed to be demolished. Major structures such as the Presidential Palace, the Cathedral, and the National Assembly all collapsed. An estimated 250,000 were injured and 1.5 million were left homeless, while almost 300,000 fled to the north and west of the country.[24] The already limited public healthcare system was badly affected by the earthquake, and eight hospitals (including the only national teaching and reference hospital), nine clinics, and 19 training institutes were destroyed. A further 22 hospitals were badly damaged.[25] Three of the country's four medical schools were damaged. A year later the situation remained desperate: 1.5 million lived in camps for displaced persons, of whom 30 percent had no access to toilets and 40 percent had no clean drinking water. And this had occurred in a country where, even before the earthquake, Haiti ranked worst of 147 countries on the Water Poverty Index.[26] Most infrastructure was destroyed or severely damaged, including the airport and the port in the capital, and most hospitals and government buildings also collapsed. Damage to the highways made them at first impassable, and obtaining emergency supplies from the neighboring Dominican Republic was difficult.

The international community responded with great generosity. Hundreds of NGOs, private volunteer organizations, aid agencies, and foreign governments sent massive shipments of supplies, and at one point there were 10,000 NGOs all elbowing for room to help Haiti's population. On January 14 the *Christian Science Monitor* published an article listing the many nations that had sent assistance. Significantly titled "Haiti Earthquake: The Nations That Are Stepping Up to Help," it mentioned that the first country to deliver aid was the Dominican Republic. Fulsome praise was given to President Barack Obama's decision to order Coast Guard cutters, an aircraft carrier, the USNS *Comfort* (a 1,000-bed floating hospital), and other vessels to transport supplies and security personnel. The Spanish newspaper *El País* printed a comprehensive list of nations helping the distraught Haitian population. The *Guardian* gave a more detailed list. Noticeably absent from all these reports was any mention of Cuba's support, a sad reflection on the enormous contribution made by Havana.[27] Fox News sang the praises of U.S. relief efforts in a January 13, 2010, story entitled "U.S. Spearheads Global Response to Haiti Earthquake." Fox also sought to issue a clear criticism of Cuba, noting, "But one geographically close country is conspicuously absent from the roster of helping hands. Cuba . . . has so far not offered any assistance publicly to its devastated island neighbor."[28] This was clearly a distortion of Cuba's actual role.

Television coverage was particularly revealing. Several key themes emerged: episodes of human suffering and adversity, individual stories of success as survivors were pulled from the rubble (sadly, less than 200), massive relief efforts, a huge presence of U.S security forces, difficulties in accessing food, water, and medical supplies, and the bravery of medical teams from around the globe. Dr. Sanjay Gupta, a neurosurgeon and the chief medical correspondent for CNN, was actually involved in some surgical operations and featured prominently in the day-to-day coverage. But remarkably little media attention was paid to the Cuban medical staff and their role in Haiti. One detailed analysis of media coverage revealed how mainstream U.S. media ignored Cuba's role. For instance, the *New York Times* and *Washington Post* had 750 posts on the earthquake and relief work, yet not one analyzed in any depth the role of Cuba, while CNN had 601 reports with only 18 brief references to Cuba's contribution.[29]

A 2012 study published by Harvard University Medical School and NATO Joint Analysis and Lessons Learned Centre illustrates the differences in approach. The United States rushed to provide "military assets," accompanied by some medical support, and the need for security was consistently emphasized as being one of the main "takeaways" of the report. Shortly after the earthquake, Washington instituted Operation Unified Response, deploying 22,000 personnel, 17 ships, and more than 100 aircraft. Appendix B of the report highlights the contributions made by U.S. forces and their allies. The Israeli Defense Forces, for instance, set up a field hospital and stayed for a 10-day mission. They set up an electronic medical records database for their 1,100 patients and an "early discharge" system ("in an effort to reduce long-term dependence on their service"), providing them with advice and medicines before discharging them. The authors of the system note, however, that this "early discharge system was not ideal, because many patients were homeless and had nowhere safe to go. Very young patients often had no adult guardian to look after them."[30] Clearly this was not a sustainable approach. Military medical support from Mexico, the United States, Canada, Colombia, France, Spain, and Italy also received compliments, although some of their contributions were of a tokenistic nature.

The U.S. 22nd Marine Expeditionary Unit and the 82nd Airborne Brigade Combat Team and the USNS *Comfort* were singled out for praise. The first two provided security at existing medical treatment facilities, while the *Comfort* spent seven weeks in Haiti, with its personnel attending 8,600 patients and performing over 1,000 surgeries. It is worth noting the philosophy behind the U.S. medical support, as seen in the discussion as to when the ship should be withdrawn. One view among the military was that it "should leave after just a few days; another view was that an abrupt departure could create a negative political image." U.S. authorities agreed on a "tacit program of 'weaning,' whereby fewer and fewer patients were accepted even though *Comfort* had additional capacity." The ship left 49 days after treating the first patients. The U.S. approach was designed to provide temporary medical aid, treating medical conditions that could be dealt with relatively easily and without any long-term goals. Projecting a political image and obtaining positive media coverage was the priority, since a sustained effort to save lives was clearly lacking. The same limited approach was common among virtually all of the other nations that provided medical aid.

An analysis of this 70-page report is useful, both because of what it emphasizes and also what it omits. It stresses the value of the 22,000 U.S. personnel deployed (almost entirely military), since they protected access to the hospitals and maintained a solid climate of order and discipline, as well as the 17 ships and more than 100 aircraft provided for transportation. It talks about the invaluable work of the military of U.S. allies. It also mentions the medical care provided by the *Comfort*, a massive vessel with 12 operating theaters and a 1,000-bed capacity that became the principal tertiary care facility—for the seven weeks it remained in Haiti. There are no references, however, to the role of the hundreds of Cuban physicians, nurses, and technicians who were already on the ground when the military personnel of the 82nd Airborne brigade arrived, much less the thousands of surgeries performed before and after the earthquake. In many ways this analysis by NATO and Harvard Medical School is a microcosm of the larger picture of U.S. media coverage of Cuba's medical cooperation role in Haiti and indeed in the developing world as a whole.

Cuba's role in the devastated country was enormous. What was not reported in mainstream media was the fact that the very first country to respond to the tragedy was Cuba—for the very reason that it had several hundred medical personnel already in Haiti, where they had been stationed since 1998. For the first 72 hours after the earthquake, Cuban doctors were the main medical support for the Haitian population, and a case can be made that their role was the most important of all nations involved in the massive rescue effort. Cuban media indicated that over 1,000 patients were seen by their doctors within the first 24 hours of the earthquake, as they turned their living quarters in the capital into the first field hospital.

Some context is needed in order to understand the role played by Cuban medical staff in promoting a sustainable healthcare model in Haiti since 1998. Mention was made earlier of Cuban medical personnel there. The future of the Haitian healthcare system lies with Haitian doctors trained in Cuba, the first of whom—132—arrived to study in Cuba in May 1999. By August 2009 a total of 544 Haitians had been trained as physicians in Cuba, and 400 had returned to work in Haiti, while others were undertaking further medical specialization both in Haiti and in Cuba. Over 200 Haitian graduates were in residency programs in their country at the time of the earthquake,[31] while a further 541 were being trained in Cuba as doctors, with 66 set to graduate in 2010 and over 100 more in 2011. When the earthquake struck, almost 1,000 Haitian doctors had either graduated or were being trained in Cuba—at no cost to the students.

At the time of the earthquake there were 340 Cuban medical personnel working on the island, in 127 of the country's 137 districts. By 2010 they had been involved in restoring sight to over 47,000 Haitians through the Operation Miracle program.[32] Perhaps most telling of all, prior to the earthquake, they had saved 230,000 lives and provided healthcare for 75 percent of Haitians.[33] Sadly most media ignored this long-standing commitment.

Prior to the earthquake Cuba, supported by Venezuela, had built five comprehensive diagnostic centers (small hospitals), with five more in various stages of completion. The Cubans immediately did all they could to make them functional in order to assist Haitians. Precise details on the Cuban medical contribution were given on January 24 by Dr. Carlos Alberto García, head of the Cuban medical brigade in Haiti. Between the afternoon of January 12 (when the earthquake struck) and January 27, more than 27,000 patients had been seen by Cuban medical staff (417), supported by Cuba-trained Haitians (240). Of these medical consultations, 2,415 had resulted in surgery.[34] The Cuban medical staff were working in three of the capital's hospitals (La Paz, La Renaissance, and Ofatma), as well as in 16 field hospitals both in the capital and in other cities. Cubans were working in the five comprehensive diagnosis centers, each with 20 beds, an intensive therapy theater, and a birthing room, while two others were expected to be ready within weeks and were also used to receive patients. There were 20 Cuban medical personnel working in the Operation Miracle ophthalmology center, which was also turned into a field hospital—and they treated

605 people within the first 12 hours of the earthquake.[35] On January 13, they were joined by some 60 emergency specialists, including personnel from the Henry Reeve contingent specialists in providing medical care in natural emergencies. Much of the damage was done outside the capital but was not featured in media reports because of the difficulties in transportation, yet that is where almost half of the Cuban medical brigade were working. These personnel would be particularly helpful, since they were in areas where people headed after fleeing Port-au-Prince. Cubans were working in 23 medical centers in the country, had formed 17 medical teams, and were running 15 operating theaters.[36]

By February 1 many foreign medical teams had returned home, and Haiti had long disappeared from the front pages of the world's newspapers. Yet the needs for comprehensive medical care were greater than ever. At that point there were some 600 Cuban medical staff working there, supported by 380 Haitian doctors trained in Cuba, and they had seen over 50,000 patients, of whom 34,000 had undergone surgery.[37] Reflecting on the role of the Cuban medical personnel, Fidel Castro spoke of the opportunity for cooperation that working to help the embattled Haitian population offered: "Our medical personnel are ready to cooperate and join forces with all other health specialists who have been sent to save lives in that sister nation. Haiti could become an example of what humankind can do for itself. The possibility and the means exist, but willingness is missing."[38]

The Henry Reeve contingent arrived within 24 hours after the earthquake, but psychological support was also needed. So two weeks later, a group of psychologists, psychiatrists, and pediatric psychiatrists arrived from Cuba. They had all taken specialized training in mental health needs in natural disasters. They remained for three months, helping the traumatized population (reaching 150,000 young Haitians) and training 350 Haitians to continue the work after they left.[39] Another invaluable addition resulted from the contribution of the Martha Machado Artists Brigade, a group of Cuban painters, musicians, clowns, magicians, and puppeteers who used various cultural media to reach the children and help them overcome their fears in the nightmarish situation that was post-earthquake Haiti. Art supplies were provided by the brigade, led by the well-known artist Kcho (Alexis Leyva Machado), again with the objective of encouraging the children to express their concerns through play and art.

One of the major problems after the initial shock was dealing with potential epidemics. Given the widespread lack of sanitation facilities as tens of thousands of people congregated in massive tent cities—without sufficient drinking water, basic sanitation facilities such as toilets and water for bathing and washing clothes, and efficient garbage disposal—the situation was grim indeed. While medical personnel continued to deal with patients badly affected by the massive collapse of buildings, resulting in a widespread loss of limbs and subsequent infections, many others were concerned at the idea of the surrounding conditions which offered an ideal breeding ground for disease. The spring rainy season also threatened to bring about a major epidemic of water-borne diseases. The main health challenges were diarrhea-related diseases (made worse by the lack of drinking water and latrines), respiratory diseases, dermatological conditions, tetanus, and meningitis. The Cubans had worked in similar conditions abroad (since 1998 responding to natural disasters in China, Pakistan, Guatemala, Indonesia, Mexico, Bolivia, and Chile) and could see the potential dangers. Their worst fears came true with the outbreak of cholera in October 2010.

Some 30 teams of Cuban and Cuban-trained Haitian personnel, four in each team, were formed to provide practical information to the population. They worked in several public health education initiatives, showing how to dispose safely of waste matter, how best to keep clean, and how to minimize their chances of becoming infected. These activities were carried out in tents and in the open air, and the Cubans worked alongside fifth- and sixth-year Haitian medical students brought from Cuba, as well as Haitians who had graduated from medical school in Cuba. Flyers and posters—all written in Creole—were widely distributed, and portable megaphones and loudspeakers were used to reach the population. They also conducted a massive tetanus vaccination campaign (using 400,000 doses of vaccines donated by Cuba for patients with lesions or wounds), held both in the Port-au-Prince soccer stadium and in the scores of parks where Haitians lived in tent cities. They were soon joined by a team of 64 colleagues, including epidemiologists, fumigators, and specialists in dealing with diseases caused by vectors. Among the horribly sad circumstances in which they toiled, there was some joy: Cuban medical staff delivered 280 babies (more than half of whom were born by caesarean procedures).

The Cholera Outbreak

Tragically much of their good work was to be undone. Just ten months after the earthquake, a massive cholera epidemic swept through Haiti, despite the campaign kept up by the Cubans for months.[40] Cholera had not been seen in Haiti for over a century, and its impact on a country still reeling from the earthquake was extreme. It broke out in an area near the Artibonite River where Asian peacekeepers were stationed and was apparently caused by waste from the base spilling into the river. Water from the river was drunk by the local population, who subsequently contracted the disease. Given the extremely limited access to both safe drinking water and proper sanitation services, the cholera spread rapidly—to all 10 departments or states within a month. By late December 2010, some 148,787 cases had been reported, with 3,333 deaths—for a fatality rate of 2.2 percent.[41] Cuban physicians sounded the alarm, after dealing with a suspiciously high number of patients with what initially appeared to be bad cases of diarrhea. Cuban and Haitian teams worked together, sending samples for testing as a precaution, and once the results were known, a nationwide alert was issued.[42] The death toll would have been far worse if Cuban personnel had not taken this initiative soon after the outbreak and helped to mobilize a national campaign against the disease.

To a large extent the vastly reduced amount of aid that now arrived from abroad could be explained by donor fatigue. People in the developed world had been swamped with images of Haiti's tragedy. Many had donated already and were suspicious about the government's probity given the rumors of corruption that circulated. Haiti was therefore largely left to its own devices as the cholera epidemic spread and as hundreds died. Cuba's reaction was the clear exception. Within weeks, reinforcements for the Henry Reeve Brigade arrived, as did scores of graduates from ELAM.

The disease spread swiftly, with two waves in late 2010 and mid-2011. By December 2010 it had killed more than 1,880 Haitians, and almost 84,400 people had been treated.[43] Cholera is a bacterial disease that can cause diarrhea and dehydration, and it is commonly spread through contaminated water. Often the water may be contaminated by sewage or feces and food handled by a person who has the disease. Given the disastrous situation of access to potable water and sewage facilities before the earthquake, compounded by the arrival of the rain that spread the contamination, in many ways the perfect conditions for the spread of cholera were present. Some 75 percent of Haitian households still lack running water, while tens of thousands remain in camps with difficult living conditions. According to the Centers for Disease Control and Prevention, by August 4, 2013, there had been 669,396 cases (including 180,439 in the capital) registered in all 10 departments of the country and 8,217 cholera deaths.[44]

While the NATO report highlights the opportunities for greater involvement in supporting the population at a time of such a natural disaster (pro-

Table 8.3. Initial response to cholera outbreak by Cuban-led medical team in Haiti

Members of Cuban-led medical team in Haiti	1,398
ELAM-trained members	234
Haitian ELAM-trained members	152
Doctors	498
Nurses	464
Countries represented in team	24 (Argentina, Bolivia, Chile, Colombia, Congo, Cuba, Dominican Republic, Ecuador, El Salvador, Guatemala, Guinea Bissau, Haiti, Honduras, Mali, Mexico, Nicaragua, Nigeria, Panama, Paraguay, Peru, Saharawi Arab Democratic Republic, United States, Uruguay)
Percent of team working in cholera-affected areas	61%
Number of cholera treatment centers staffed by team	59
Results	
Cholera patients treated	47,537
Cholera fatalities	270

Source: Conner Gorry, "Haiti One Year Later: Cuban Medical Team Draws on Experience and Partnerships," *MEDICC Review* 13, no. 1 (January 2011): 53.

tecting the supply chain for resources, using engineering assets to provide water and sewage infrastructure, ensuring stability, and disposing of cadavers), NATO countries chose not to become involved. In contrast, the Cuban medical mission established separate cholera treatment centers and oral rehydration posts, distributed public health messages in creole, and set up detailed tent-by-tent examinations of Haitians. Mobile units visited rural areas, taking Aquatab to treat drinking water. Teams of Cubans and Haitians traveled throughout the country taking with them oral rehydration salts and basic medicines. One article in the *New York Times* praised the Cubans: "As the epidemic continues, the Cuban medical mission that played an important role in detecting it presses on in Haiti, winning accolades from donors and diplomats for staying on the front lines and undertaking a broader effort to remake the country's shattered healthcare system." Cuba "took the lead" in the fight against cholera for one basic reason: nobody else was. Indeed, the UN's Paul Farmer put this succinctly: "Half of the NGOs are already gone, and the Cubans are still there."[45]

As a result of epidemiological research, community contacts, a well-established tradition of popular education on health topics, and the support of hundreds of Cuba-trained Haitian doctors, the Cuban strategy was successful. After a year of treating patients—an estimated 76,000 according to Archibold—the fatality rate of 0.36 percent (in all, 272 deaths) was significantly lower than the national average of 1.4 percent.[46] The cholera epidemic rate in Haiti amounted to 57 percent of all cholera cases and 53 percent of related deaths in the entire world reported to the World Health Organization in 2010. By late October 2012, 604,634 cases had been reported, as well as 329,697 hospitalizations and 736 deaths.[47] The rates finally became manageable, mainly because of the role played by Cuban medical personnel throughout the country.

Evaluation of the Cuban Contribution

While international media may have ignored or downplayed Cuba's role in Haiti, it is significant that members of the Haitian government did not.[48] Fully aware of 11 years of solid cooperation with Haiti, they emphasized the importance of Cuba's medical contribution. Jean-Renald Clerismé, principal adviser to President René Préval, for instance, remarked how the Cubans had been the first to assist the Haitian population.[49] This point was made clear by Prime Minister Jean-Max Bellerive in a conference held in Montreal among major industrialized nations to plan for the rebuilding in Haiti, when he noted that the first three countries to help were Cuba, the Dominican Republic, and Venezuela. Unlike all other nations that came to Haiti's assistance, Cuba did not need to send doctors to help out, as some 340 medical staff were already there and had been for 11 years. In addition to the dozens of members of the Henry Reeve contingent from Cuba, the hundreds of Haitian graduates of Cuban medical school, and the 240 Haitian interns and students still in medical school in Cuba who returned to their country, Cuban doctors are the unsung heroes of the rescue efforts in Haiti. With some justification, the Haitian ambassador to Cuba, Jean Víctor Généus, wrote, "Every time a disaster has hit Haiti, Cuba's response has been immediate and altruistic, despite its own scant resources and the unjust, illegal, and inhumane blockade imposed by the United States over the last 50 years."[50]

Cuban foreign minister Bruno Rodríguez provided data on the Cuban medical role in a speech delivered at the UN conference on international donors for the reconstruction of Haiti. Between the earthquake and March 31, 2010, Cuban medical personnel had provided almost 260,000 medical consultations, undertaken 7,000 surgeries, attended almost 1,400 births, and vaccinated 100,000 people. More than 50,000 patients had been seen for rehabilitation treatment, and 75,000 children had received psycho-social therapy. In terms of the personnel delivering this care, Cuba clearly had a major role: 783 Cuban medical personnel, supported by 481 Haitian doctors trained in Cuba, and 278 medical staff from 28 countries all trained by Cuba had assisted the beleaguered Haitian population.[51] Efforts were redoubled by Cuban medical staff after the cholera outbreak, and no other country or organization had provided anything approaching this level of medical care to the stricken country. Media coverage of these achievements was sadly lacking, however.

Data from December 2012 show that Cuban medical cooperation continues to improve the health of the Haitian people, according to Dr. Michel Escalona Martín, deputy director of the Cuban medical contingent in Haiti. During 15 years of uninterrupted medical support, Cuban personnel gave 20,946,428 consultations and treated one-third of all patients (6,792,394) in their own homes. There were 373,513 surgeries, of which 140,191 were major, and Cuban staff assisted at 150,336 births (including 16,481 caesarean deliveries). Operation Miracle improved or restored the sight of 60,281 Haitians, and examined 322,753 patients. In the cholera outbreak, Cuban personnel treated 76,897 patients. An estimated 314,363 Haitian lives were saved as a result of Cuban medical attention. Cuban medical school professors had also trained 878 doctors, of whom 367 specialized in general medicine, under the supervision of the Cuban medical brigade. And Cubans were working in 96 healthcare centers in Haiti, of which 65 units including the 23 national reference hospitals were part of the Cuba-Venezuela program designed to support the Haitian national health system.[52] This is an extraordinary contribution made by Cuba, a small developing nation.

Plans for the "New" Haiti

The healthcare situation in pre-earthquake Haiti, while improving in those areas served by Cuban medical personnel and Haitian graduates of ELAM, was still poor. The country had the lowest number of health workers per population (mainly concentrated in urban areas), and the health sector was notoriously underfunded. There were major divisions between the delivery of healthcare, with the private sector, public health (supported by Cuba), and NGO-funded groups all delivering medical services. A widespread lack of supplies, coordination, and personnel all made for a poor situation. And this was before the earthquake, followed by the cholera epidemic.

On March 31, 2010, a significant gathering took place at the United Nations headquarters, the International Donors' Conference towards a New Future for Haiti. The spirit was relatively upbeat, with official government clichés about "new beginnings" and "opportunities for growth" shared widely. Capacity building, government effectiveness, and disaster mitigation were concepts bandied about by delegates of developed countries. Significant emphasis was placed on the "importance of the private sector to catalyze sustainable economic development," although few chose to reflect on the limited impact that this traditionally had had in Haiti.[53] Perhaps most important of all, commitments were made by many countries and organizations to support the promise of this "new future." In all 59 pledges were made by a number of countries, regional blocs, and financial institutions. The largest donation came from the United States, which pledged $1.51 billion. Among other members of the G-8 industrialized countries, France pledged $188.93 million, Germany $53.17 million, Italy and the United Kingdom were not listed (although a $203.19 million donation was made in the name of a generic "EU Remaining" group of countries), Japan pledged $75 million, Canada $375.23 million, and the Russian Federation $8 million.[54] In-kind contributions were also made by Colombia, Cuba, Mexico, Slovenia, Thailand, and Venezuela (although Venezuela had also pledged $2.14 billion, roughly twice that offered by the United States).

Unfortunately, pledges given at a time when popular sentiment is urging governments to assist the victims of natural disasters are not always delivered after media coverage has died down, and the case of Haiti was no exception. Fully 18 months after the earthquake, and despite a flurry of media reports on U.S. support, Washington had disbursed less than 14 percent of its pledge. By the end of 2011, most donors still had not released two-thirds of the funds promised, and only 12 percent of the funds that had actually arrived had been channeled through the government. Instead, the vast majority sent their (severely reduced) contributions through NGOs, reducing the influence of the Haitian government in directing the funds where they were most needed.[55] Donors had been interested in emergency aid, but not so much in rebuilding the country, and even the ravages of cholera appeared to exert little influence now.[56]

In analyzing the significance of the Cuban contribution (made with the notable assistance of Venezuela, Brazil, and Norway), it is worth noting the value and nature of the pledge. Cuba's pledge was clear and concrete, as noted in the conference communiqué detailing its commitment: medical services for the construction and strengthening of the national health system in Haiti (39 health centers, 30 community hospitals, 30 rehabilitation facilities, three electro-medicine centers, one orthoprosthesis lab, a program for hygiene and epidemiology, and 80 specialists for the projected national specialties hospitals). The above is valued at $690,540,739 in four years. With the exception of the U.S. contribution, this represents more than the rest of the G7 countries combined and 35 percent more than the contribution of the World Bank ($479 million). More pertinent, however, is the nature of the commitment. With the medical coverage pledged, the primary healthcare centers (101, and not 39, according to Cuban documentation) would care for 2.8 million patients annually, deal with 1.3 million emergency cases, attend 168,000 births, and provide 3 million vaccinations. At the secondary level there would be 30 community hospitals distributed throughout the country. These would have a high degree of technology and would annually treat 2,154,000 patients, perform 54,000 surgeries, deal with 1 million emergency cases, and provide 276,000 electrocardiograms, 144,000 ultrasound diagnoses, 43,000 endoscopes, 181,000 X-rays, 107,000 dental examinations, and 487,000 lab tests. In the 30 rehabilitation centers (necessary because of the high number of victims of the earthquake) it was projected that there would be 520,000 patients annually who would receive 2.3 million treatments. In addition to these primary (healthcare centers) and secondary (community hospitals) levels of medical care, at the tertiary level there would also be a national specialist hospital, in which 80 Cuban specialists would work. Finally, 312 additional scholarships would be given to Haitian medical students to continue their studies in Cuba.[57] The two ophthalmological missions of Operation Miracle would continue, one being based in Port-au-Prince while the other tours the interior, recruiting patients for surgery.

Salaries are a major factor. This was included in the Cuban pledge for the reconstruction of Haiti (significantly calculated at half the international rates) and would include payment for Cuban medical staff and the training of 312 more Haitian doctors in Cuba. It does not take into account, of course, the training of 1,000 Haitian doctors in Cuba in the past decade or that of more than 6,000 Cuban medical personnel who had worked in Haiti since 1998. Cuba has been assisted in this ambitious endeavor by financial support from Norway, which has pledged to provide $800,000 annually from 2013 to 2016 in order to assist the work of Cuban medical professionals. Venezuela and Brazil have also been major financial backers of Cuba's role, with Venezuela committing to build a new $80 million hospital in the capital. This follows an initial pledge of $2.4 billion from Venezuela after the 2010 earthquake and its ongoing financial support for Cuban medical assistance.

An Overview of Cuba's Role in Haiti

Since 1998, when Cuba first became involved in a medical internationalism program in Haiti, several themes have stood out. Above all is the importance of a focused and targeted emergency response to massive humanitarian emergencies. The international response to the 2010 crisis was enormous, although too often the best of humanitarian intentions did not translate into effective medical support for those who most needed the support. Often lacking basic medicines, and without sophisticated operating room equipment, the physicians who came from developed societies were often at a loss as to how to deal with traumatized patients. For the most part they came alone or in small groups, volunteering out of the most basic and laudable humanitarian spirit. But often these groups floundered, basically out of a manifest lack of organization on the ground in Haiti, a lack of experience and training in such appalling conditions in this immense catastrophe, or an inability to adjust to the tragic conditions. Many of the 10,000 NGOs who flocked there were not particularly helpful, often marching to their own drummer and ignoring the overall needs of the grief-stricken population.

Moreover, after the initial stage of rescuing and treating earthquake survivors (a process that lasted two to three weeks), it was then necessary to start a radical public education program for the population, showing them how to avoid—or at least reduce—the dangers of living under such squalid, vermin-infested conditions, where hygiene was so limited. Most foreign staff were unprepared to meet this need and returned to their regular medical practices. By contrast, in both the response to the emergency and the subsequent health education campaign, the Cubans took the lead.

Many spoke creole after working there for several years and, aided by Haitian students studying in Cuba, lost no time in starting such invaluable campaigns. Despite being a poor developing nation, Cuba possesses a far better emergency response capacity than many developed countries, in no small degree because of many years of experience dealing with hurricanes on the island. The head of the Cuban medical mission, Dr. Carlos Alberto García, summed up the situation just two weeks after the tragedy: "Many foreign delegations have already begun to leave, and the aid which is arriving now is not the same as it used to be. Sadly, as always happens, soon another tragedy will appear in another country, and the people of Haiti will be forgotten, left to their own fate. . . . However, we will still be here long after they have all gone."[58]

A second major theme is the need to recognize that emergency aid, while extremely important, has to give way to a sustainable public health system, accessible and free to all, with a focus on prevention (rather than cure) of disease. This takes nothing away from the invaluable efforts to help in a crisis. But preventive medicine is far more cost-effective than a curative approach, particularly when it is financially out of the reach of most Haitians. It took a massive crisis in Port-au-Prince for the world to see how much help Haiti really needed. It could be argued that Cuba saw this in 1998 when it initiated its medical support in Haiti.

The Cuban role in Haiti is respected by the local people. Most of the hospitals in which U.S. medical personnel worked at the time of the earthquake were guarded by some of the estimated 15,000 American military who had landed, while none of those run by the Cubans needed armed guards. This illustrates the acceptance of Cuban medical staff by Haitians. The main thrust of the U.S. aid effort was to provide military security, while that of Cuba was to provide medical support. Haitians are aware of the importance of the Cuban public health contribution to their country, appreciate the fact that Cubans live in extremely poor housing in the midst of the community, and do not charge for their services. Furthermore, unlike foreign NGOs that are totally independent, the Cubans work in public hospitals run by the Haitian government and at the request of Haitian officials. They take courses in creole, are active in the local communities, and are available day and night. The Cuban medical personnel and their approach to public service are key aspects of any sustainable public health service. In an interview with Marcel Young, the Chilean ambassador to Haiti, the diplomat emphasized this point clearly: "The work undertaken by the Cubans is of fundamental importance. They are working in all regions of the country, and the most admirable aspect of their role is that they didn't just arrive after the earthquake—they have been working here for many years. All of the embassies here recognize that, if we want to do anything important in terms of public health, we have to involve Cuba. There is an example of a truly exemplary solidarity. . . . Ever since I have been in this country, whenever a problem arises, the only people whom everybody respects and listens to are the Cuban doctors."[59]

A comparison of attitudes is perhaps pertinent here. On January 14, 2010, Québec premier Jean Charest announced that the Canadian province (with a large Haitian population) would send a delegation of medical personnel, firefighters, and police to help Haiti. The president of Québec's orthopedists' association then requested that the health minister, Yves Bolduc, pay these "volunteers" the $850 daily wage they would normally receive.[60] This attitude is worth comparing with that of Cuban pharmacist Dr. Idilisa Núñez, who reflected upon the suffering that she saw around her after the earthquake. The recipient of a monthly salary that was one-quarter of the Canadian per diem, she noted the reason why she had volunteered to work in Cuba: "We in Cuba have a strong culture of help and education. Wherever we're needed we must go to help humanity."[61] By 2010, Cuban medical personnel had established themselves as the frontline of medical support for Haitians. They were present in "127 of the 137 Haitian communes, had saved 223,442 lives, offered more than 14 million consultations, performed 225,000 surgeries, assisted 109,000 child deliveries, and recovered or improved the sight of 46,000 Haitians through the Miracle Operation."[62] By July 2012, these figures had increased, and according to Haitian government minister Marie Carmelle Rose-Anne Auguste, 331,724 surgeries had been performed, 140,589 births had been attended by Cuban medical staff, and 312,584 lives had been saved.[63] In 2013, it was noted that Cuban medical personnel were working in 24 community reference hospitals. A national prosthesis, orthotics, and orthopedic laboratory was being constructed to assist those who had lost limbs in the earthquake, Operation Miracle ophthalmology clinics were active, and more than 1,100 Haitian medical students had graduated in Cuba.[64] Raúl Castro has summed up the essence of this approach. Accompanied by vice presidents, government ministers, and the leaders of the Cuban army, Castro visited the Haitian embassy in Havana to sign the book of condolences there in the wake of the earthquake. He noted: "We have accompanied the Haitian people, and we will continue with them whatever time is needed, no matter how many years, with our very modest support."[65] To date, as can be seen in the Cuban response to hurricanes, flooding, a massive earthquake, and the world's largest cholera epidemic, as well as the "regular" medical treatment of the majority of Haitians (approximately 7 million), the Cuban medical brigade has delivered on this commitment.

9

Cuba's Medical Internationalism in the South Pacific

> The Cubans taught me many things. They taught me to be independent; they taught me to love people more than simply as human beings; they taught me to embody this great love and to express it in the treatment of my patients; they taught me how to live among the people; and they taught me how to make the most of the scarce resources available to them.
>
> Dr. Merita Armindo Monteiro, East Timorese graduate, quoted in Cameron, "East Timor"

At first glance the idea of Cuba having any role in this exotic area of the world seems strange. After all, Cuba has no strategic interest here, virtually no trade, and definitely no investment. It is also a poor corner of the world, with little to offer. Yet Cuba has been providing medical care to Timor-Leste since 2004, with Cuban doctors making up about two-thirds of the physicians in the country. Moreover, Cuba has trained approximately 1,000 physicians and set up a medical faculty in Dili, the country's capital, where it is now also training scores of young people from other small South Pacific island communities and has sent its own physicians to several of them to improve access to healthcare of their people.

It is difficult to imagine why Cuba would take so much interest in Timor-Leste, a small (pop. 1.14 million) and poor ($1.27 billion GDP) country. The amount received for the services of a relatively small number of Cuba's army of physicians abroad in this poor country cannot be great, while the medical students are taught for free by Cuban professors. According to the logic of a developed nation, this role seems inexplicable, given the limited benefits that could accrue. This chapter seeks to shed light on this situation, analyzing Cuba's medical missions in the South Pacific with a particular focus on Timor-Leste (also known as East Timor), which is the largest medical cooperation project of Cuba outside Latin America and the Caribbean. It is in this region that Cuban medical internationalism has continued to spread, training students from Timor-Leste and increasingly its South Pacific neighbors.

Cuba's medical collaboration in Timor-Leste is the first of its kind in the South Pacific, and it has evolved since Cuba first responded to a call for support from the newly independent leadership in 2004. This chapter starts with an analysis of the implementation of the Cuban medical model in Timor-Leste in order to highlight some of the characteristics of this approach, as well as its successes and its challenges. The chapter will then analyze some of the problems facing the South Pacific region as a whole and conclude by examining Cuba's role in other South Pacific island states. The extension of Cuban medical internationalism from Timor-Leste to other South Pacific nations is important, since it shows the widespread regional adaptation of the Cuban medical model. Many of these small, sparsely populated countries will soon have more Cuban-trained medical personnel than doctors prepared under any other medical models by the time their graduates return from Cuba and Timor-Leste. This is already the case in Timor, where there is a state-led preventive, participatory medical model. If it is true that ELAM graduates are changing the face of medicine in Latin America and the Caribbean, the same is also true in the South Pacific.

The Cuban Role in Timor-Leste

When the Cuban medical staff first arrived in Timor-Leste, they found a desperate situation. The country became independent from Portugal in November 1975, yet nine days later was invaded by the Indonesian military who took control of the country and claimed it as a province. For the next quarter-century the country was ruled with an iron fist, and massive human rights abuses occurred. Almost 25 percent of the population died through conflict, forced migration, malnutrition, and disease.[1] Following a national referendum in 1999, the Timorese voted for independence, which was finally obtained in May 2002.

Major health problems remained, however. Between 1999 and 2002, for example, the number of healthcare workers fell from 3,540 to 1,500 as the Indonesians left. There had been 135 physicians in 1999—yet three years later only 20 remained, to tend to a population of approximately 1 million. It was then that the Cubans arrived at the request of the new government, and a dramatic increase in personnel working within the public healthcare system resulted. Official data reveal the growth in this field since independence. According to the Ministry of Public Health in 2001, there were only three general practitioners in 2001 (but 75 in 2011 after the Cubans arrived), no specialists (9 in 2011), one dentist (7 in 2011), no pharmacists (15 a few years later), nor were there any junior pharmacy technicians (but 95 a decade later). Nursing staff had also increased from 462 to 1,252, as had the number of midwives (151 to 398).[2]

This poor patient-to-physician ratio in 2002 after independence was relieved somewhat by the arrival of the first 16 Cuban doctors in February 2004. They came at the request of the country's president, who had met with Fidel Castro at a meeting of the Non-Aligned Movement.[3] The impact of the new physicians was immediate, and by 2008, with the arrival of more Cuban medical personnel, "more than 2.7 million consultations had taken place, and an estimated 11,400 lives had been saved because of their medical interventions."[4] By 2008 there were almost 300 Cuban healthcare workers in Timor-Leste, yet far more significant was the contribution by Cuban professors in training Timorese medical students. By that time, some 700 Timorese were studying medicine in Cuba, and 150 were studying in the newly created Faculty of Medicine in Timor, where the teaching was carried out by Cubans. As is the case elsewhere, the Cuban government sought to develop a sustainable public healthcare system and to gradually replace the Cuban medical personnel when there was enough local capacity to take over medical care.

While many of the Cuban physicians were initially attached to the National Hospital in the capital, the vast majority were sent by the government to rural areas, at both the district and subdistrict levels. This decision was important, since it initiated the policy of healthcare delivery to areas of the country that had been traditionally neglected. There had never been resident doctors at the subdistrict level, for instance, nor were people accustomed to the daily house calls that were an essential component of the Cuban medical practice. Despite the influx of Cuban physicians, however, living conditions remained extremely poor. The country was 120th out of 177 countries in the 2010 UNDP Human Development Index. Moreover, in 2007 nearly half of the population lived on less than $0.88 per capita per day, the official national poverty line. Government spending on health increased 109 percent from 2006 to 2011, yet was still only $38.2 million or less than $60 per capita.[5] The increased presence of the Cuban medical personnel helped the population, but in light of the deeply rooted poverty it would be a slow, steady process before an acceptable standard of living could be established.

As to be expected, the Cuban doctors have been steadily replaced by Timor-Leste graduates from ELAM and the new faculty of medicine at the National University of Timor Lorosa'e (NUTL), which Cuba helped establish. The latter development was particularly important because since 2006 all incoming students now entered NUTL for medical studies instead of going to Havana. The graduates emerge from a curriculum that emphasizes "responsibility to society, critical thinking, flexibility and openness to knowledge exchange, quality with equity, long life education." Thus the teaching and learning processes are based on the approach of "'learning how to learn,' creativity, innovation and solidarity with the changes and transformations in scientific knowledge, research, social insertion, inter- and trans-discipline thinking, inter-relation and inter-dependence with other professions, and education on good and productive citizenship."[6] This is a local initiative, supported by Cuba and designed to focus on local healthcare needs, with training now done in Timor.

The Cuban doctors have been continually reinforced by local graduates each academic year as Timorese students graduated. In 2010–11, for example, 64 Timorese doctors trained by Cuban professors graduated, with 501 in 2011–12, 245 in 2012–13, "and 17 in 2013–2014, with an average of 50 students being admitted in each subsequent year."[7] At the National University of East Timor, it is also interesting to note the number of students now being trained locally, with 55 admitted in 2006 (after the medical faculty was inaugurated), 47 (2007), 47 (2008), 19 (2009), 60 (2010), and 42 (2011), for a total of 270 new doctors studying in East Timor under Cuban professors. The number of nursing and midwifery professionals has also grown, with 40 starting their studies in Dili in 2007, 75 in 2008, and 75 in 2010 and 2011.[8]

Timor-Leste will shortly have 17 times the number of doctors it had in 2002—a truly remarkable achievement in such a relatively short time.[9] This will, of course, lead to a major challenge, as the government strives to absorb this wave of over 1,000 newly minted doctors. It is also clear that, in the spirit of preventive medicine developed by Cuba for decades, a concept which was an integral part of their training, most of the new graduates will work at the grassroots level in the countryside, where the need for effective health promotion is the greatest. One recent graduate outlined the significance of the training she had received and how she perceived her mission: "In Cuba they taught us to work, but to work with love—as a doctor, a scientific doctor but a doctor with a heart. More than the work to cure illnesses, we have the responsibility to prevent it, to teach people so they can participate actively in the prevention of illness."[10]

Another challenge will be for the public healthcare service to compete with the private sector, largely composed of urban clinics run by religious groups, international NGOs, and coffee cooperatives, who together deliver 25 percent of medical care in the country. In Dili and Baucau, for instance, they own 26 private clinics. The greatest need for healthcare, however, is in the rural areas, where private clinics have little interest in working because it is not profitable. In order to meet this need, the government introduced the Integrated Community Health Service (SISCa is the Portuguese acronym) in 2008, with the objective of improving health conditions in rural villages. These are similar to the ECOS, rural clinics established in rural El Salvador, an area that faces similar problems—and where many of the ELAM graduates are also working. In Timor-Leste this farsighted government approach has resulted in the creation of just over 600 SISCas in recent years, the principal goal of which is to promote medical care within the community in a cooperative fashion, emphasizing a preventive approach to healthcare. It is hoped that this strategy will ultimately be both cost-effective and successful in eradicating avoidable diseases.

Early results are encouraging: between 2003 and 2009, for instance, under-5 mortality rates decreased from 83 per 1,000 to 64, while infant mortality rates during the same period have fallen from 60 per 1,000 live births to 45. Likewise, there has been a huge increase in immunizations, while assisted deliveries have increased from 27 to 30 percent.[11] Rural Timor-Leste is the logical place for the graduates of the Cuban program (from both Havana and Dili) to be placed, in no small part because this is where the need is greatest. So far their work in underserved communities has paid off.

The new hands-on approach to providing the appropriate medical services, emphasizing a preventive strategy to delivering public healthcare, working with the community to improve local conditions, and promoting a greater knowledge of health issues, is exactly what the Timorese medical graduates will have trained for in their six-year program under the Cubans. It was summarized well by one recent graduate: "We do not seek wealth for ourselves but rather to serve the people with a dedication and a spirit of humanism that does not see race, locality, religion, gender, or political parties, but which services all people according to the teaching of God . . . and so once more we as doctors declare that we are ready to receive orders and work in any part of the country."[12]

Graduates of the NUTL Medical School in Dili receive the title of Médico Geral Básico/Basic General Doctors upon graduation, and follow an integrated medical training that is similar to that given in Cuba. These new medical professionals are expected to have

> skills in diagnostics and therapeutics, able to provide comprehensive medical services through promotional, preventive, curative, and rehabilitative interventions on individuals, families, communities, and their living environment, by applying clinical and epidemiologic methods, with a profound social focus, embedded in ethical and humanistic values, solidarity, and good citizenship, called upon to transform the health situation in accordance with the expectations of the society.[13]

The NUTL medical school is on its way to becoming a smaller-scale regional version of ELAM in the South Pacific, having now expanded to take in students from several small island countries. By 2009, for example, there were 186 students registered at the "Medical School of NUTL (from year 1 to year 6), and 658 at various medical schools in Cuba (from year 1 to year 5)."[14] In addition there has been a small but significant increase in the number of Cuban medical personnel working in small island communities throughout the region. In all cases the role of Cuban medical personnel is clearly defined. They are there to establish solid medical traditions in the country and to strengthen the teaching of a new generation of physicians for both Timor-Leste and a number of small island countries, after which they will return to Cuba. They work where the government sends them, invariably the area of greatest need, usually rural underserved communities. In terms of their educational role as medical professors/mentors, the goal of the education process created at Timor-Leste has been summarized concisely:

> Timorese students have either been trained in Cuba or in small groups by Cuban physicians working at local hospitals and district health centers. Increasingly students from the region will be trained locally, instead of travelling to Cuba. Cuban medical personnel will also gradually withdraw, as the need for their cooperation decreases and their role as physicians and educators is filled by Timorese—who in turn will be able to use their Faculty of Medicine to train medical students from several South Pacific islands. The multiplier effect of medical personnel is thus the goal, with the intention of gradually reducing the number of Cubans as local practitioners fill the vacuum.[15]

Cuban medical professors conduct the basic hands-on training to the students at NUTL and act as mentors. All 13 districts of Timor-Leste have district team lecturers with training locations onsite. They are supervised by a coordinator, who oversees 13 districts, and reports directly to the dean of the NUTL medical school. In other words, there is a direct connection between the medical school and the Cuban personnel working at the grass-roots level. In terms of personnel in 2009, there were "78 certified lecturers distributed throughout the 13 teams, and 146 medical doctors, nurses, and health technicians holding a certificate in pedagogy, who are also part of the district teams."[16] In this way medical coverage for previously underserved areas is implemented, while Timorese medical students receive hands-on training. This is the antithesis of the traditional approach in developing countries, an urban-based system that is costly to maintain and uses a technology-based pedagogy which is often rendered ineffective in areas with limited access to reliable electricity.

Despite the progressive approach to medical training, as well as the opportunities given to hundreds of young people who otherwise could not dream of becoming physicians and the clear need for their services, problems remain. The rapid development of the Cuban-sponsored program, and the addition of over 800 physicians within a decade, will understandably pose many problems for the Timorese government as it deals with this massive scaling-up. Part of the challenge facing medical authorities in Timor-Leste is resolving the differences between the public sector Cuban-trained doctors and those (educated abroad) from earlier medical training programs who emphasize private practice. The latter are few in number but traditionally have held positions of influence within the national healthcare system. By contrast, in addition to working at hospitals performing functions at outpatient and inpatient settings, the Basic General Doctors are "prepared to work at the facilities of the national health system and particularly those of primary care such as health posts and villages, health centers at sub-districts and districts, which are the main venues to provide comprehensive health services."[17] Australian academic Tim Anderson quotes the perspective of Ildefonso Da Costa Nunes, one of the first graduates of the Cuban-Timor-Leste medical program. Da Costa Nunes explains this challenge, noting that medical practitioners from the traditional system

> don't want to work in the sub-districts, they all go to private clinics. . . . But we can't think just of money, but rather how we can develop this country. . . . Those [patients] who go to a private clinic have money, and those who don't have money have to go to the public

> system. . . . There has to be a balance between the private clinics and the public health system. . . . We eighteen, we're going to do a project . . . which is social, which is human for this country.[18]

Clearly many medical personnel trained in traditional capitalist models find the challenges of working in distant rural areas or with impoverished populations hard to bear, and they prefer working in more lucrative urban locations. Anderson has explained the context of the sweeping changes that are occurring in Timor-Leste:

> Almost a thousand new doctors are emerging in a system which has less than one hundred, and they have been trained with a public health service ethos which has begun to confront a system dominated by a small, established profession embedded in an elite culture and a network of private clinics. This clash of cultures, in terms of vision and ethos, is quite similar to that seen in many other countries—such as Bolivia, Venezuela, and Honduras—with large Cuban health training programs. In Timor-Leste, as in those other countries, jealousy and obstruction have at times undermined the potential for collaboration and cooperation.[19]

It is a familiar debate in several Latin American countries, where graduates of ELAM face major obstacles placed in their way by members of the established medical elite and its traditional approach to medicine.

Regardless of these tensions, however, as well as the different models of medical training, the stark health problems of Timor-Leste remain as major challenges. The country is extremely poor, and it faces many health challenges, as data from 2010 reveal. Life expectancy at birth was 60.2 for females and 58.6 (males). The maternal mortality rate was 557 per 100,000 live births, while the infant mortality rate was 44 per 1,000 live births and the under-5 mortality rate was 64 per 1,000 live births. The total fertility rate was high at 5.7 per woman. The lack of adequate nutrition resulted in 53 percent of children under five with stunting conditions, while 52 percent were underweight.[20]

The main causes of morbidity and mortality were acute respiratory tract infections, malaria, diarrheal diseases, and tuberculosis, all of which could be avoided or at least drastically reduced with better living conditions, improved sewage disposal, and access to safe drinking water. The same Ministry of Health report noted that 27 percent of the population did not have access to safe water, while 57 percent had no access to safe sanitation facilities. More than one-third of the Timorese population lived at least 10 minutes away from a safe water source. The 850 medical students trained in Havana and Dili thus faced major health challenges. The context was explained clearly by a Timorese doctor who graduated in 2011 and who is the head of the Department for Control of Contagious Diseases at the national health ministry: "There's a lot of ignorance in rural areas. People don't know about hygiene, about clean water, about hand-washing and wearing shoes."[21]

While the Cuban medical cooperation program in the South Pacific region is concentrated in Timor-Leste, it has had a multiplier effect, and its impact has steadily spread throughout the region among the smaller islands, which also faced the problems of insufficient medical personnel and inadequate public healthcare. While still not large, the combination of medical training (both in Cuba and increasingly in the NUTL medical faculty in the Timorese capital, Dili) and provision of Cuban medical personnel is having a notable impact on several other small island communities where the Cuban medical role is steadily increasing.

Java

In 2006 the Cuban medical response to a devastating earthquake in Java became so popular that locals asked Cubans to stay on. The medical team of 135 Cubans saw up to 1,000 patients a day at two field hospitals during the first two months after the earthquake. Within this crucial period, the Cuban medical team treated 47,000 patients, immunized 2,000 people against tetanus, and performed 900 operations. One of the more interesting aspects of this medical cooperation is that approximately half of the Cuban doctors were women. This has proven a great advantage because in Muslim countries women are often reluctant to be examined by a male doctor. A UNICEF worker witnessed that the Cuban teams "treat patients like people, not just cases"—an aspect of the ethos embedded in the Cuban medical training.[22]

Pacific Island Countries (PICs)

There is no doubt that there is a need for an increased medical presence in the small islands of the Pacific, as can be seen from a comparison of the significant vital statistics of several of them with Australia. The need is particularly acute in rural areas. The situation is further exacerbated by the decision of qualified medical personnel to leave for more lucrative positions in developed countries. Given these pressures, the role of Cuban-trained doctors is significant, filling a pressing need. The contrast between Australia, the wealthiest country in the region, and all others in the area, is stark indeed. For example, the infant mortality rate is nearly 10 times greater in Kiribati, while the maternal mortality rate (4 per 100,000 live births in Australia compared with a shocking 470 on Papua New Guinea) reveals a massive gulf. The amount spent per capita on healthcare also illustrates the great divide between a wealthy country and seven others that are in the same geographical area but that, in terms of access to public health, might as well be on a different planet. While in Australia the figure is $3,357 per annum, one should not expect much attention in Vanuatu ($111), the Solomon Islands ($113), Fiji ($118), or Papua New Guinea, where a paltry $65 is spent.

The situation is complicated by the trend of many medical graduates from the South Pacific to head north to obtain far better salaries in industrialized countries. Many Pacific Island Countries (PICs) have had extreme difficulties in retaining medical personnel and not losing them as part of the "brain drain" phenomenon—mostly to Australia and New Zealand. As Negin highlights, in the 2006 census data there were 652 "Pacific Island born doctors and 3,467 Pacific Island born nurses and midwives . . . [that were] working in Australia and New Zealand, more than half of whom [were] from Fiji with significant numbers from Papua New Guinea, Samoa, and Tonga as well."[23] This brain drain occurs despite the incredibly low health workforce density in their home countries—a situation that is particularly bad in rural areas.

The former health minister of Timor-Leste has compared Australia with select PICs in terms of medical personnel and illustrated some of the clear differences.[24] For instance, the density of doctors per 10,000 people for Australia was 33, with Tuvalu coming the closest at 9 and Nauru at 8—while the rest of the PICs were between 5 and 1 doctor per 10,000 people. The number of nurses fared little better. While Australia, for example, has 130 nurses per 10,000 population, Nauru was the next closest PIC at 48 and Tuvalu at 45. The rest of the countries in the region were between 30 and 13. The worst distribution was Papua New Guinea, which has an atrocious ratio, with five nurses per 10,000 people to go along with its one doctor per 10,000 people ratio.[25] Clearly the situation for access to medical care in the region is extremely poor and is made worse with the exodus of local personnel.

Another challenge for these countries is the high cost associated with importing medical personnel from abroad, a process which has reinforced issues of dependency due to the exorbitant costs incurred. The response in many South Pacific countries in the last 10 years has been to gradually move away from the traditional models of western medicine and toward a Cuban model of sustainable social medicine, as is well documented by Anderson in some of his research.[26]

Cuba's regional cooperation has now extended beyond Timor and the Java region of Indonesia to a number of small Pacific Island nations where it is training medical personnel and providing support to address key health issues. In their findings, Asante et al. track the evolution of Cuban health assistance.

> Diplomatic relationships between Cuba and the countries in the Pacific were largely initiated in the early 2000s, except for Vanuatu, where such relations began in the early 1980s. In 2004, cooperation between Nauru and Cuba led to the arrival of 11 Cuban doctors. However, their contracts were terminated ahead of schedule due to language difficulties. Over the next few years, bilateral agreements between Cuba and a few PICs were signed and some Cuban doctors arrived in the region. However, these relationships were made more concrete in September 2008 when the first Cuba–Pacific Islands ministerial meeting was held in Havana and representatives from ten Pacific countries—Fiji, the Federated States of Micronesia, Kiribati, Nauru, Papua New Guinea, Samoa, Solomon Islands, Tonga, Tuvalu, and Vanuatu—attended.[27]

At first glance the numbers of Cuban medical personnel look small, and compared with medical cooperation programs in Latin America or even Africa, they are. Their impact, however, is great indeed. To put this in context, the 33 Cuban medical personnel account for one-quarter of the 120 medical workers found in the Solomon Islands, Kiribati, Tuvalu and Vanuatu.[28] Asante et al. provide the most recent account of Cuban medical personnel working in PICs. By 2010, Tuvalu had 5 Cuban doctors, the Solomon Islands had 10, Kiribati had 16, and Vanuatu had 2.[29] The numbers of Cuban medical personnel in the area, although small, show a clear trend, as does the number of students being trained by Cuba.

Data for 2012 illustrate this growing role of Cuban doctors in the region. In Timor-Leste the government had approved 200 medical personnel, of whom 159 were already in the country. Comparative figures for Kiribati showed 10 and 6 who were already working, for Tuvalu 5 and 2, and Vanuatu 5 and 5. Perhaps more significant was the number of students from the area studying medicine under Cuban medical professionals: 922 from Timor, 31 from Kiribati, 90 from the Solomon Islands, 19 from Tuvalu, 25 from Vanuatu, 9 from Mauru, 8 from Fiji, 3 from Palau, and 6 from Tonga. They were to graduate between 2010 and 2016.[30]

As can be seen, Cuban medical personnel are offering a significant service for these low-populated and geographically small PICs. More importantly they are training hundreds of doctors from the region. This is the core of what may be considered the first replication of the Cuban medical approach to become the dominant medical model for many countries in a region. Within 10 years of their return from Cuba's ELAM program and increasingly from medical training in Timor-Leste, where they will follow a Cuban approach, these doctors will become the majority of local personnel. They will also shape their previously understaffed medical systems, especially in rural, marginalized areas. A new type of doctor and a new approach to community health will eventually be found throughout this region.

Introduction of ELAM in Pacific Island Communities

Asante et al. document that 177 Pacific Island students were studying medicine in Cuba in 2010.[31] Thus the relatively small number of Cuban doctors in the region is supplemented by the training of a new generation of local students. This is a microcosm of the policy that Cuba is implementing in Timor-Leste. In Cuba's western ELAM campus located in Sandino, the number of medical graduates from PICs will undoubtedly result in a major improvement in the delivery of medical care to their relatively small populations. As of 2010, in terms of students on full Cuban government scholarships, there were 75 from the Solomon Islands,[32] 20 from Kiribati,[33] 30 from Tuvalu,[34] 9 from Nauru,[35] 37 from Vanuatu,[36] three from Tonga,[37] and 6 from Fiji.[38] Some case histories are worth examining to illustrate the significance of Cuban cooperation.

Kiribati

The impact of the work of Cuban personnel has been noted throughout the region. In 2007, for example, Radio New Zealand reported how the arrival of 10 Cuban doctors in Kiribati had reduced the child mortality rate by 80 percent—from 50 in every 1,000 to 9.9.[39] Six more doctors were to arrive at the request of the Cuba-Kiribati cooperation committee's request. The increased medical personnel's efforts are noted in an April 2012 Cuban diplomatic report. The report shows that between 2006 and 2011, Cuban doctors

> made 329,303 physician visits, dealt with 127,089 cases of pediatrics, 43,019 children under one year, and 27,975 obstetric cases. In the same period, 411 lives have been saved, [Cuban medical personnel] opened 21 new services, and were given 11 training courses to national staff. 4,610 surgeries have been performed and have attended 1,922 births, including 286 cesarean surgeries.[40]

Community care is noted as one of the key aspects of this Cuban medical involvement, and in this report it was noted how Cuban doctors had treated 71,363 patients in 10 communities they oversaw. This effort has seen a marked reduction in infant mortality, falling from 16.5 to 6.9 per 1,000 live births. The addition of the Kiribati medical graduates trained by Cuba,[41] whose numbers are estimated to be between 20 and 31, will result in an important increase of the number of doctors (only 20 in 2009), improving the physician-patient ratio of two doctors per 10,000 population.[42]

The Solomon Islands

After seeing the success of medical programs in Timor-Leste and Kiribati, the Solomon Islands also began recruiting Cuban doctors. The Cubans have had a notable impact on the health profile of islanders, and the graduation of physicians from the medical school in Dili will continue to improve accessibility to healthcare. Prior to 2007, the Solomon Islands had approximately 10,000 patients for every doctor.[43] With 80 percent of the population in rural areas among its 350 islands, medical accessibility has been a challenge for this nation of 500,000. The country's training of doctors (5 to 10 annually) has only kept pace with the number of doctors leaving for more lucrative posts abroad. As a part of the Solomon Islands bilateral agreement with Cuba, 10 Cuban doctors arrived in May 2007 in an effort to help with the poor doctor-per-patient ratio that improved to 1:3,300 by 2012.[44] The first cohort of 25 Solomon Island medical students departed for Cuba in February 2008, with the remainder (25 each year) following in July 2008 and December 2009, bringing the total to 75, which was 25 more than the initial agreement of 50.[45]

Until these medical students graduate, the Solomon Islands' public healthcare system depends largely on the services of Cuban physicians. The Health Minister of the Solomon Islands, Clay Forau, noted that the cost of employing Cuban doctors was much less than recruiting doctors on the international market. The local government pays approximately $300 a month as an allowance to the Cuban doctors, as well as their living expenses and return airfare. (An undisclosed retainer is also paid to the Cuban government.) This has turned out to be a much cheaper alternative to the reliance on other doctors employed locally who were currently earning $170,000 per year. What was even more unaffordable was the cost of bringing in doctors from the international market, a process that, according to the Ministry of Health, used to cost taxpayers approximately $400,000 each per year. Apart from the financial advantage that resulted from employing Cuban physicians, it is also worth noting that the Cuban doctors have substantial experience in dealing with certain diseases such as malaria which are problematic for many South Pacific nations, and are accustomed to working in underserved rural communities.

In the Health Ministry's 2007 budget documents, it was noted that there were 196 vacancies in the country. Clearly, considering the cost of doctors on the international market as well as those from the traditional medical system, importing doctors from developed countries would have been prohibitively expensive. At the Solomon Islands' largest hospital in Honiara, for example, there were 11 such vacancies for doctors and an additional 20 more vacancies in other provinces. The situation was much worse in rural areas, one example being the Malatya region's hospital, which was supposed to serve 122,620 people but which had only three doctors prior to the Cuban medical accord.[46]

The Cuban Cooperation agreement shows no signs of letting up in the face of the ongoing health challenges faced by Solomon Islanders, and recently a request was made for a further 40 Cuban specialists.[47] With the return to the country of 75 Cuban-trained doctors in 2013 and the medical agreement in place, the Solomon Islands will finally be able to provide sustainable medical accessibility for its rural population.

Fiji

For a nation which has almost as many of its Fijian-born doctors working in Australia and New Zealand as there are working in their home country, Fiji clearly has its share of personnel challenges.[48] In addition to the staggering effects of the brain drain on Fiji's ability to develop its medical workforce, it has also had trouble in encouraging the remaining medical personnel to work in rural areas. Fiji's ambassador to Cuba, Peter Thomson, has noted that eight Fijian students in Cuba were "making good progress."[49] In 2012, four of the "Fijian students [were] in the first year of the six-year course to qualify as medical doctors. The other four [were] working through the Pre-Med year, which includes learning to speak and read Spanish."[50]

In addition to the return of these future graduates, the bilateral medical cooperation agreement between Cuba and Fiji is expected to expand. In April 2012, it was reported that the Cuban first deputy foreign minister, Marcelino Medina González, would lead development cooperation talks with Fiji regarding the possibility of recruiting Cuban doctors:

> Fiji's New York Mission was provided with a mandate in October 2011 by Fiji's Foreign Affairs Ministry, the Ministry of Health, and the Public Service Commission. The discussions with the Cuban authorities were about the recruitment by Fiji of Cuban medical doctors to serve in Fiji's rural areas. Minister for Foreign Affairs and International Cooperation Ratu Inoke Kubuabola said talks and negotiations were currently under way and a draft agreement should be finalized this year. Cuba is recognized globally as a medical powerhouse, especially in fields of child maternal health and groundbreaking surgery. Cuban medical specialists have been working in the Solomon Islands and Kiribati in recent years and have brought immediate improvements in health services and systems there.[51]

Australia might also participate in the program. Anderson, who has written extensively about the Cuban role in Timor-Leste, has noted that the Australian government had traditionally chosen to ignore the Cuban role in the region, despite it being by far the largest medical cooperation program ever in the South Pacific region. However, the Australian government has taken notice that Cuban internationalism may actually constitute a major contribution to solving complex medical issues and medical personnel shortages within the region, as the specific case in Fiji may come to highlight.

In 2011 Australia's parliamentary secretary for Pacific island affairs, Richard Marles, said in an interview with ABC Radio Australia that Australia was engaged in a "scoping study of Cuban experts and Australian experts." He believed that Cuba's effort at improving healthcare was crucial because a healthy population is "probably the key social indicator." As a response to Cuban success, Marles said the Australian government wanted to look at ways in which they could "leverage the Cuban [medical] expertise against our presence in the South Pacific to do something really important" since "they are engaged in developing assistance for the same reasons we are."[52]

If this triangular cooperation is ever established, it will lay the groundwork to establish "the provision of medical training for Fijian students, the reciprocal visa agreement between Fiji and the Republic of Cuba, and draft Article of the Agreement from the Cuban National Institute of Sports in 2011" between "the Republic of Cuba, AusAID, and Fiji."[53] Hopefully the expansions of Cuban involvement will help to meet the challenges facing the Fijian people. Support from Australia, the country that most benefits from Fiji's brain drain, would be beneficial. As of 2014, however, and following the election of a Conservative government there, apart from drafting a program to teach English to Cuban doctors, little of consequence has been accomplished to support Cuban medical training in the Pacific community.

Nauru

Although Nauru was the first PIC to benefit from the Cuban health assistance program, the initial 11 Cuban doctors who arrived in 2004 had their contracts ended 18 months later due to language difficulties. However, as noted above, Nauru currently has 9 students abroad studying at ELAM who, upon graduation, will be a huge boon to healthcare for the 11,218 island residents, as well as the two Cuban doctors working there.[54] With a male life expectancy of 56, well below the regional average of 72 years, Nauru has significant health challenges. Jonathan Hopper of 3rd Degree writes that only "seven per cent of Nauru's population was over the age of 60 in 2009." The 3rd Degree article highlights a conversation with the acting secretary of health and medical services in Nauru, Dr. Lepani Waqatakirewa, who noted there were "14 [local] doctors in Nauru servicing an estimated population of 10,582." Thus the two additional Cuban doctors scheduled to arrive would equate to roughly "one doctor looking after 661 people each."[55] Thus the return of 9 to 14 medical graduates will cut the patient-to-doctor ratio by half for this country—a country that is the second smallest nation in the world next to the Vatican.

Tuvalu

As Julie Feinsilver explains, even though the numbers of Cuban doctors working in PICs is relatively small, their impact is great. For instance, the original three Cuban doctors who arrived in Tuvalu on October 2008 "attended 3,496 patients [and had] saved fifty-three lives" by February 2009.[56] In addition to this, doctors had delivered 76 babies, including the first 11 caesarean sections, and 47 major surgical operations—the first ever to take place on the small South Pacific island.

Doctors have also opened up abortion services as well as specialized consultation services dealing with diabetes, chronic diseases in children, and hypertension. In the hopes of developing long-term capacity for the small island nation, Cuban doctors implemented a family medical model in order to train local staff as well. Cuban specialists developed several courses in primary healthcare so that the local population would be able to provide medical access for Tuvalu's previously underserved population.[57] In the Tuvalu Ministry of Health Strategic Health Plan, they note that with the "addition of four doctors from Cuba, the recently built Princess Margaret Hospital, strong senior leadership, and new analytic equipment due to be installed, [Tuvalu] could provide an example of [the] best Pacific small country health practice."[58] Once again, the basic Cuban model of working with the local community, of developing a preventive healthcare model, and of grassroots campaigns in public healthcare have proved successful, particularly for the traditionally underserviced sectors of the population.

Vanuatu

In 2010 the Vanuatu Ministry of Health noted that there were only 29 local doctors who were aided by three doctors from Cuba. A comparison with Australia is pertinent in order to illustrate the context, for while Australia has 33 doctors and 130 nurses/midwives per 10,000 inhabitants, Vanuatu has only 1 doctor and 17 nurses.[59] With the return of their 24 to 37 medical graduates from ELAM, Vanuatu will have doubled their number of doctors.[60] Understandably this development will have a major impact on the health profile of this small country.

Cook Islands

On June 1, 2012, the Health Minister Nandi Glassie met with the Cuban ambassador to New Zealand in order to discuss possible health scholarships to Cuba for young Cook Islanders. Minister Glassie noted in the report that resulted that, given the "continued decline in the number of scholarships available to Cook Islands over the years [from other nations], the scholarships offered by Cuba [were] particularly welcome and [the Cook Island]

Government look[s] forward to bringing these opportunities to fruition through Ambassador Caseiro and our High Commission Office in Wellington."[61] Cuba is thus not only supplementing current efforts to capacitate the local medical system but also stepping into traditional aid roles that have been vacated by other developing countries which continue to address global economic issues and tightening of fiscal budgets. Cuba's role in training physicians in the area has become increasingly important, especially for Timor-Leste, a process which started in 2003. By September 2013, the country had seen 486 doctors graduate (with a further 500 in various stages of their training). Many students from other communities were also being trained by Cuban professors: 90 from the Solomon Islands (since 2008), 31 from Kiribati (2005), 25 from Vanuatu (2008), 9 from Nauru (2009), 19 from Tuvalu (2008), 6 from Tonga (2012), 3 from Palau (2012), and 8 from Fiji (2012).[62]

Concluding Thoughts

South Pacific countries, poor, small, and with significant geographic obstacles, can ill afford to adopt a western healthcare system while providing medical accessibility to their rural and vulnerable populations. There is a desperate need for qualified medical personnel, particularly doctors and nurses who will stay in their communities. A focus on curative healthcare with accompanying higher wages and utilizing large amounts of resources, advanced technology, and expensive imported drugs is unsustainable for these countries. Moreover, often the most basic services are unavailable. Former president of Timor-Leste José Ramos-Horta put it well: "Now at least basic services are available, but we still don't have enough equipment. . . . For decades we've not resolved the problem of electricity. How can you have even a functioning hospital if electricity always breaks down?"[63] In addition, the continued exodus of talented doctors and nurses to more lucrative positions in Australia is a major blow to any attempt at stable planning for the delivery of healthcare services. Particularly affected are rural and marginalized populations who are often overlooked and underserved.

The Cuban approach to healthcare is radically different. The case history presented here (of Cuban medical cooperation in developing healthcare service delivery in several countries of the South Pacific region) reveals an interesting development, however, since the Cuban medical model will become the dominant paradigm for the many countries in the region within the next few years. Cuban medical personnel, bolstered by the training of indigenous students (taught by Cuban professors, both in ELAM and locally at the Dili campus) have developed a model that is clearly adaptable and increasingly established in the South Pacific. It is also clear that this approach has had a major impact on the health of people from the region, as well as on the model of basic healthcare delivery. For the first time, too, there is a cadre of doctors trained in the Cuban tradition that is choosing to stay in their homelands, since Timorese graduates make a commitment to work for at least six years in their home country.

This is an important development, since a brain drain of medical personnel continues to plague developing nations that wish to retain their healthcare workforce. In Fiji, for example, despite its repeated attempts to scale up its workforce under the traditional medical model, it has continued to lose more doctors and nurses abroad than are willing to stay in the country, let alone work in rural areas. Even though Fiji has received much support from Australia and has one of the most advanced western medical models in comparison with other Pacific Island neighbors, it continues to struggle with the basic notion of "health for all." This support from Australia is sadly lacking in its dealings with other countries in the region, even though it gains significantly from the importation of medical professionals from the region. Lee Rhiannon, speaking in the Australian Senate in March 2009, noted how the government had decreased the number of university scholarships to students from Timor-Leste from 20 to 8 between 2002 and 2007. During the same time, the senator noted, Cuba increased its scholarships from 50 to 1,000.[64]

The cost of importing doctors from abroad is also incredibly prohibitive as a reliable means to solving the health workforce shortage, most aptly illustrated in the Solomon Islands example by Wasuka.[65] Importing expensive doctors for low-GNI countries has only been shown to reinforce the dependency on foreign medical personnel, further driving up the need for aid or "handouts" from developed neighbors. Before Cuba's response to requests for help in the South Pacific, the importation of expensive foreign doctors has been the norm—a policy which has yielded poor results and is clearly unsustainable. That has now changed.

Of particular importance to this discussion is the Timor-Leste example. The radical adaptation of the Cuban medical model, on a scale not seen anywhere else outside of Latin America, is unique. In addition, the adoption of the Cuban medical education model at the new faculty of health at NUTL is already showing impressive results regarding its contribution to the development of its medical workforce, especially in rural areas. In areas where the Cubans work, for example, child mortality has been reduced to 27.5 per 1,000, more than 50 percent lower than other regions of the country.[66] With further measures in place to support its most vulnerable and rural populations, the decentralized healthcare model's adaptation has been successful. The training of the students, both in Havana and in Dili, has also produced a new type of activist, community-oriented physician to meet the challenge. As Maria Monteiro, a 2011 graduate from Timor-Leste, noted: "It's a tropical, underdeveloped country. We can't just sit there in the hospital waiting for the patients to come to us. We have to go where the people live. And the doctors who go to the rural districts are the ones who were trained in Cuba—because we made this commitment to our government."[67]

Even though the most significant long-term aspects regarding the retention of the workforce and further evaluation of health indicators of this particular adaptation have yet to be seen, this may become the most promising and comprehensive way to combat brain drain in the region. That said, the government will have to face a major challenge in paying salaries for the wave of Cuban-trained physicians now flooding back, a task that will not be easy. In addition, resolving tensions between physicians trained in the traditionalist school and the ELAM graduates, who have a clearly different approach, will also be a challenge.

Each adaptation of the Cuba medical system throughout the South Pacific highlights a larger significance of the "healthcare for all" problematic. With traditional medical models failing to provide this basic service, especially in rural and marginalized areas, the expansion of Cuba's preventive community-oriented primary care medical model seems poised to become the dominant model for many countries in the South Pacific region. A generation of Cuban-trained medical personnel will soon be providing medical care throughout the region and providing evidence of a successful alternative to the traditional public health model. Tim Anderson puts this contribution in perspective:

> Without doubt the most powerful cooperation program in the region in recent years has been the Cuban health cooperation. Placement of Cuban doctors in many of the islands . . . has been impressive, and their house visits and emphasis on preventive health is new to the region. Yet even more impressive is the huge training program. Almost 1,200 students from the islands have been studying medicine with the

> Cubans, either in Cuba or under Cuban supervision. No other health aid program has helped build human capacity like this.[68]

Much like the arrival of a few dozen Cuban family doctors in Venezuela in April 2003 developed into a massive medical cooperation program with some 30,000 Cuban personnel now working there, the Timorese example has also flourished. Nobody could have imagined the arrival of 16 Cuban doctors in Timor-Leste in 2004 would have developed so successfully. By September 2013 a total of 891 Cuban healthcare personnel had worked in Timor-Leste since 2004, mainly in remote areas of the country, with 148 there in late 2013.[69] In Timor-Leste, the focal point of Cuban medical cooperation, nearly 3 million consultations had taken place by mid-2012, and over 11,400 lives had been saved between 2003 and 2008.[70] The development of an innovative patient-centric health paradigm, soon to be run by young local physicians trained in the Cuban mold, has also prepared the way for a totally new approach to healthcare delivery. It will bear watching.

10

The Children of Chernobyl

25,000 Treated

> While many other countries, rich countries, have shown pity, Cuba has shown its solidarity, helping to increase health and save thousands of children and young Ukrainians.
>
> Leonid Kuchma, former president of Ukraine, 2010

The Nuclear Meltdown

On April 26, 1986, an explosion occurred at the Number 4 reactor at the nuclear power plant of Chernobyl in Ukraine, some 80 miles northwest of the city of Kiev. This led to a steam explosion and fire, resulting in the meltdown of the reactor and a huge release of radioactive material into the atmosphere. The temperature rose to 2,500 degrees, melting everything nearby, and a cloud of radioactive dust spread. Radioactive pollution was released, 500 times the amount resulting from the atomic bomb in Hiroshima. While many countries in northern Europe experienced the fallout from the explosion, those most affected were 2 million in Belarus, 3.5 million in the Russian Federation, and 2.7 million in Ukraine.[1]

So immense was the impact on the surrounding area that 350,000 people from all over the former Soviet Union came to help. Given the potential for massive health problems, the nearby town of Pripyat (pop. 45,000) was immediately evacuated, and within three weeks 116,000 people living within a 30-mile radius were relocated. A further 220,000 were subsequently resettled, and local authorities increased the initial exclusion zone to incorporate 4,300 square kilometers.[2] In all, 8.4 million people were exposed to abnormally high levels of radiation. Approximately 150,000 square kilometers were contaminated, and 52,000 square kilometers of agricultural land were ruined.[3] The average life span of Cesium 137 (a radioactive isotope) is between 20 and 50 years, and so it will take decades for the area to return to normal—so great was the nuclear tragedy.

The impact on the health of the surrounding population was immediate and devastating. Between 1987 and 2004 half a million people died in the Ukraine, with 2.3 million suffering health problems, including 500,000 children.[4] Life expectancy plummeted to just over 50 years for men in surrounding towns, and cancer rates soared. Ionizing radiation has resulted in significant increases of leukemia among those most heavily exposed to the radiation. There has also been a rise in the number of people with cataracts and an increased risk of cardiovascular disease. Of particular concern to medical officials was the large number of children with thyroid cancer, the result of drinking milk that had been contaminated with radioactive iodine (which had settled in pastureland). Indeed, 5,000 cases of thyroid cancer have been diagnosed in children who were under 18 at the time of the nuclear accident. To place this in context, this represents a 30-fold increase in thyroid cancer. Other radioactive nuclides found in the environment are cesium, strontium, and plutonium, all of which have had major impacts on health.

The World Health Organization concluded that an additional 4,000 cancer deaths were to be expected.[5] This does not take into account the many other long-term medical problems also caused by radiation. The impact on mental health was also great, given the stress about health problems, relocation (and destruction in many cases of traditional family and friendship ties), unemployment, and feelings of frustration and sorrow. This was, of course, taking place just as the Soviet Union was starting to collapse, resulting in mass confusion and uncertainty about the future. Yet there are limited data on such unseen mental health concerns.[6] Perhaps most troubling is the fact that nowadays some 270,000 people still live in areas with high radioactive levels, clearly an unhealthy situation. On April 26, 2012, UN secretary-general Ban Ki-moon summarized the extent of the disaster, remembering "the more than 330,000 people who were evacuated from surrounding areas with little hope of return; the thousands of children who later contracted thyroid cancer; and the six million still living in the affected areas of Belarus, the Russian Federation, and Ukraine."[7] Put simply, this nuclear disaster was the greatest since the bombing of Nagasaki and Hiroshima in World War II, and its impact will be felt for decades.

The International Response to Chernobyl

The gravity of the Chernobyl accident was clear, and the government immediately appealed for international support. Until the fall of the Soviet

Union, the most significant support came from the socialist countries in the region. When the Soviet Union imploded in 1989–90, the situation became much worse, since there was little funding to alleviate the problem in these impoverished regions. People in the countries affected still suffered from profound health issues, but there was no longer any command structure in place: the Russian volunteers no longer came, nor was there any financial support from Moscow. Several international organizations began to participate tentatively in programs to assist the population, but little of substance was accomplished in the years immediately following the collapse of the Soviet Union. The most common form of assistance was for associations of expatriates to bring children from the affected areas to the West, where they usually spent short vacations with families of Ukrainian origin.

There were, however, several international conferences that talked about the need for concerted action, as the medical problems continued to mount. In April 2011, one of the major conferences on the lessons to be learned from Chernobyl was held in Kiev. Sponsored by four UN agencies, there were many sessions on the impact of the explosion 25 years earlier. According to official documents, the objective was to "provide scientifically sound information for Chernobyl-affected communities" and "sound practical advice for residents of the affected territories." The repetition of the "sound" nature of their conclusions in the press release in many ways sums up the empty rhetorical approach of UN agencies, which have talked a lot about the need to help those affected but have not actually been overly supportive.

The release noted how the UN Children's Fund (UNICEF) and the European Union (EU) "have been helping children in Ukraine since 2006" (i.e., fully twenty years after the reactor meltdown, but not before). The EU ("one of the largest donors of UNICEF in Ukraine") was supporting projects in Chernobyl and the Khmelnitsky region "to the amount of almost U.S. $2 million."[8] In 1997, together with Israel NGO Chabad's Children of Chernobyl, UNESCO issued a commemorative stamp to draw attention to the plight of children in the affected region. Some 11 years after the nuclear meltdown, the total budget of UNESCO in Chernobyl was $2 million.[9] Given the hundreds of thousands of people affected by the events of Chernobyl, this was clearly a minimal contribution—a useful token of support, but a token nonetheless.

A significant contrast can be drawn between money provided for the people of the affected region by UN agencies and funds given by governments and international banks to contain the damaged reactor. The EU gave $2 million to help children in the affected region, whereas the European Bank for Reconstruction and Development donated a staggering 550 million Euros to build a protective shell over the remains of Reactor 4 measuring 275 meters wide and 105 meters high. In another international conference in Kiev on the same anniversary, 28 nations contributed to a fund that would encase the failed reactor and deal with nuclear waste for the other three reactors (the Shelter Implementation Plan and the Spent Fuel Storage Facility for the other three units, which had been decommissioned). The total cost of the Shelter Implementation Plan would be 1.54 billion euros, of which 990 million had been received by 2010.[10] While it is hard to argue against the goals of the New Safe Containment facility, the differences between the amount of money spent on this building and that given to the care of the hundreds of thousands of people affected directly by radioactivity seem extraordinary, and they illustrate the priorities of governments and international banks.

On a smaller scale there have been dozens of initiatives undertaken to assist the people of this region. In 1990 Israel offered to provide medical assistance to 50 Jewish children affected by the disaster. In North America two basic approaches have been implemented, both sending material aid to the affected region and also bringing children for respite vacations to Europe and North America. The Chernobyl Children's Project International, based in New York, has focused its efforts on sending humanitarian aid to Belarus. In 2005, for instance, a convoy of trucks and ambulances and 60 volunteers brought $3.2 million of material support to the region. In 2004, two medical missions had been sent to Belarus, one to evaluate 200 children for cleft lip/cleft palate surgeries, while the other provided cardiac surgery for 25 children.[11] Another organization, the Friends of Chernobyl Centers in the United States, was established in 1996 and by 2010 had sent over $500,000 in financial support, training, and medical supplies to the areas affected.

Perhaps the most successful of these grassroots organizations was the Irish NGO, Chernobyl Children International, set up in 1996, which has provided over 91 million Euros in aid and has brought 22,000 children to Ireland for two-week respite stays in their Rest and Recuperation program. Less successful have been smaller activities undertaken by celebrities, such as those of Irish rock star Bono, English fashion designer Stella McCartney, and Danish model Helena Christensen, which were individual events designed to raise funding for Chernobyl projects. While they generated attention to the needs of the region, they only resulted in limited financial support.

Given the high rates of thyroid cancer that have resulted in the region, the International Federation of Red Cross and Red Crescent Societies has concentrated its efforts in dealing with thyroid cancer screening, principally for people under 40 years of age. Using six mobile diagnostic laboratories, they have screened more than 1,230,000 people since 1997 and have detected 171,000 patients with thyroid pathologies, resulting in 2,050 operations.[12] Their budget for 2010–11 was $883,039, which is sufficient to screen 180,000 people and provide multivitamins to 60,000 children.

After the reactor meltdown, the Soviet Union and the socialist countries of Eastern Europe came swiftly to the assistance of the affected areas. Later, with the fall of the Soviet Union, western nations took up the initiative. Several programs resulted, mainly at the level of smaller NGOs (implementing people-to-people exchanges) and at the multinational level (especially with extensive funding being awarded for the encasement of the Chernobyl reactors). The latter strategies can perhaps be seen as being less altruistic, since one of the goals was to prevent the spread of nuclear contamination outside the affected zone to other countries. Comparatively little has been spent on helping the thousands of people affected by this tragedy. Moreover, after the initial years following the Chernobyl implosion, other natural disasters elsewhere became the new focus of the international community, and as a result initiatives to help the victims petered off. Political tensions between the Ukraine and Russia and a subsequent increase in military spending further reduced any funds available for those affected by the nuclear meltdown.

The Cuban Response

The Cuban approach was very different. At the time when Havana drew up its program to treat victims of Chernobyl, its economy was in freefall following the collapse of the Soviet Union. Preferential prices paid for Cuban exports had disappeared, as had oil supplies from the former Soviet Union (which had accounted for approximately 90 percent of Cuba's fuel needs). Cuba's capacity to import fell by 75 percent with resulting shortages of food, spare parts, and energy, since some 80 percent of its trade had been with the (now defunct) Soviet bloc. GDP fell by 35 percent, hundreds of factories closed, and tens of thousands of Cuban workers were left unemployed. For anybody traveling in Cuba at this stage of what the government called the "Special Period in a Time of Peace," it was a depressing picture indeed. The average Cuban male lost 20 lbs. in weight, and 52,000 Cubans went blind (mainly on a temporary basis) because of a vitamin deficiency. It was clearly not the best time to launch a costly venture of humanitarianism to support a poor country in Eastern Europe, particularly when the former socialist countries of Europe were turning their backs on Cuba.

Despite being in dire economic straits, Cuba pushed ahead with its Chernobyl initiative. The first victims arrived in March 1990 and were received in Havana by Fidel Castro. They would continue to come to Cuba for medical treatment until December 2011, 21 years later. About 25,000 people were treated, most of them children. Between 1990 and 1992, some 2,700 children and 213 adults from Russia, as well as 671 children and 59 adults from Belarus, came to Cuba. However, the vast majority of patients throughout this period were Ukrainian children. For several years the Cuban program received 2,000 patients each year, although in most years this was reduced to an average of 700 to 800 and only from the Ukraine, all of whom were required to belong to a family from within the area affected by the Chernobyl disaster.

In early 1990, the Cuban government sent a group of medical professionals to investigate the health problems in the Ukraine and to see how Cuba could be of assistance. During their assessment, 139 children suffering from the effects of the nuclear explosion were selected for treatment in Havana. These children mainly had cancer-related conditions, some extremely serious. From the outset, the Cuban program was intended to be a humanitarian mission, providing medical care as well as compassion. The patients paid nothing for their medical care, accommodations, food, or any activities during their stay on the island. They were only expected to pay for their transportation or have the Ukrainian government pay for it. In the cases of the younger children, they were required to bring a close relative to ensure that they did not feel too isolated or lonely, and their living costs were also covered by the Cuban government.

Cuban solidarity was now put to the test as it pushed ahead with this program to assist thousands of very sick children—at a time when many of its own were going to bed hungry. The place chosen for this exercise in humanitarianism was Tarará, some 10 miles east of Havana, which in prerevolutionary times had served as a place for the Cuban middle class to seek refuge from the stifling summer heat on its nearby beaches. Hundreds of summer homes had been built there. In the early years after the Batista dictatorship was overthrown, Che Guevara also convalesced here, recovering from asthma. After the revolution, when most of the owners left for the United States, it was used by the Pioneros youth organization as a summer camp, and an estimated 2 million children stayed there over the years. When the town was turned into a camp for the Cuban youth organization, a polyclinic was established, and in the 1980s, when there was a dengue epidemic in Cuba, this clinic was expanded to become a midsized hospital.

Now the Pioneros were asked to forego their summer camp and turn it over to the children who started to arrive from Eastern Europe in March 1990. It was in many ways an ideal place for the children (and a small number of adult patients) who came to Cuba for treatment. Tarará has just over 500 homes, a cultural center, a movie theater, two large sports fields, a store, and a school. It also had a stretch of beach about a kilometer long. The central hospital there had a 350-bed capacity as well as other treatment centers and laboratories. At the height of the "Children of Chernobyl" program, 400 people worked there, including 50 doctors and 80 nurses.

In the spring of 1993, I visited the camp for the children of Chernobyl for the first time. It was a very moving experience to meet and talk with dozens of children suffering from a variety of diseases, from cancer to alopecia. The director at the time was Dr. Carlos Dotres (later to become minister of health), and I was visiting the camp with a group of my students from Dalhousie University in Canada. In addition to talking with the children who were residing there, we also met with their parents and several members of the Cuban medical staff. Fortunately we had some students among our group who were able to interpret our conversations with the Ukrainians. One key memory from that encounter of twenty years ago stands out, the result of a private conversation with Dr. Dotres about this ambitious program.

The context of this conversation was important, because Cuba suffered the worst moments of its economic crisis in 1993–94 after the fall of the Soviet Union. It was a depressing time to be in Cuba, and signs of hunger and frustration were clearly visible. How could Cuba undertake such a venture when the economy was in such disastrous shape, following the recent implosion of the Soviet Union and the virtual rupture of ties with its major trading partners in the socialist COMECON common market? The Cuban economy was in tatters, there was massive unemployment, food supplies were scarce, and transportation was badly curtailed following the end of oil imports from the Soviet Union. Perhaps more pertinent, there were also major shortages of medicines for the Cuban population. So how could the medical treatment of foreigners be justified? I remember clearly

Dotres's emotional reply to my questions: "These are children, extremely sick children. How could we **not** treat them?" He added that, because of his medical training, every instinct told him that these children had to be cared for, whatever the cost. "Until the Comandante en jefe tells me otherwise, the doors will not be shut to sick children, wherever they come from."

Speaking at a celebration to commemorate the seventh anniversary of the arrival of the first group of victims from Chernobyl on March 29, 1990, Dotres reflected on the significance of the Cuban reaction at the time. He referred to Cuba's spirit of cooperation in the affected area in 1986, citing Ukrainian press reports of Cuban students who traveled to a Kiev hospital and offered blood and plasma for the victims, immediately after hearing of the accident at the nuclear reactor. Ukrainian ambassador Oleksandr Taranenko noted how many foreigners fled the country fearing for their health, while the Cubans were examples of heroism and solidarity, remaining and offering to help. For Carlos Dotres, the Cuban role illustrated how always "true solidarity is more profound, of greater value, when the challenge is so great."[13]

It is important to note that most of the approximately 26,000 patients who took advantage of Cuba's invitation were not mortally ill. In addition to the medical treatment provided, the main advantage of their stay (usually about six to seven weeks) was to offer them respite in a warm climate, with cultural and educational activities, excursions, and general child-related activities in a region that, unlike their home region, was uncontaminated. Other patients, however, with more serious diseases such as lymphoma, cancerous tumors, and serious kidney problems, spent months and in some cases even years in Cuban hospitals receiving treatment. Significantly almost all of them suffered from medical conditions that had developed several years later in the aftermath of Chernobyl and not at the time of the actual reactor meltdown, illustrating the long-term effects of the accident. All of the children were tested for levels of Cesium 137, and almost two-thirds had relatively high levels, a factor which could lead in later life to the risk of congenital malformations. DNA testing and cytogenetic studies were carried out in cases of high levels, to both treat the patients and determine a prognosis.

In an article published in 1995 in the Revista Cubana de Pediatría, Dotres and several colleagues spoke about the early stages of planning for the arrival of the children and the treatment provided at Tarará.[14] When Cuba decided to begin treatment of the children, they sent to the affected area a team composed of an interpreter, hematologists, pediatricians, psychologists, and endocrinologists in order to assess the health condition and needs of the children. (A small Cuban medical team remained in the area, working in a Ukrainian sanatorium, throughout the 21 years that Cuba provided medical care for their patients.) On average between 5,000 and 6,000 potential patients were assessed by this team each year, and at its peak every two months some 250 children were selected for the trip to Cuba. Many were orphans or came from extremely poor families and were selected on the basis of their medical needs.

While the patients had already been examined in their home countries by a team of Cuban physicians, and basic medical information on their condition had been provided to colleagues at Tarará, they were submitted to a battery of tests during their first week in Cuba. The medical team sought to determine the general health condition of the children, outline actions for their treatment, implement a program of physical and mental care, develop a prognosis, and plan a strategy for follow-up treatment. A detailed clinical history was prepared, and laboratory specimens were taken, particularly focused on ascertaining the impact of the iodizing radiation received. An integrated program of treatment and rehabilitation was then drawn up for each patient. They were treated not just for the specific pathology that had been identified when they had been initially screened in the Ukraine, but also for any and all medical conditions that were discovered following their thorough examination in Tarará. In addition detailed care was given to ensuring proper dental care. This was important because cavities among the children were a common problem, due to the limited availability of dental services in the Ukraine, and basic dental hygiene was also taught to the children.

The first 139 children to arrive in Havana on March 29, 1990 were seriously ill and had a variety of cancer- and blood-related disorders. They were examined at the Institute of Hematology and the oncology service of the Juan Manuel Márquez pediatric hospital in Havana. Several thousand children were suffering from major medical conditions in the affected areas, and in July the intake of patients increased. The Pioneer camp at Tarará was rapidly turned into a place to receive hundreds of children.

Cuban Ministry of Public Health (MINSAP) officials classified the patients into four basic groupings. The first group included those children with severe problems. After their arrival in Cuba these patients were transferred to one of the major tertiary care hospitals for specialized medical treatment. These included the William Soler and Juan Manuel Márquez pediatric hospitals, the Hematology Institute, the Frank País Orthopedic

Hospital, and the Hermanos Ameijeiras Hospital, as well as centers specializing in pediatric cardiology and radiation pathologies. These children with life-threatening conditions represented 3 percent of the total number of patients. They traveled with a family member or guardian to provide moral support and, depending on their recovery, generally stayed in the hospital for long periods, sometimes years. Patients with chronic pathologies, but who could be cared for in the 355-bed hospital located at the Tarará camp and various hospitals and clinics in Havana, made up the second group of patients. They represented 17 percent of patients. If they were under eight years of age, they were required to travel with a close family member.

The third group treated at Tarará were children with clear medical conditions but who were ambulatory and could receive treatment in primary healthcare facilities (approximately 60 percent of all patients). They were treated through the Tarará outpatient services, and they generally stayed in the cottages at the resort for 45 days. If required, they returned to Tarará on an annual basis. The final group were children who were relatively healthy but who lived in the contaminated zone and needed further medical screening to determine if there were any residual conditions that needed to be treated (20 percent).[15] Many of the illnesses related to the disaster do not show symptoms until later—such as leukemia, heart disease, and thyroid cancer. More than anything else, this latter group received respite care. (Based on a sample of 8,000 children at Tarará, 27 percent came from areas that had not been affected by radiation, 25 percent were from areas with different levels of radiation, 23 percent from areas that had been evacuated, and 25 percent from areas in which the level of contamination was unknown. Levels of internal contamination were noted in just over 60 percent of this sample.)

Children in the latter two groups who required primary healthcare attention lived in residences in Tarará, where their medical needs were provided by a family doctor and nurse for each 50 children, supported by specialists in comprehensive general medicine, pediatrics, and psychology, as well as a team of hygienists, epidemiologists, nurses, and interpreters. At its peak there were 50 doctors and 80 nurses (as well as a support staff of nearly 300 more) working in Tarará. Particular attention was paid to children with dermatological conditions (such as vitiligo, alopecia, psoriasis, and dermatitis) and to patients with cancer-related pathologies. A specialized computer division was also established, and it maintained a thorough clinical history of each patient. A battery of detailed medical tests was prepared for each patient, and in particular the impact of exposure to nuclear contamination was investigated. To place this in context, there were 174,992 laboratory analyses carried out on the patients, as well as 15,937 microbiological studies and 50,788 imaging tests.

For the vast majority of the children (most of whom were between 9 and 14 years of age), the experience at Tarará provided them with the opportunity to rest and relax after the major disruptions and significant health difficulties that they had faced at home. They received excellent medical care, and the treatment in Cuba also provided an opportunity to escape from the various tensions at home. At the Tarará camp there were several activities provided for the children, in addition to time on the beach and sailing. These included access to the library, discotheque, cinema, and theater. Excursions were also provided to the zoo, aquarium, museums, Lenin amusement park, and the Botanical Garden. Children were allowed free telephone calls to relatives in the Ukraine, and those remaining in Cuba for long-term care received schooling from a team of Ukrainian teachers. On average, at any given time there were 160 patients at Tarará, supported by 17 interpreters.

While most of the children did not suffer from life-threatening conditions, and while all benefited from the stress-free conditions living next to a tropical beach in an area that was contamination-free, all had been badly affected by the nuclear meltdown. Ukrainian children, for example, faced a 30-fold increase in thyroid cancer. One journalist in 1991 summarized the major conditions: "More than half have thyroid problems; about 20 percent have digestive problems from contaminated food, and equal numbers have glandular problems or 'Chernobyl syndrome' (generalized symptoms including nausea, headaches, and constant fatigue.)"[16] They may have enjoyed playing on the beach, but they were clearly sick.

Most of the patients had suffered enormous psychological trauma. As a result, particular care was given to their emotional needs by a team of psychologists, and of course having a close family member present was of great assistance. (As noted, all accommodation costs for accompanying relatives were paid by the Cuban government.) The mental health problems of the children should not be underestimated, as they were in the midst of tremendous stresses back home, as the Soviet Union steadily disintegrated, and their family members in the Ukraine faced an uncertain future. Dr. Xenia Laurenti, deputy director of the program at Tarará, placed this in the appropriate context when she explained, "If you ask a Ukrainian child what he or she would like the most, the answer is not 'toys' but rather 'to be healthy.' That aspect has been fixed in their psychological makeup. And so part of our program here is focused precisely on psychological rehabilitation, on not rejecting any kind of pathology. Our goal is to heal."[17]

The children had indeed been through major trauma. Many were sick and had relatives back home who were also ill or who had died. They had all been forced to evacuate their homes, leaving their entire belongings behind. There was the uncertainty about what they would do afterwards, where they would live, or even how long they would live. Their parents were also under extra stress, having left their homes, family ties, and possessions, and most were without employment. Additionally, this was happening against the backdrop of the dismantling of the government and the sense of security under which they had lived for decades. Now it was unclear what the future would bring. Significantly these mental health concerns of the patients evolved in time, as the extent of the societal changes in the former Soviet Union unfolded. In the first decade of treatment, for example, most of the children suffered from post-traumatic stress disorder, along with feelings of anxiety, depression, and low self-esteem. In the second decade of the program, problems with adapting to the new economic order following the collapse of the USSR were far more common.

Throughout the two decades that the program operated, very sick children continued to arrive in Cuba. So while most came for shorter respite programs, it is also true that many also came for specialized medical care. A detailed internal study prepared in early 2012 by the staff in Tarará indicates the origins of the patients and the medical conditions from which they suffered. In terms of the origins of the patients, it is clear that the vast majority (86 percent) came from Ukraine (18,477 children and 3,964 adults), while there were 2,715 children and 213 adults from Russia. There were 730 patients from Belarus (671 children and 59 adults), with a small number from Armenia (9 children and 2 adults) and Moldavia (2 of each group). In all 26,114 patients were treated between 1990 and the end of 2011.[18] Of the pediatric patients (21,874), most were under the age of 14 (2203 were younger than 5, while 4,814 were between 5 and 9 years of age, 12,480 were from 10 to 14, and 2,377 were over 15).

It is important to emphasize that the program in Tarará was an integrated medical treatment plan, which followed a detailed assessment in the affected area and a week of medical tests and assessments when the children arrived. Unlike other approaches used in different countries which offered two-week programs of respite care with local families, the Cuban strategy emphasized an integrated medical and psychological approach for the patients. This can be seen also in terms of the medical conditions diagnosed by the medical staff at Tarará. In terms of chronic morbidity, several conditions clearly predominated. The most common medical conditions were related to endocrinology (12,822 cases diagnosed), gastroenterology (10,634), dermatology (9,225), and dentistry (7,346), although typically many patients suffered from more than one chronic condition. A sample of the first 18,910 children at the camp revealed that 59 percent had endocrine system problems (thyroid hyperplasia being the most common), followed by digestive tract disorders (57.6 percent), adenopathies (30.4 percent), and nose/throat conditions—mainly chronic tonsillitis (29.3 percent). In later years a variety of genetic malformations, especially in the kidneys, and a variety of skin disorders (such as alopecia and vitiligo) became more common.[19]

It is also useful to remember that Cuban medical personnel carried out 1,687 major surgeries and a further 5,466 surgical procedures during the course of the program. In all 7.7 percent of patients were operated on. Of the 1,687 in the first group, the majority (780) underwent general surgery (most commonly involving operations on the thyroid gland), with 343 being for orthopedic surgery. In particular scoliosis (an abnormal curving of the spine) was a major pathology, and a program of physiotherapy and rehabilitation (with the supply of appropriate equipment) as well as surgery when necessary, were provided at no cost to the patient. The surgery was carried out in several tertiary care Havana hospitals and often involved subsequent operations, with the support of surgeons from differing specialties. There were also 18 complex cardiovascular operations, as well as 300 on children suffering from leukemia, 99 to remove malignant tumors, with six receiving bone marrow transplants and two kidney transplants.

In terms of patients suffering from endocrinology conditions, hyperplasia of the thyroid was the most common (affecting 23.1 percent of patients). Many children (48.6 percent) suffered from problems with the digestive system, and 60 percent of the children had endoscopy tests to diagnose conditions. Some 54.8 percent of children showed evidence of chronic gastritis, with 39.5 percent suffering from chronic duodenitis, while many (34.5 percent) suffered from giardia (infection of the small intestine). Many children, exposed to high levels of radiation, had major dermatology conditions (22.2 percent suffered from vitiligo, and 14.3 percent from alopecia). Children with hair loss received a daily treatment of the application of a lotion made from human placenta, followed by daily infrared light sessions. Hair loss was understandably a major concern, particularly for adolescent girls, who were treated with particular sensitivity. It is worth noting that patients with these severe health problems stayed an average of six months, receiving frequent treatment. In the case of patients suffering from vitiligo, there was a noticeable improvement—90.3 percent saw the pigmentation grow back—while 86.4 percent of alopecia patients experienced a regrowth of hair.

Perhaps the most serious medical condition of the Ukrainian children were cancer and hematological illnesses (122 had different types of leukemia, and 6 required bone marrow transplants). The others were treated with radiotherapy and chemotherapy, according to the needs of each case. A further 267 had major hematology-related problems. In some cases these cancer patients spent several years in Cuban hospitals (mainly at the Juan Manuel Márquez and William Soler pediatric hospitals), receiving specialized care.

In Synthesis

In October 2011 Ukrainian president Viktor Yanukovych visited the Tarará site and announced that in the future his government would pay for medical costs of children from the affected area. This commitment was well received in Cuba since, despite crippling economic circumstances, for over twenty years the Cuban government had offered a high quality integrated approach to all of the patients affected by the Chernobyl tragedy. As Dr. Julio Medina, director of the medical program at Tarará, explained to me in a December 2012 interview, from the moment that patients arrived in Cuba, all costs—food, accommodation, and medical treatment—were borne by the Cuban state as were those of accompanying family members.

These costs have been extensive, and of course there has been no economic gain to Cuba. While Cuban government officials have not provided data on the expenses incurred, in 2010 the International Fund for Chernobyl (a Ukraine-based NGO) estimated the cost in medications alone for patients as being $350 million. That is certainly an underestimate, yet it gives some idea of the contributions made by Cubans, particularly at a time when their own economy was crumbling and they were facing severe hardship. The costs of the medical treatment of these thousands of patients over two decades has never been published, but would be in the billions of dollars. One mother of a patient at Tarará noted that medical care for her son (with a rare hearing disorder) at home in Ukraine would cost over $105,000.[20] And this as a time when less than 10 miles away habaneros were going hungry, struggling to make ends meet in a hostile economic climate.

Not surprisingly, there were mixed emotions in Cuba about this example of medical internationalism. Cuba was caught in the fierce grip of blackouts and food shortages as people sought medicines for their own relatives, while knowing that the "Chernobyl children" were being treated so well for their own medical conditions.

"Cuba has borne the great financial burden carrying out the Children of Chernobyl Program, but today it's time to offer you appropriate remuneration for these services," noted Yanukovych.[21] He added that his government "did not have the right" to close the program, and despite Ukraine's own economic challenges, "We will maintain it. We will not abandon it—and you will have our complete support."[22] His comments mirror those of former Ukrainian president Leonid Kuchma, who had visited the children in Tarará in 2010 and made a similar commitment: "The new government will provide assistance for this program. The most important aspect is to have the financing in place, and I am absolutely convinced that we will receive it."[23] He conferred the Order of Merit (First Degree) upon Fidel Castro and the Order of Prince Yaroslav the Wise (First Degree) on Raúl Castro—appropriate recognition, although the Cuban government would undoubtedly have preferred more tangible benefits.

To date, however, the Ukrainian government has not delivered the promised economic support, and in early 2013 the last of the Ukrainian children left Tarará to return home. The hospital and houses remain active, and medical services are now focusing on the needs of foreign students housed in the Tarará area as well as of the local population. However, in many ways it is an unbecoming and rather disappointing end to a program that had been so successful—and for which the need clearly still exists. Indeed the impact of radiation on the area surrounding the defunct reactor will be felt for decades to come.

There are several reasons that help to explain the Cuban government's decision to develop this ambitious program of international cooperation. As is obvious, there has been no economic gain for Cuba in this 20-year process. Rather, this has been a huge drain on the country at a time when it was facing an enormous financial challenge, a struggle for survival. There is no doubt that political considerations were an important element in the decision to make this magnanimous gesture in 1990, since in many ways it represented a significant and symbolic manner of thanking the Soviet Union and its socialist allies for 30 years of support in the face of U.S. aggression. The maintenance of the program at Tarará may also have been a despairing gesture to its former allies to not forget Cuba as it faced an extremely uncertain future in 1990 and, if circumstances in Eastern Europe stabilized, to reconsider a working relationship with its erstwhile comrade.

The program also fell victim to its own success, a beacon of international cooperation against all odds, making it difficult to close once it had become such an example of humanitarianism and such a major success. Finally the role of Fidel Castro is also important, since he visited the children at Tarará on many occasions and, according to the hospital director, frequently called to follow their progress. As in so many diverse aspects of Medical Internationalism, his strong personal interest had a major impact.

Useful medical lessons were learned. For example, the treatment of the victims of Chernobyl offered Cuban researchers an excellent opportunity to learn about illnesses caused by radiation, and the collection of primary data on the impact of radiation was an invaluable by-product of the decades of care. For instance, this experience helped Cuban officials to treat some 50 people in Goiana, Brazil, who had also been exposed to Cesium 137. New medications and approaches to cure illnesses of the patients were developed, such as pilotrofina (used to treat alopecia) and coriodermina (an effective treatment for psoriasis).

The Cuban support for the Children of Chernobyl was an exceptionally magnanimous gesture, and undoubtedly would have been appreciated by the governments in the areas affected. But Cuba's role goes far beyond being a "gesture," and its continuation for over two decades—a period when Cuba was passing through an excruciatingly difficult period, and its own people were suffering badly—shows a significant humanitarian dedication. Dr. Julio Medina, director of the medical program at Tarará, has explained this well: "Many people who are unaware of our ideals still wonder what Cuba might be after. . . . It is simple: we do not give what we have in excess; we share all that we have."[24]

It is wrong to dismiss the Cuban humanitarian offer to the victims of Chernobyl as a cold political gesture, undertaken to curry favor with its former trading partners. If the Chernobyl program had been in effect just from 1990 to 1994 (when it was manifestly clear that there would not be any return to the Soviet past), then there might be some potential value to that argument. After all, there were no benefits that could accrue to revolutionary Cuba after the former socialist countries deliberately turned their back on Cuba and demanded hard currency for goods and services—money which Cuba clearly did not have. In fact, some of the most strident critics of Cuba since that time have been former allies, most notably Poland and the Czech Republic.

So if we are to search for an explanation as to why Cuba maintained this program until December 2011, we have to go beyond questions of simple geopolitics and some unusual international political strategies. Rational political explanations alone clearly do not explain the exceptional degree of humanitarianism shown by Cuba for over 20 years (in exceptionally difficult economic circumstances) to these victims of the Chernobyl nuclear explosion, children after all. Indeed, as other examples of medical internationalism in this book illustrate, there is a complex amalgam of factors at play. Here we see one major component of that program—the treatment of approximately 23,000 children between 9 and 14 at an enormous cost to Cuba, but without charging the victims of Chernobyl. In March 1990, as he received the first seriously ill contingent of children, Fidel Castro commented, "They are going to have the best doctors, the best medical care, the best hospitals, the best medicines that exist in the world. This cooperation of ours is a very basic duty."[25] It is also a fitting explanation which illustrates many other facets of medical cooperation a la cubana, which are studied in this book and for which logical First World explanations do not always apply. Julio Medina's summary ("We do not give what we have in excess; we share all that we have") is a mantra often repeated to summarize Cuba's medical internationalism. At times we fail to grasp its full meaning, influenced by our own experiences and sensitivities and limitations, because we cannot imagine such a magnanimous gesture being taken by our own governments. The Cuban response to Chernobyl illustrates that, in fact, another response is possible.

11

Cuba's Medical Internationalism in El Salvador since Hurricane Ida

> That degree of solidarity which has been generated by the Cuban medical personnel . . . that unquestioning support which they have shown to our people—these are qualities which we would like to see spread to all our countries in Latin America.
>
> Dr. María Isabel Rodríguez, minister of public health of El Salvador, interview, February 25, 2010

Former Cuban foreign minister Felipe Pérez Roque has summed up Cuba's approach to the basis of solidarity contained in medical internationalism: "We don't give out our leftovers; instead, we share what we have."[1] This sentiment echoes the opinion of Dr. Julio Medina, director of the Chernobyl children's program studied in the previous chapter, and illustrates the widespread acceptance of medical internationalism in government circles. This chapter focuses on the role of the Cuban medical brigade in El Salvador since its arrival in November 2009. It begins with an analysis of the actions of the medical personnel in the face of the natural disaster caused by Hurricane Ida—the original motivation for the arrival of the brigade. In the first three months after its arrival, the Brigada Médica Cubana Salvadoreña Mons. Oscar Romero saw some 50,000 patients, visiting half of them in their homes. But the multifaceted nature of the work undertaken once the immediate health needs had been met is also exceptional, and the second half of this chapter studies the evolution of this contribution to improving the health of the population of El Salvador. The objective is to evaluate the Cuban contribution to both emergency medicine and public health needs in this country.

It is surprising that Cuba would become involved in El Salvador, given the animosity that existed between Havana and the right-wing government in San Salvador. During the Salvadoran civil war (1980–92), which led to the death of 75,000 people in a country the size of the state of Massachusetts (just over 8,000 square miles), Cuba was often vilified. The war had been fought between the United States–supported military government and five left-wing guerrilla groups (later united as the FMLN), and after the war the right-wing party ARENA held power until 2009, when it was defeated in elections by the FMLN. Death squads, torture, and disappearances had been the order of the day for many years, as had rule by the military and right-wing governments. Not surprisingly, Cuba was identified as one of the principal enemies of the country.

Yet despite the lack of diplomatic relations with the Salvadoran government of the day, Cuba provided medical support on various occasions. For example, a large Cuban medical mission came in 2000 and stayed for two months to participate in the nationwide campaign against dengue. Two years earlier, the devastation of Hurricane Mitch in 1998 was in many ways a watershed in bilateral relations. It resulted in the death of 240 people and severe damage to 10,000 homes. Cuba responded by inaugurating the Escuela Latinoamericana de Medicina (ELAM) in Havana, designed primarily to train doctors from the populations of the Central American countries most affected by Mitch. As a result, in the early years of ELAM, most of the graduates were Central Americans. Again it should be remembered that, despite not having diplomatic relations with several of the countries in the region, hundreds of Cuban doctors came to Central America in the aftermath of Mitch. Cuba trained more than 1,000 physicians from the region (at no charge to the medical students) during a period when diplomatic relations had still not been established between Havana and El Salvador, Guatemala, and Honduras. The situation improved in 2009 with the election of journalist Mauricio Funes of the FMLN as president, resulting almost immediately in the normalization of relations with Cuba. Since then medical cooperation, reflecting improved diplomatic ties, has grown. This chapter examines the experience of Cuban medical support following Hurricane Ida and the impact that it has had since then.

The Cuban Response to Hurricane Ida

Hurricane Ida arrived on the morning of November 8, 2009. The communities of San Vicente and Verapaz were the worst affected. In Verapaz alone, some 355 millimeters of rain fell in just four hours, the same amount that fell when Hurricane Mitch devastated Central America in 1998. This occurred at the end of the rainy season, when the ground was already sodden and therefore incapable of absorbing more water. Twelve rivers overflowed their banks, 200 mudslides occurred, over 2,000 homes were destroyed or severely damaged, 77 bridges and 117 schools were damaged, crops were devastated, and over 200 people were killed (some bodies were never recovered). Others were swept 20 kilometers away by the force of the rivers. Damage was estimated at $2.5 billion, and approximately 14,000 people were forced to seek refuge in schools and churches. For miles the jagged sides of the mountains revealed where boulders had crashed down onto the village below, destroying everything in their way.[2]

The Salvadoran government declared a state of emergency and appealed for international support. Following the report from Cuba's ambassador, Pedro Pablo Prada, Havana responded within days, sending a brigade of 18 specialists in disaster medicine (all members of the Henry Reeve contingent). Their medical background was a microcosm of the training needed for natural disasters of this kind, involving specialists in epidemiology, pediatrics, obstetrics and gynecology, internal medicine, and public hygiene. They arrived on the morning of November 13 and headed directly to San Vicente. Shortly afterward the earthquake in Haiti resulted in the head of the Cuban mission being sent there in a supervisory role, while one of the epidemiologists was seconded to the Salvadoran Ministry of National Public Health and Social Assistance as an adviser to the national dengue program, at that point facing a potential epidemic. The rest remained based in San Vicente (about 1.5 hours from the capital), where they continued to work—attending to patients on a daily basis but increasingly involved in other public health activities. The Cuban medical brigade set up a field hospital in one of the principal town squares of San Vicente as soon as they arrived and received their first patients that afternoon. By the end of the day, they had seen 215. They remained working in the town square, seeing 250–300 patients a day. The team consisted of four general medicine specialists, three epidemiologists, a pediatrician, a gynecologist, two hygienists, three nurses, a laboratory specialist, a logistics technician, and the head of the mission.

Cuba's prompt response to the request for international assistance by the Salvadoran government, as well as the length and nature of the mission, was summed up by Ambassador Prada: "We have responded to the request of the Salvadoran government, and we are prepared to collaborate until the president of the Republic, Mauricio Funes, decides otherwise."[3] Healthcare was thus to be provided at no cost to the Salvadoran people, Cuban medical staff were to be located where the government of El Salvador indicated that they were needed, and they would remain for as long as the government wanted them to stay. In an extremely polarized society such as that of El

Salvador, the conservative media lost no time in criticizing Cuba's medical role, forcing the ambassador to clarify the strictly humanitarian goal of the mission.[4] The support given by Salvadorans to the role of both the Cuban staff and the hundreds of Cuban-trained medical graduates from El Salvador has been a telling response to media manipulation.

The Initial Tasks of the Brigada Médica Cubana Salvadoreña Mons. Oscar Romero

The primary objective was to help the tens of thousands of displaced people directly affected by the hurricane, and several steps were taken simultaneously. The field hospital (stocked initially with medicines made in Cuba, soon to be supplemented by medical supplies from the Salvadoran government) was the clearest and most obvious symbol of Cuban cooperation. All were welcome to seek free medical treatment, and the first patient was the mayor of the town, a member of the political opposition, ARENA. He and other local authorities emphasized the medical, humanitarian objectives and thanked the Cuban brigade for their support. The common theme stressed by Cuban medical staff was their focus on cooperation and their desire to serve the people. Meanwhile, diplomatic and medical leaders met with local officials (hospital and clinic directors, functionaries of the state government, the mayor and members of the council, and local directors of health) to emphasize their commitment to serve where they were most needed. By the second day of their arrival, together with local officials, they had drawn up an integrated health plan for the affected regions. Later as their medical mission intensified, they widened the circle to meet with officials from other states and the national government. At all times the Cuban medical personnel worked where they were requested by local health officials—usually where the needs were greatest.

It soon became clear that there was danger of a major dengue outbreak. Dengue has long been a problem in El Salvador, and in September 2000 it reappeared, with almost 3,000 cases being diagnosed and 32 people dying of hemorrhagic dengue. At that time 37 Cuban specialists flew to El Salvador to participate in a massive national campaign and stayed for two months.[5] Almost a decade later, their expertise was again called upon.

While the majority of the Cuban staff remained at the San Vicente field hospital, others fanned out, offering care wherever it was needed. Accompanied by Salvadoran health promoters and medical volunteers (including dozens of Salvadoran doctors trained at ELAM), the Cubans visited every home. This extensive visitation, which took place in 23 communities and for which a detailed checklist of every family was completed, formed the basis for a comprehensive diagnosis.[6] The checklist, found in table 11.1, illustrates the organized nature of the Cuban strategy. Each member of the Cuban medical staff carried a large backpack, full of the most common medications, as they visited each home in order to provide immediate relief where it was needed.

Cuban medical training emphasizes the need for an integrated approach to treating patients, who are seen as unique socio-psycho-biological beings. It is thus crucial to understand the patient's environment, since it could have a major influence on any resultant pathology. This includes everything from their diet to family relationships, from the level of domestic hygiene to alcohol consumption. All elements are considered in order to determine an accurate diagnosis. The home environment is thus carefully observed and analyzed. In the case of the medical survey in San Vicente, patients were asked about medical conditions, but other elements were also assessed such as sewage facilities, garbage disposal, access to water and food, and the presence of vectors. This helped Salvadoran officials to understand the nature of challenges awaiting them so they could prepare an appropriate strategy.

Cuban medical officials, together with their Salvadoran counterparts, also visited on a daily basis the emergency shelters now occupied by local inhabitants whose homes had been destroyed. Approximately 1,400 people were evacuated, and 600 chose to stay in local emergency shelters (mainly schools), while others moved in with friends and relatives. These people faced different challenges, and Cuban medical personnel provided first aid and ongoing medical care and assessed everything from access to latrines to proper food preparation. A major concern was the need to avoid the spread of infectious diseases, particularly with hundreds of people sharing such cramped living quarters. They continued to visit these shelters twice weekly for three months.[7]

Cuban medical personnel are trained to maintain rigorously detailed records. This was also clearly the case with the Henry Reeve Brigade in El Salvador, and a perusal of their data illustrates the extent of their collaboration. Table 11.2 covers the period from November 13, 2009, to February 22, 2010, with data obtained from the interim brigade leader, Dr. Eduardo Ojeda.

A useful point of comparison can be made between the medical cooperation of Cuban personnel and that of other nations, especially the approach

Table 11.1. Form used by Cuban personnel to evaluate health profiles in areas affected by natural disasters

Municipality_________ District_________ Date_________
Address of the dwelling_________________________________
Name of head of family_________________________________
Number of family members_________________________________
Sex: M___ F___
Age groups of family members: Under 15______ Under 1______
Over 15______ Over 60______
Pregnant women: Yes___ No___ Receiving medical attention: Yes___ No___
Trimester of pregnancy: First___ Second___ Third___
Suffering from any medical conditions: Yes___ No___

Medical Conditions Noted

Condition	Yes	No	Under 15 (No.)	Over 15 (No.)	Total
Acute respiratory infections					
Fever					
Diarrhea					
Diabetes mellitus					
Arterial hypertension					
Asthma					
Dermatosis					
Anxiety					
Other conditions					
TOTAL					

Current state of Dwelling
Habitable______ Inhabitable______

Water Consumption
YES NO
Bottled water
Piped in
Rain water tank
From other source

Disposal of Human Waste
YES NO
Solar latrine
Over a dug hole
Toilet
In the open air
Common latrine

Food
YES NO
Donation
Own supply

Garbage Disposal
YES NO
Regular collection
Buried
Burned
Not disposed of

Presence of Vectors
YES NO
Flies
Rodents
Mosquitos
Mosquitos bite during the day

Table 11.2. Accumulated data on the work of the Cuban medical brigade in El Salvador, November 13, 2009, through February 22, 2010

Medical consultations	<15 years	>15 years	Total
No. of cases seen	16,234	33,036	49,270
(Of these, no. seen at home)	10,249	15,035	25,284
Pediatric consults	16,233	0	16,233
(Of these, <1 year old)	1,144	0	1,144
Obstetric patients	5	272	277
No. of lives saved	13	11	24

Source: "Brigada Médica Cubana en El Salvador," internal report produced February 22, 2010, by the Henry Reeve medical brigade in El Salvador.

used by their U.S. counterparts. The Canadian government, which has a rapid response team (DART) for such emergencies, decided not to send it, but instead offered $40,000 to the International Red Cross Federation and $50,000 through the Canada Fund for Local Initiatives at the embassy.[8] Medical delegations from Guatemala and Spain came to help, according to CNN.[9] The U.S. military also assisted: 45 members of U.S. Southern Command's Joint Task Force Bravo, located at the Soto Cano Air Force base in Honduras, sent four helicopters, a medical assessment team, and engineers. In terms of the Medical Civil Action Program (MEDCAP), this was scheduled to run from November 19 to 23, with 10 U.S. doctors, and at first glance their goal sounded like that of the Cubans: "Our main focus is going to be primary care and preventative medicine," noted their liaison officer.[10] This, however, was to be accomplished in just four to five days and was clearly more of a token than anything else.

It is interesting to compare the medical cooperation of the Cuban approach with the aid provided by U.S. forces. The rather paternalistic approach can be seen in one of the bulletins from the U.S. military summarizing their contribution: "The first stage of medical care provided during the MEDCAP was health and hygiene education where all 2,987 people learned proper hand-washing techniques and received multi-vitamins."[11] In all, these 2,987 patients were seen by the MEDCAP team over a five-day period. Dental hygienists also provided 416 screenings, and children were given "preventative dentistry instruction to teach them proper brushing techniques." Finally, about 60 children received vaccinations. One brief reference in an online newspaper summarizes the differences between the Cuban and U.S. approaches to disaster relief: "The Cuban Medical Brigade that will provide medical consultations in the emergency shelters within

Table 11.3. Principal medical conditions of patients seen by Cuban medical brigade

Medical condition	<15 years	>15 years	Total
Acute respiratory infections	5,871	5,043	10,914
Acute diarrhea-related diseases	353	204	557
Dermatitis	271	483	754
Arterial hypertension	3	2,705	2,708
Urinary tract infections	247	1,490	1,737
Intestinal parasites	1,471	674	2,145
Other infections	591	1,252	1,843
Gastritis and/or ulcers	71	1,559	1,630
Damage to skeletal structure	127	3,713	3,840
Psychological trauma	114	983	1,097
Other diseases	6,035	11,488	17,523

Source: "Brigada Médica Cubana en El Salvador," internal report produced February 22, 2010, by the Henry Reeve medical brigade in El Salvador.

the communities of Verapaz and Tepetitán will be there 'for an indefinite period' until the medical needs have been met. . . . Meanwhile Bravo Task Force of the U.S. South Command will provide medical attention for three days, together with local personnel, in the municipality of Guadalupe, also in the province of San Vicente."[12] The Cubans had made it abundantly clear that they were there to provide medical support for as long as the host government regarded it as being necessary—and as of the time of writing (early 2015) they are still there, although in larger numbers and in different roles.

The challenges of the almost 50,000 Salvadorans treated by Cubans during the initial emergency period were severe. Massive quantities of mud and boulders had been displaced, forced miles down the mountainside into the nearby plains, with soil being whipped around by the wind. A visit to the site three months later revealed the extent of the disaster. The denuded side of the nearby volcano that stretches for miles to the plain below, the line showing the height of the mud (almost five feet high) in those houses in Verapaz that had not been swept away, and the clearly changed river courses flowing through San Vicente and for miles around, illustrate the forces of nature. The impact on neighboring communities was also disastrous. Described to me by one villager as "the perfect storm," the combination of heavy rain off the Pacific coast of El Salvador, massive rainfall in San Vicente and the surrounding area, and flooding in the southern flatland coastal area combined to form a raging torrent. The most common conditions treated by Cuban medical personnel in the immediate months after the hurricane are listed in table 11.3.

Cuban-Salvadoran Medical Cooperation

From a dozen interviews with hospital managers, local politicians, and provincial public health directors, as well as with the Salvadoran minister of health, I learned that Cuban medical personnel worked closely with local hospitals. While the Cubans were often the first line of medical contact with people affected by Ida, any patients requiring diagnostic services such as EKG, X-ray, or USG were sent directly to the hospitals. In addition, members of the Cuban medical staff were frequently called in as consultants in local hospitals to provide advice. The medical cooperation was exemplary, according to information shared in several meetings with three provincial health directors, the head of the hospital in San Vicente, and Dr. María Isabel Rodríguez, El Salvador's minister of public health and social assistance.

The contribution of Salvadoran volunteers was an extremely important factor in the success of the Cuban medical mission. The day after the Cuban brigade began its work, they were joined by Salvadoran doctors (graduates of ELAM in Havana), and soon there were 34 working alongside the Cuban medical staff. Some left after volunteering to work in Haiti following the earthquake there, and in January most of the 2009 graduates from ELAM left in order to start their obligatory year of social service in the public health system of El Salvador. Other Salvadoran doctors who had graduated locally also volunteered their time, coming to help after finishing their shifts at local hospitals and clinics. Mutual respect and cooperation were commonplace.

In their earlier work on the dengue campaign in El Salvador, Cuban doctors had summarized the basic premises for their work in that country, and these concepts remained pertinent. Of essence was the need for Cuban humanitarian cooperation to respect local customs, ideology, religion, and institutions. The means to ensure these goals can be summarized in the following manner:

To be assigned to the most difficult areas, where the need was greatest
To work together in order to ensure unity
To utilize scientific methods as the principal tools of their trade
To exchange knowledge and experiences[13]

The name chosen for this combined medical team in 2009/10—the Brigada Médica Cubana Salvadoreña Mons. Oscar Romero—honored the memory of the assassinated archbishop of San Salvador, and it illustrates the respect for Salvadoran traditions and Cuban desire to cooperate with local medical staff.[14] As one health promoter in San Ildefonso explained to me, "When I heard that Cubans were participating, I expected something quite different—a form of supervision or control by them. I did not expect to find a team in which we were all fully integrated, working side by side as we went door to door together advising people about the means of eradicating dengue."[15]

Of particular note is the role played by Salvadoran graduates of ELAM. This medical school had been founded directly after the devastation caused in Central America by Hurricane Mitch in 1998 and was intended specifically to help the people of the region. The largest contingent of the first intake year a few months later were Hondurans, Guatemalans, and Salvadorans. This first cohort of Salvadoran doctors graduated in 2005, and by 2009 some 515 had graduated, while 742 more were still studying at ELAM.[16] The largest single graduating class of Salvadoran doctors was in 2013, with almost 400 newly minted physicians returning to the country in August, following seven years of study in Cuba. Under the previous right-wing (ARENA) government, several obstacles had been placed in their way following graduation, while the national medical association had criticized the value of their professional qualifications. It had also proved difficult to receive an internship for the obligatory social service, without which their medical degree was invalid. The election of the FMLN in 2009 facilitated the reintegration of ELAM graduates, and their track record in Salvadoran hospitals following this service requirement has been exemplary.[17] ELAM graduates have been particularly active in the frequent Jornadas de Acción Social, where they arrive on weekends at a traditionally underserved community in order to provide basic medical care to the community. I participated in one of these on February 20, 2010, held in a rural Lutheran church in Cantón Platanillos, Quezaltepeque. A dozen medical personnel—almost all of whom were ELAM graduates—spent five hours tending to some 250 patients. Some of these doctors also worked with the Cuban medical brigade following their own shifts at local hospitals.

This cooperation between Salvadoran and Cuban personnel was particularly noticeable in the campaign against dengue. Cuban and Salvadoran medical staff visited homes in the affected communities to ensure that standing water (the ideal breeding ground for the mosquitoes responsible for the transmission of dengue) had been treated properly. People were also advised on basic hygiene and how to dispose of garbage safely.

The overall Cuban strategy in El Salvador was straightforward—to offer their experience and services in any way that Salvadoran officials requested, and for as long as was necessary. At all times it was clear that the Cuban role was to be supportive. Their participation in the campaign against dengue was noticeable. In the three-stage fumigation process to kill mosquito larvae, four Cuban personnel planned the operation, with the bulk of the work being carried out by Salvadorans. On the weekends, their efforts were visibly strengthened by the support from the ELAM graduates.

The Goals of the Cuban Medical Brigade in El Salvador

The essence of the Cuban approach to public health is the need for prevention rather than the application of curative medicine, a strategy that is both cheaper and more effective. In Cuba massive public health campaigns—with the use of media and support from schools, NGOs, and government agencies—are usually well developed. Some of this experience was implemented in the large information campaign undertaken by members of the Cuban medical team to make Salvadorans aware of public health challenges. Within the first year of the arrival of the Cuban mission, some 49,137 face-to-face meetings had taken place (mainly in home visits), and an estimated 22,017 people had participated in public presentations, which ranged from roundtable discussions in public fora to presentations at church services. In addition, 11,984 flyers were distributed, advising people on public health concerns.[18] The objective was to encourage Salvadorans to become protagonists of their own development process, turning the disaster of Ida into an opportunity for a fresh approach to long-standing health challenges. Cuban medical staff participated in many sessions with local high school students, training them (in a "multiplier" effect) to provide practical health information to Salvadorans.

What was also noticeable in the affected communities was the role of Cuban medical personnel in supporting local communities to develop their potential, particularly in terms of public health issues. For instance, the small coastal community of Las Moras (73 dwellings and 231 inhabitants) was badly affected by the floods that swept ashore when Ida struck. This is a low-lying region bordered by the Pacific coast and with several rivers nearby, and flood waters rose to more than four feet when the hurricane hit. A major flood pushed water several kilometers inland. Farm animals were lost, homes were flooded (although fortunately nobody died), and residents were forced to flee the community within a two-hour period.

The support of the Cuban medical contingent started as soon as the flood waters receded. Asked by the Salvadoran government to participate in restoring hygienic conditions in the community, and aided by ELAM graduates, the Cuban staff started the long process of helping the community to return to normalcy. Dr. Mayra Fontes, an epidemiologist, played a major role in this transformation, visiting every home on several occasions to offer advice on domestic and personal hygiene, living conditions, natural medicine, and avoidance of vectors—in addition to providing medical consultations. She worked with women in the community and was instrumental in forming a youth group. Certificates were awarded to the homeowners whose homes showed the greatest improvement in hygiene and cleanliness, and follow-up visits by Dr. Fontes provided ongoing support to the community. This cooperation resulted in the community organizing to deal with improving hygienic living standards, to prevent the spread of disease, and to prepare for future natural disasters.

This crucial role of the Cuban medical delegation in the community was summed up well by Dr. Eduardo Ojeda, interim director of the Cuban Medical Brigade. Referring to the noticeable change in mentality of the communities in which the Cubans worked, he summarized the Cuban role: "We came here not to bring material goods to the affected communities but rather to accompany them as they rebuilt."[19] In this regard the combination of Salvadoran graduates of ELAM and Cuban medical personnel has been successful, helping impoverished communities to improve their level of hygiene, fumigating areas where mosquitoes bred, and in general supporting them as they gradually took control of their shattered lives.[20] As these communities developed self-confidence, Cuban medical staff visited less, although they continued to work with local health promoters and offer advice where needed.

It is clear that the 17 members of the Brigada Médica Cubana Salvadoreña Mons. Oscar Romero had a strong multiplier effect after they arrived in November 2009. From emergency relief, they became involved in a variety of activities, including support for the Salvadoran government in its dengue campaign, ongoing medical treatment for the communities affected by the natural disaster (most visible at the field hospital in San Vicente), monitoring the health of evacuees in temporary housing, public health campaigns throughout the affected areas, and widespread support for activities undertaken by the communities as they sought to recover from Ida.

Two other important Cuban public health initiatives in El Salvador deserve to be mentioned. Neither is related to the efforts of the Henry Reeve Brigade, yet both illustrate Cuba's commitment to supporting the Salvadoran people in public health matters. The first is focused on the Lower Lempa area of El Salvador, where acute renal failure led to an extremely high morbidity rate. Dr. Carlos Manuel Orantes, a Salvadoran graduate from ELAM, has taken the lead in analyzing the causes of this pathology. He specialized in nephrology in Cuba and brought several Cuban specialists to the region to work with Salvadoran medical students. By 2010 more than 8,000 people had been examined and 971 samples had been taken. It was discovered that over 600 suffered from chronic renal conditions and 103 from moderate conditions. This is three times the normal profile.[21] Research into the high incidence of acute renal failure continues in Havana at the Institute of Nephrology, while preventive measures and an active public education campaign involving Cuban and Salvadoran medical personnel has started in the Lower Lempa region, as illustrated by the March 11, 2010, celebration of World Kidney Day, complete with workshops on kidney care, early detection of acute renal conditions, and factors contributing to kidney deterioration. The motto for the day's activities—"from studying molecules to applying this knowledge to our society"—is a fitting summary of the campaign's objectives.

The other Cuban initiative has to do with Operation Miracle, a program initiated by the governments of Cuba and Venezuela in July 2004. In the case of El Salvador, 6,106 patients were operated on between June 19, 2006, and June 6, 2009.[22] Patients were also seen in neighboring Guatemala, where the José Martí Hospital in Jalapa received busloads of Salvadoran patients each week for eye surgery. Several flights took patients from El Salvador to Venezuela for surgery.[23] A future ophthalmology clinic could be opened in El Salvador, similar to the four already in existence in Guatemala. More than 10,000 Salvadorans have had their sight restored by Cuban specialists—again at no cost to the patients.

In April 2010, the Ministries of Health of both Cuba and El Salvador drafted a fundamental agreement under the rubric of naming it a "Project of Technical Cooperation between Countries" and "The Strengthening of Local Health Capacity." It has formed the basis for a stronger bilateral relationship. The document emphasizes the role of the Pan American Health Organization (PAHO) in supporting these agreements, recognizes Cuba's wealth of medical experience abroad, and analyzes the situation of El Salvador's public health needs. It draws attention to the priority assigned to it by the FMLN government as well as the need for a fundamental restructuring of the national healthcare system, and recommends the need for a strategy of Primary Health Care (Atención Primaria de Salud, or APS), focused on a preventive public health approach, based in the community.

Great attention has been paid to the contribution of the Cuban medical brigade since its arrival after Hurricane Ida, emphasizing its role in the national campaign against dengue and subsequent public health programs. Given that the Cuban system is based on APS, and in light of the approximately 1,000 Salvadoran medical graduates of ELAM familiar with the Cuban system, it seems that there are many advantages to be gained by working with this strategy. The basic objective is to strengthen the Salvadoran public healthcare system, incorporating Cuban specialists in restructuring the national system and basing it on a primary care focus. The budget for this first year of cooperation was $99,500, a remarkably modest sum for the amount of work involved.

In July 2011, a delegation of PAHO specialists met in San Salvador to assess the previous year's technical cooperation program between the two countries. The minister of public health, Dr. María Isabel Rodríguez, noted the integrated approach of Cuban professionals and their Salvadoran counterparts. Given the impressive results in terms of the delivery of healthcare, PAHO encouraged an increase in the scope of Cuban cooperation. The most vocal support was expressed by the deputy minister of public health, Dr. Violeta Menjivar, who emphasized the professional role of the 20 Cuban advisers and noted that their experience and scientific training had been decisive in the improvement of the Salvadoran health system. For her part, Dr. Argelia Dubón, director of the national primary care program, referred to the huge improvements since the arrival of the Cubans: "Our country has waited many years to construct a model of public health delivery like the one we are building, and which has advanced since the arrival of the Cuban medical mission. We have worked together as a team, and it is this integration which has allowed us to advance so much."[24]

Concluding Remarks

The Cuban role in El Salvador has developed significantly in recent years. From its modest beginnings as a small Henry Reeve contingent that arrived in late 2009 to help after Hurricane Ida, its role has increased significantly. It is now involved in several healthcare initiatives, ably assisted by approximately 1,000 Salvadoran physicians who were trained in Cuba and are familiar with the Cuban approach. In many ways the role of Cuban medical personnel in El Salvador is a microcosm of its medical internationalism. Starting with support to the anti-dengue campaign, and then the response of the Henry Reeve Brigade in 2009, its role has increased. Its responsibilities range from supporting the National Health Service to providing specialized assistance on specific medical challenges. Meanwhile, Cuban-trained doctors continue to graduate from ELAM.

In an interview on February 25, 2010, with Dr. María Isabel Rodríguez, she and I discussed the Cuban role in her country in detail. Rodríguez, a cardiovascular physiologist by training and former president of the National University of El Salvador, emphasized the solid scientific basis of the Cuban medical system and the high quality of public healthcare in Cuba.[25] She also dealt in some detail with the impact that Cuban medical personnel had caused in El Salvador and not just in terms of public health. Referring to the outbreak of dengue in 2000 and the support of Cuban medical professionals at the time, she noted how "the Cubans showed us a new form of medical commitment. . . . Not only do they have an enormous amount of medical ability (which clearly has a major influence on the public health situation), but they also have a major impact on the community members who come in contact with them—and in whom we see a clear change of attitude."[26] Dr. Rodríguez also praised the very different medical training provided in Cuba and the manner in which patients were treated by Cuban medical personnel: "The Salvadoran people realize that the Cubans treat them as individuals, recognizing their human quality and spending time with them. Their medical training is different—the Cuban doctors respect their patients and listen to them." This opinion was in many ways reflected in interviews with three dozen Salvadoran graduates of ELAM whom I met and by patients treated by the Cubans in several locations.

A common theme of the Cuban approach to medical internationalism—the ability to do more with less—proved extremely successful in El Salvador. The Cuban approach to MI is difficult for medical personnel in an industrialized country to understand, since they lack the experience that results from Cuban training. The pragmatic Cuban approach is particularly well suited to conditions in the developing world, since for decades the Cubans have learned how to adapt to economic difficulties, to "make do" in extremely difficult circumstances. This approach is implemented wherever they work.

In the case of the emergency humanitarian work carried out during their first five months after Ida, and according to confidential Salvadoran and Cuban sources, the entire cost of the Cuban medical brigade (including transportation, maintenance, and all public health activities) was less than $60,000. However, the impact of these many medical interventions in terms of benefits and outcomes is half a million dollars.[27] Despite limited resources, much can be achieved when there is political will, combined with a high degree of solidarity and commitment. The success of the emergency mission of the Henry Reeve Brigade in just a few months revealed the potential of this medical cooperation in El Salvador and in other countries where conditions allow.

Cuba's role in El Salvador has made a significant contribution on several levels to the public health of people there. In October 2010 Salvadoran president Mauricio Funes visited ELAM where he noted that 575 Salvadorans had already graduated at no cost to the students or the government. In 2013 a further 386 graduated from ELAM. Cuban advisers have also been extremely important in providing support and guidance in developing an ambitious reform of the country's national healthcare system. With an emphasis on primary healthcare and the establishment since July 2010 of 517 community health centers (Community Teams of Family and Specialized Health, or ECOS in the Spanish synonym), and a further 36 specialized community health teams, much has been accomplished. Within two years of their establishment, staff at the ECOS (many of whom had studied in Cuba at ELAM) had given 2.5 million medical consults, and in 2012 alone they attended 1.6 million patients. The role of the ECOS is particularly important in the program of preventive healthcare that is the hallmark of the Cuban system. Healthcare is now brought to the communities, instead of making individuals seek it out through a maze of private and public clinics, and each ECO serves an average of 200 families. President Funes praised the significance of the healthcare reform in his preface to the annual report (Informe de Labores) of the Ministry of Public Health and Social Assistance for 2012/13: "The most transcendental reform that we have initiated is the creation of our new National Integrated System of Health. This is a revolutionary initiative, a profound change that will deliver medical care to every Salvadoran." He is correct, and in no small degree the success of this approach is the result of Cuban cooperation.

What started out as a series of isolated humanitarian gestures (e.g., thousands of Salvadorans traveling to Guatemala for cataract surgery under the auspices of Operación Milagro, assistance during a major dengue outbreak, the Henry Reeve brigade helping after Hurricane Ida, and the graduation at ELAM of some 1,000 doctors) has now evolved into a program of cooperation between Cuban and Salvadoran medical personnel. Despite a lack of diplomatic relations for over 50 years, Havana has provided Cuban medical support and saved many lives. The victory of FMLN presidential candidate Salvador Sánchez Cerén in 2014 will in all likelihood continue the reform process, along with Cuban support for the revamped public health system and will improve the health of this Central American nation of 6 million.

Conclusion

No Longer the World's Best-Kept Secret

> Graduating as a doctor is like opening a door to a long road leading to the noblest action that a human being can do for others.
>
> Fidel Castro, September 19, 2005

This book has attempted to illustrate the role played by Cuba in medical internationalism, principally among countries of the Global South. Certainly there is an enormous need for such initiatives in medical cooperation, given the many profound health challenges facing the billions of people in the developing world. These include a shortage of medical personnel, a massive "brain drain" of qualified physicians to the industrialized North, the lack of affordable medicines, and rapidly growing populations. To take just one example, over half a million women die in childbirth every year—all from treatable complications. A comparison is pertinent here: women in northern Europe have a 1 in 4,000 chance of dying from pregnancy, yet for women in Africa it is 1 in 16.[1] In an article by Clare Nullis-Kapp in 2005 it was estimated that 1 million additional health personnel were needed in Africa over the next decade.[2] However, these badly needed doctors and nurses are leaving in droves, mainly to five industrialized countries: Australia, Canada, Germany, the United Kingdom, and the United States. The impoverished populations receive short shrift.

The case of Ghana is illustrative of this exodus. There are more Ghanaian doctors working abroad than in the country itself, with 50 percent of its professional nurses working in Canada, the United Kingdom, and the United States. While they flee to the industrialized North, the situation for medical care in Ghana remains desperate, where there is one doctor for 17,489 patients, compared with one for 300 in the UK.[3] Sub-Saharan Africa as a whole has 11 percent of the world's population and 25 percent of global disease, yet it has "only 3 percent of the global health workforce and accounts for less than 1 percent of health expenditure worldwide."[4] The flight of medical personnel is the root of this problem. Zimbabwe, for instance, trained 1,200 doctors during the 1990s, yet by 2000 only 360 remained. In Ghana, a similar phenomenon can be found, since 604 from a total of 871 medical officers who had trained between 1993 and 2002 left to work abroad.[5] This situation is repeated throughout the developing world. As can be seen, there is an immense need for a more just and equitable system to ensure access to healthcare there. Cuba's approach to medical internationalism does, however, make a contribution to resolving that enormous imbalance as well as offering a distinctive alternative. It shows that the adage about steady economic growth being required before healthcare can be provided is not necessarily the case: health before wealth is indeed possible. It also shows that where there is solid political will and commitment to help those who cannot help themselves, accessible, affordable healthcare can be made available, even in developing and underdeveloped countries.

As noted in the introduction, Cuba's contribution to global health is one of the world's best-kept secrets, despite the fact that this process has been in existence for over five decades. Media in the industrialized world have long ignored it. Yet even allowing for some exaggeration by government bureaucrats, the facts are undeniable, as supported by data from PAHO and the WHO among others. The medical internationalism program has been so successful that the administration of George W. Bush sought to embarrass the Cuban government by encouraging Cuban medical personnel to defect and come to the United States through its Cuban Medical Professional Parole program (CMPP), inaugurated on August 11, 2006.[6]

So have Cuban physicians defected in droves? An editorial published in the *New York Times* on November 16, 2014, "A Cuban Brain Drain, Courtesy of the U.S.," noted that there had been 1,278 defections by Cuban medical personnel that year. The irony of the U.S. position in this strategy to tempt Cuban doctors from their missions in developing countries should not be ignored. At the time of the earthquake in Haiti, and particularly during the Ebola outbreak in West Africa, U.S. ambassador to the United Nations Samantha Powers and Secretary of State John Kerry had expressed support for the work of Cuban medical staff. Yet, at the same time, the government was seeking to take that medical care away from those who needed it most by offering a "parole" program to Cuban doctors, encouraging them to defect. This was indeed a contradictory, hypocritical position.

As in so many things to do with Cuba, understanding the size of Cuban defections depends on where the individual's perspective lies. Perhaps useful in this regard is a study of the Cuban role in Brazil, where in 2013–14 the government of Dilma Rousseff imported the services of some 11,400 doctors on three-year contracts. The physicians were criticized for their poor language skills and the fact that they lacked the approval of local medical federations. Indeed, these federations have actually offered to help the Cubans defect. Conservative media have painted a picture of mass desertions, basing their case on the well-publicized case of Ramona Matos Rodríguez, and claimed that the Cuban contribution to healthcare was a disaster.[7] The Brazilian government showed, however, that the rate of defections by the Cubans (14 had left the program by June 4, 2014, including 5 who defected) was in fact low: 0.1 percent of the 11,400 Cuban professionals, compared with the 131 Brazilians who left "Mais Médicos," or 8.4 percent of their group.[8] After one full year of the program, only 19 Cubans out of 11,429 had left. And while the medical federation condemned the role of Cuban physicians, the response of their patients was overwhelmingly positive, with polls showing support ranging between 70.3 percent and 84.3 in the first months after their arrival.[9] A year later, a survey of 4,000 people in 200 cities where the program had been introduced was carried out by the Federal University of Minas Gerais. It showed that 95 percent of people interviewed were either satisfied or very satisfied with the program.[10]

In sum, as in so many Cuba-related matters, there is a wide polarization in analyzing the question of Cuban MI. This lack of interest in any form of balance can be explained by the confidential report of June 5, 2006, by Michael Parmly, head of the U.S. Special Interests section in Havana, which stated that "USINT is always looking for human interest stories and other news that shatters the myth of Cuban medical prowess."[11] In terms of promoting defections, Erisman criticizes the CMPP program, calling it "exaggerated at best and duplicitous at worst," claiming that only 2 percent of Cuban physicians defect.[12] Lost in the polarized media frenzy about the U.S. government program encouraging defections is the fact that the greatest losers in the process are the underserved, generally poor social groups in developing societies who have now lost their medical support system.

While the numbers of Cuban *internacionalistas* are changing continually, and the administrators of this huge, multifaceted program of medical internationalism face a daunting task of keeping in touch with 50,000 medical personnel, there are key points to be made. Clearly, over the past five decades Cuban medical internationalism has saved millions of lives. In addition, millions of lives more have been improved. In a recent visit to the nerve center of the Cuban MI missions, the Unidad Central de Colaboración Médica in Havana, the statistics (which were being updated on that day, October 16, 2013) are revealing (see table C.1). But they were already badly out of date, since they did not take into account many of the thousands of physicians who had started work in Brazil in the Mais Médicos program, nor did they include the departure from Venezuela of many others, some of whom had gone to Brazil. Nevertheless, they did provide a valuable insight into the "big picture" of Cuba's medical internationalism program. The fact that they were out of date just a few months after being posted illustrates the fluidity of Cuba's medical support overseas.

It is important to reflect upon the impact that the numbers in table C.1 signify for the millions of patients whose lives have been changed by these programs. They are mainly poor people living in underserved areas in what is termed the developing world, most of whom in the past were unable to receive basic medical services. In many cases these were simply unavailable or unaffordable. Rather than become numbed by the broad sweep of these overwhelming figures, however, it is instructive to examine the specific examples of two developing countries that have benefited. In this way it is possible to appreciate the impact of medical internationalism and how this translates into the lives of the people there. One of the poorest countries is Guatemala, where Cubans first became involved after Hurricane Mitch in 1998 and where they are still working. Between 1998 and late 2013 there had been 35,431,805 medical consults for Guatemalan patients. (Just as the Cubans prefer the term *medical cooperation* to *aid*, they also refer to their *patients* as opposed to *clients*.) Operación Milagro staff had performed 122,658 ophthalmology operations.[13]

So in practical terms, what do these figures mean for the people in Guatemala? Quite simply, millions now have the basic human right to visit a doctor and not have to pay for the service. Given the distribution of the Cuban physicians—in rural and underserved areas where most Guatemalan doctors prefer not to work—this is a rare privilege. Having the money to pay for surgery would have been even more unlikely, yet surgeries are now performed at no charge by the Cuban doctors. Operation Miracle will also have brought tremendous relief to over 120,000 Guatemalans who can now see to work and enjoy life in a way that only a person with vision can. The presence of over 1,000 Guatemalan physicians trained at ELAM is significant, illustrating the commitment to sustainability in the system. They will undoubtedly change the delivery of healthcare in their country, making it more accessible to those who have been traditionally ignored.

On the other side of the world, in the small country of Timor-Leste, we can see a similar situation where Cuba has provided accessibility to, and

Table C.1. Cuban medical internationalism statistics presented by the Unidad Central de Colaboración Médica in Havana, October 16, 2013

Form of cooperation	Total collaborators	Including physicians	No. of countries	No. of patients	No. of surgeries	No. of births attended	No. of lives saved
Venezuela program	32,514	11,416	1	868,501,538	1,720,734	73,800	1,746,417
Cuban medical services (private)	2,422	1,426	11	20,509,835	1,534,869	346,961	262,335
Paid cooperation	3,253	1,804	16	27,267,341	694,645	339,913	645,312
Comprehensive Health Program	2,630	1,427	32	206,121,781	3,357,907	1,310,862	2,416,983
Operation Miracle	322	88	14		2,519,534		
Henry Reeve contingent				76,202			75,930
Mental and physical disabilities program				2,211,566			
Doctor training							
Total	**41,239**	**16,259**		**1,124,688,263**	**9,827,689**	**2,071,536**	**5,146,977**

sustainability of, healthcare. In November 2013 a graduation ceremony took place in Dili, the country's capital, for 246 Cuban-trained physicians. They were accompanied by 71 nursing students. From having just 47 doctors when the country became independent, the country now had 798 doctors who had graduated following training first in Havana and subsequently in Dili.

Common to both these case histories are some fundamental tenets of the Cuban philosophy of MI and public healthcare. First is the premise that access to healthcare has to be seen as a basic human right.[14] The Cuban constitution itself insists on the need to ensure that that there shall be "no sick person who does not receive medical attention." From the Cuban perspective, the state has a fundamental and permanent obligation to ensure that all citizens have access to public healthcare, free of charge, and not just in wealthy sectors of major cities. Hence the significance of the role of the Cuban doctors in rural and underserved communities. Moreover, while the use of medicine to treat illness is often necessary, for Cuba there is an overarching emphasis on a preventive—rather than curative—approach to public health. Related to this is the holistic approach employed by Cuban physicians, who view their patients as bio-psycho-social human beings, influenced significantly by their environment and by their social interactions as well as by disease. Moreover, members of society are also required to participate in this process and be responsible partners.

Cuba's commitment to international development is also seen in the preamble to the national constitution, which emphasizes the need for Cuba to look beyond its borders. In particular it states the fundamental concern of helping others in the developing world on the basis of "fraternal friendship, aid, cooperation, and solidarity"—a commitment made decades ago. It is this premise which lies behind all of the actions and policies analyzed in this book. The constitution thus formalized a policy that Cuba had been carrying out since the first emergency physicians went to Chile in 1960 and that continues today.

The training of doctors who will stay in their underserved communities is a key component of the Cuban approach to ensuring a sustainable healthcare system, as the references above to the situation in Guatemala and Timor-Leste attest. The same need is true, however, for any developing country seeking desperately to retain its medical personnel, who are often attracted by the siren call of higher financial rewards in the industrialized North. In many ways the Cuban approach to training thousands of physicians from developing countries—now being replicated in several of them—has been able to make up for the exodus of trained professionals in many countries of the South. Theirs is a totally different, pragmatic form of training doctors, and it is badly needed.

The success of ELAM since it first opened its doors, the establishment of medical schools with Cuban professors in several countries, and the training program in Venezuela all herald a radically new approach to medical education from which a very different physician is emerging. It is largely for this reason that traditional medical federations in several Latin American countries have been so critical, fearing this radically different philosophy of medicine, as well as a potential decrease in their influence (and income).[15] They have reason to be concerned as the model of the "new physician" committed to the right of all patients to receive free, accessible medical care, emerges and spreads across Latin America.

The nature of the medical training that is provided is in many ways the most crucial element. At their graduation ceremony the newly minted doctors take an oath "to strive always to be worthy representatives of Cuban health professionals, devoting ourselves with true love to our profession, with a profound respect for human life, feeling the pain of others as our own, seeing in each patient and their family our own loved ones, and working tirelessly toward excellence in health services." One further aspect of this oath is pertinent, since the graduating physicians also pledge "to serve the revolution unconditionally wherever we are needed, with the premise that true medicine is not that which cures but that which prevents, whether in an isolated community on our island or in any sister country of the world, where we will always be the standard-bearers of solidarity and internationalism."[16]

This commitment to internationalism has been consistent for more than five decades, with differing approaches and emphases employed as the support for MI has evolved in the context of Cuban reality. The most recent stage under the government of Raúl Castro has maintained the core elements of this approach while also using this abundance of human capital as a means of generating funding for the economy. This has been successful, with the exportation of medical services now constituting the single largest form of income for the country—worth almost three times the amount generated annually through tourism. For some this selling of medical services is a clear departure from the traditional model espoused by Fidel Castro and practiced for decades, and it is not defensible. Yet this is not completely correct, since as early as 1978 Fidel Castro himself had indicated the potential for the exportation of medical goods and services, which he termed "an important factor for the economic development of the country."[17] Cuba currently has more physicians than Canada, a wealthy, industrialized country with three times the population. Given those circumstances, why not use the surplus of medical talent to bring in funding for Cuba's other programs? Or, as is the case with Venezuela, barter the surplus of oil for medical cooperation? In an interview in 2007 Dr. Yiliam Jiménez, the person in charge of Cuba's medical internationalism program, outlined Cuba's position: "We believe in fair trade. If that means that we export a product that we have a surplus of—in this case medical and educational goods and services—to a friend at a reduced price, and they export to us at favorable conditions something that they have in abundance—petroleum—what is wrong with that?"[18]

In an interview ("Jorge Rodríguez: 'Cuba no exporta armas, exporta salud, un servicio para el planeta,'") in January 2015 in the Ecuadoran newspaper *El Universo*, Jorge Rodríguez, Cuban ambassador to Ecuador, explained the government rationale in exporting medical services. In Ecuador, Cuban medical personnel (approximately 800) receive a monthly salary of $800 of the $2,641 paid by the Ecuadoran government to Havana. For many years this medical cooperation had been offered at no charge to Ecuador. In recent years, however, Cuba had started to charge for medical services. Both governments agreed on an amount that Ecuador could pay but that was still significantly less than the international rate for medical services. When asked if this was "good business" for Cuba, Rodríguez replied: "If it were a question of business, we would send our doctors to another country where they pay more. . . . We are not a country with large oil deposits or great natural resources. Instead we have developed an important scientific capacity, and we have to live from this talent. . . . Cuba exports health, not weapons."

The Rationale for Cuban Medical Internationalism

So why has Cuba pursued this decades-long policy of medical cooperation, one which has been applied in dozens of developing countries? In the last analysis it can be reduced to the desire to replicate in developing countries the same philosophy of healthcare found in Cuba. There is a fundamental belief that all should have access at no cost to medical care, since this is the most valuable human right, especially for people in developing countries who often see this as an unaffordable luxury. It is also important to recognize that the prime mover behind medical internationalism is Fidel Castro, who since 1960 has seen the need to link public health as a domestic right with its application in developing countries. Over the course of the research for this book, and in dozens of interviews, I have constantly been made aware by doctors and academics of the many initiatives of Castro.

A study of his many speeches on the question of medical internationalism reveals several core ideas, all revolving around issues of fairness and social justice, particularly for people who had traditionally been denied access to healthcare. At the founding of the Henry Reeve Brigade in September 2005, he explained with clarity and passion the major differences between rich and poor countries in terms of the accessibility of public healthcare: "Although every person has the right to a healthy life and to enjoy the privilege of a long and useful existence, the richest, most developed societies, ruled by consumerism and a thirst for profit, have made the health service into a common business, inaccessible to the poorest sectors of the population. In many Third World countries this service barely exists, and between developed countries and the euphemistically called 'developing countries' the differences are vast."[19]

Many Cuban exiles and conservatives strongly disagree. One of the most outspoken is María C. Werlau, an exile who claims that the low wages paid to Cuban health workers violate the Trafficking in Persons Protocol and the ILO Convention on the Protection of Wages.[20] With reference to the Cuban role in Haiti she notes how "these accords exploit Cuban workers and contribute to the continued oppression and impoverishment of the Cuban people."[21] For her, Cuba is involved in Haiti because it is a "very profitable subsidiary in Cuba's global multi-billion dollar 'humanitarian' enterprise. Most of its profits come off the backs of Cubans indentured as 'collaborators.'"

Werlau also maintains that many *internacionalistas* are "trained by Cuban intelligence to monitor the host country and diffuse opposition to Cuba or the revolutionary project," adding that hundreds of the armed forces and paramilitary groups have trained in technical medical specialization so that they can serve the revolution abroad.[22] For her, medical internationalism is a cynical ploy on the part of Havana to make money, burnish the government's revolutionary credentials, carry out acts of espionage, and exploit "the highest qualified slave-labor force in the world."[23] A similar note is sounded by a *Miami Herald* reporter who feels that the Cuban government is pursuing its MI programs for political propaganda: "After relying for decades on guerrillas and guns to export his Marxist model, Cuban president Fidel Castro has found another tool: 'doctor diplomacy.'"[24]

In a 2005 article, "Slaves in White Coats," Cuban exile Carlos Alberto Montaner denounced Cuba's MI program on several grounds. Fidel Castro's offer of some 1,500 medical personnel to the United States after Hurricane Katrina was merely a "gesture," he claimed, and should not be taken seriously. In the wake of the Bush administration's refusal to accept Cuban support, notes Montaner, the "truly humiliated and offended people" were not the poor and overwhelmingly black victims of Katrina but rather the Cuban doctors. He explains: "They are the *comandante's* favorite slaves: He rents them out, sells them, gives them away, lends them, exchanges them for oil, or uses them as an alibi to justify his dictatorship."[25] The rather crude ad hominem attacks on Fidel Castro (whom Montaner describes as commanding "an army of sad-eyed slaves in white coats") are disappointing and clearly driven by his ideological position. While there is no doubt that the role of Fidel Castro is enormously important in the development of Cuba's medical internationalism, Montaner's claim that Castro sends medical personnel abroad solely for profit does not bear examination, as the people of Haiti, Niger, or Vanuatu among dozens of developing countries can attest. A more balanced perspective has been presented by a group of epidemiologists: "Like all foreign aid programmes, it assumes that some political benefits will be forthcoming in return. However, most of the countries that have been assisted, for example, Ethiopia, The Gambia, and Haiti, have nothing to offer in return. Unlike many donor programmes, placing physicians where none have practiced before has been overwhelmingly well received by the local communities."[26] The same authors note that the assignments abroad "are accepted as a professional obligation by the vast majority of the Cuban practitioners."[27]

Over the past eight years, I have interviewed 270 *internacionalistas*, mainly doctors who have served in Africa and Latin America. Almost all served for two-year periods, with a monthlong vacation back in Cuba every 11 months. About 35 percent of those I interviewed served on at least two missions abroad. For six weeks I accompanied many of them in Central America, while in Cuba I have interviewed formally and met informally with scores of others. For both the structured and informal meetings I have usually inquired about the motives for participating in these difficult overseas missions and how they have been affected. Their responses have been very similar.

Most admit that they were attracted to the idea of working abroad mainly for financial reasons. After all, the average salary for a physician on the island is poor (even with the recent increases in the spring of 2014, physicians are only earning $60 to $90 monthly).[28] The salaries abroad—even though the living and working conditions are often extremely poor—are significantly better. In the spring of 2014, for instance, it was decided that the 11,400 Cuban doctors in Brazil would earn $1,400 monthly, payable there rather than in an account in Cuba. Many of the medical personnel I interviewed also noted that, particularly on their first mission, they went as a "rite of passage," because it seemed the "right thing to do" at that stage of their lives. Some went out of a spirit of adventure, to have the opportunity to explore another culture. Others went because of the medical experience that it offered, the opportunity to learn about new diseases and medical conditions and to further their training in a challenging environment.

While financial motives were often the main reason for their participation (and most saw a significant improvement in their standard of living upon returning with goods and money), there were other benefits. Almost everybody commented on the medical experience. One family doctor who told me that she had never witnessed infant malnutrition before, and seeing the swollen bellies of children in Gambia had shocked her. Others remarked on diseases that they had read about in medical textbooks but had never experienced before, and all emphasized that they were far better medical practitioners for the experience. Many became quite emotional when reflecting on the appalling conditions in which their patients lived, especially those who suffered from conditions that were preventable. Almost all came back changed, more committed to their humanitarian vocation. One of the aspects that surprised me was the way in which many expressed a greater level of patriotism in the wake of their experiences abroad and an appreciation for the quality of life in Cuba. "I thought things were bad in Cuba, but you should see just how atrocious things are in rural Niger" (or any of the dozens of countries in which they had worked) was a common reaction.

It is clear that the Cuban government has pursued a policy of MI since 1960 for a variety of motives. There is no doubt that their policy has helped to win the hearts and minds of many countries, and for many this will be a textbook case of the exercise of "soft power." After all, many countries that were fervently opposed to Cuba have normalized diplomatic ties after receiving substantial medical support for many years. Others will point to the "medical tourism" services being offered in Havana for foreigners and the commercialization of the Cuban healthcare system and wonder whether Raúl Castro has gone too far in seeking compensation for Cuba's human capital.[29] The mutually beneficial ties with Venezuela, receiving approximately 100,000 barrels of oil per day at subsidized rates in exchange for extensive medical services, will also be criticized by some who will claim that the doctors should remain with their patients in Cuba.

Lost in this analysis, however, is the fact that Cuba has been pursuing these initiatives since 1960 and has done so in a fashion that is far less Machiavellian than might be supposed. The use of medical cooperation as a form of "soft power," for instance, was never a primary goal. Indeed, the votes of support for Cuba at the UN and the normalization of relations with Cuba were seen in Havana as principally a welcome but not totally expected benefit. The Cuban government did not have as its main objective the normalization of relations with Guatemala and Honduras when it sent hundreds of medical staff there after Hurricane Mitch in 1998. In addition, on a cost/benefit basis, many of its cooperation programs are financially unviable. The case of Pakistan is worth noting. Having some 2,500 medical personnel work for seven months in appalling conditions after the earthquake, and then donating 32 fully equipped field hospitals and training 1,000 Pakistani doctors at no charge, Cuba's Henry Reeve mission was a massive financial failure. The same can be said about sending thousands of civilian personnel to countries in sub-Saharan Africa, the decision to treat 25,000 survivors of the Chernobyl nuclear meltdown, and Cuba's Operation Miracle ophthalmology program. None of these made any real economic sense but were carried out in a basic humanitarian spirit.

Diplomatic support, the generation of badly needed funding, and international recognition have all been significant gains for Cuba. But they were not the original goals of the medical internationalism program or its principal objectives. Far more important was the fact that Cuba had the political will and the capacity to help people in far worse situations—and this was largely because of the initiative of Fidel Castro. It is important to remember that until the turn of this century Castro was a larger-than-life political figure, a leader with enormous natural charisma. He also had a broad international vision in which public healthcare was always a major consideration. And the Cuban people overwhelmingly supported those initiatives.

The end result of this complex amalgam of Fidel Castro's charisma and vision, popular support for an activist foreign policy in which Cuba identified with Third World struggles, and a medical system that graduated tens of thousands of doctors at home and abroad is medical internationalism.[30] It has evolved dramatically from that first small delegation to Chile in 1960 to the present when a quarter of all Cuban physicians are working abroad. Between April 1963 and March 2014, 131,933 medical professionals have worked as medical *internacionalistas* and have served in 120 countries around the world.[31]

It is often difficult for us in the "developed world" to understand this approach. After all, in many industrialized countries the provision of medical services is a business. As a result we are understandably skeptical when we see a model which is so radically different from anything that we are accustomed to. Moreover, the idea of providing long-term support to ensure a sustainable approach to preventive medicine (and at no cost to the patient) to people in developing countries is also virtually unknown. Yet this is what Cuba has done since 1960. We therefore need to challenge ourselves to consider medical care for developing nations through a totally different optic.

Medical internationalism *a la cubana* has saved millions of lives in scores of countries and at no cost to the patients. Nowadays Cubans are well aware of the contributions of the *internacionalistas*, but back then they must have been surprised at the claims made by their leader. In June 1965 Fidel Castro predicted: "So never, looking ahead to the future decades, will we have too many doctors or dentists, teachers, engineers, or technicians. . . . We will need them all, and if we don't need them, other countries with greater needs than ours will. So we should prepare ourselves to meet our obligations to other peoples, since otherwise our concept of human solidarity will remain limited by our own needs and by our own borders."[32] Fifty years later, there is significant truth to his claims.

This particular blend of nationalism, ambitious planning, resources, and a conviction that anything was possible led to medical internationalism, a process that continues today, now with a grander vision and a solid financial basis. This process requires "great long-term vision, a sense of humanitarian ethics, and a commitment to the well-being of others. It means placing value on human capital rather than in the marketplace."[33] And finally, as the title of this book suggests, it is predicated on the conviction that there are no borders to this decades-old program.

Notes

Preface

1. "La participación cubana en el enfrentamiento al ébola en África Occidental no es un hecho aislado." See *Juventud Rebelde*, September 12, 2014. This is the transcript of the joint press conference between the director general of the WHO and the Cuban minister of public health which took place in Geneva.

Introduction: Setting the Scene

1. Fonticoba, "Cuba tiene médicos por todo el mundo."

2. Vázquez García, "La escuela médica más avanzada del mundo."

3. Data found at data.worldbank.org/indicator/SH.MED.PHYS.ZS. An article in 2013 provided slightly different information, noting that Cuba had more than 85,000 doctors, or a doctor for every 137 people. See "Más de 37000 cubanos y 10000 extranjeros estudian medicina."

4. Collazo Montano, "Cuba, por incrementar los servicios médicos."

5. Data found at CIA, *World Factbook.*

6. Souers, "Cuba Leads the World in Lowest Patient per Doctor Ratio."

7. Fariñas Acosta, "Cuba ha demostrado que es posible tener salud y bienestar para todos."

8. Data from the National Office of Statistics, Havana, found at www.one.cu/aec2011/esp/19_tabla_cuadro.htm.

9. De la Osa, "A las aulas casi 86 mil estudiantes de Ciencias Médicas."

10. Souers, "Cuba Leads the World in Lowest Patient per Doctor Ratio."

11. "La Salud Pública cubana apuesta a más calidad y más eficiencia."

12. It is worth noting that this first medical mission took place at a time of social polarization in Cuba, with a significant number of the urban bourgeoisie leaving. This included medical personnel, and by the end of 1961 almost half of Cuba's 6,000 doctors had left the island.

13. José Manzaneda, "Why You Will Not Be Told about This Miracle."

14. The preamble of the 1976 constitution (amended in 2002) refers to the need for "proletarian internationalism, by the fraternal friendship, aid, cooperation, and solidarity of the peoples of the world, especially those of Latin America and the Caribbean."

15. "Speech Given by Dr. Fidel Castro Ruz, President of the Republic of Cuba, at the Celebration of the 40th Anniversary of INDER and the Dedication of the International School of Physical Education and Sports, on February 23, 2001."

16. Riverry, "Misión Milagro de dos fronteras."

17. As was noted in a recent article, "In essence it comes down to political will, combined with a determination to provide support—cooperation—to the world's impoverished and marginalized populations. . . . It requires great long-term vision, a sense of humanitarian ethics, and a commitment to the well-being of others. It means placing value on human capital rather than in the marketplace." Kirk and Walker, "Moral Medicine, the Cuban Way," 27.

18. Delgado Legón, "Massive Graduation of Doctors in Cuba."

19. Kirk and Kirk, "Cuban Medical Aid to Haiti: One of the World's Best-Kept Secrets."

Chapter 1. Origins and Evolution: From "Beggar's Helper" to a "White-Jacketed Army"

1. Information taken from the CIA's *World Factbook*.

2. See the section on the Cuban economy in the summary published by the Heritage Foundation at http://www.heritage.org/index/country/cuba.

3. Feinberg, "Reaching Out," 14.

4. Domínguez, *To Make a World Safe for Revolution*, 115, 172.

5. "During the 1970s and continuing into the mid-1980s, the combination of these two elements—establishing a highly lucrative coalition with the socialist bloc that also included large infusions of military aid and expanding dramatically its relations with developing nations throughout the Southern Hemisphere in an effort to bolster its Third World leadership aspirations—was the defining hallmark both of Havana's overall foreign policy and of its counterdependency agenda." See Erisman, *Cuba's Foreign Relations in a Post-Soviet World*, 78.

6. Domínguez, *To Make a World Safe for Revolution*, 7.

7. Erisman, *Cuba's Foreign Relations in a Post-Soviet World*, 98–99.

8. Ibid., 221.

9. Cited in Reed, "Cuban Medical Teams in Global Disaster Relief."

10. "The majority of the doctors in Algeria were French, and many have now left the country. The population of Algeria is four million greater than that of Cuba, and there are many diseases that have been left by colonialism. Yet they have only a third—and maybe less—of the doctors that we do. In matters of health their situation is really tragic."

"That's why I said to the students that we need 50 doctors to volunteer to go to Algeria.

"I am sure that there will be many volunteers. Today we can send only 50, but in 8 or 10 years, who knows how many we'll be able to send. And we will be helping our brothers and sisters, because the revolution has the right to gather the fruits that it has sown." Cited in Gleijeses, *Misiones en Conflicto*, 29–30.

11. Ibid., 31.

12. López Blanch, *Historias secretas de médicos cubanos*, 102.

13. Ibid., 191.

14. Gleijeses, *Misiones en Conflicto*, 31.

15. Erisman, *Cuba's Foreign Relations in a Post-Soviet World*, 99–100.

16. In 1991 Nelson Mandela traveled to Cuba to thank the Cuban people for their sup-

port in southern Africa. He referred to the military victory over South African forces in Angola: "The decisive defeat of the racist army in Cuito Cuanavale was a victory for all Africa. This victory in Cuito Cuanavale is what made it possible for Angola to enjoy peace and establish its own sovereignty. The defeat of the racist army made it possible for the people of Namibia to achieve their independence. The decisive defeat of the aggressive apartheid army destroyed the myth of the invincibility of the white oppressor. The defeat of the apartheid army served as an inspiration to the struggling people of South Africa." See "Nelson Mandela on How Cuba 'Destroyed the Myth of the Invincibility of the White Oppressor.'"

17. Edmonds, "Cuba's Other Internationalism."

18. Weaver and Owens, "Nelson Mandela's Memorial Service."

19. Brooke, "Cuban Doctors and Builders Also Aid Angola."

20. Garófalo Fernández and Gómez García, eds., *Pensamientos de Fidel sobre la salud pública*, 50.

21. Domínguez has summarized well the essence of Cuba's approach: "Within the context of Soviet hegemony, Cuban foreign policy is very much its own. . . . The Cuban government decided on its own to deploy troops in Angola in 1975; . . . Cuba led the USSR in fashioning policies toward Central America. . . . Overall, there is little evidence that Cuba acts in international affairs simply at the bidding of the USSR. Fidel Castro's Cuba is no one's puppet." Domínguez, *To Make a World Safe for Revolution: Cuba's Foreign Policy*, 4.

22. Kirk and Erisman, *Cuban Medical Internationalism: Origins, Evolution, and Goals*, 68–69.

23. Feinsilver, *Healing the Masses*, 160–61.

24. Domínguez, *To Make a World Safe for Revolution*, 155.

25. Feinsilver, *Healing the Masses*, 170.

26. For further information, see Gorry, "Joining Forces to Develop Human Resources for Health."

27. Menéndez Cabezas, "Experience of Cuban Faculty in Establishing a Medical School in the Republic of The Gambia."

28. Feinsilver, *Healing the Masses*, 157–58, 160.

29. These were Botswana, Burkina Faso, Burundi, Chad, Eritrea, Gambia, Ghana, Equatorial Guinea, Guinea Bissau, Guinea Conakry, Lesotho, Mali, Namibia, Niger, RASD, Rwanda, Sierra Leone, Swaziland, Tanzania, and Zimbabwe. Other forms of Cuban medical cooperation were found in Angola, Algeria, Cape Verde, Congo, Djibouti, Mozambique, Sao Tomé and Principe, South Africa, Seychelles, and Uganda. See http://www.saludthefilm.net/ns/Cuban%20Cooperation%20in%20Africa.pdf.

30. See "Asume nuevo coordinador de brigada médica en Guatemala."

31. Data taken from Kirk and Erisman, *Cuban Medical Internationalism: Origins, Evolution, and Goals*, 135–36.

32. "Speech Given by Dr. Fidel Castro Ruz, President of the Republic of Cuba, at the First Graduation of Students from the Latin American School of Medicine, Karl Marx Theatre, August 20, 2005."

33. Raúl Castro, "Cuba no teme a la mentira ni se arrodilla ante presiones."

34. "Información sobre el resultado del Debate de los Lineamientos de la Política Económica y Social del Partido y la Revolución."

35. Feinberg, "Soft Landing in Cuba? Emerging Entrepreneurs and Middle Classes," 2.

36. "La Salud Pública cubana apuesta a más calidad y más eficiencia."

37. Raúl Castro, "Intervención del General de Ejército Raúl Castro Ruz, Presidente del Consejo de Estado y de Ministros en la sesión plenaria de la Cumbre de América Latina y el Caribe, el 23 de febrero de 2010."

38. Kupferschmeidt, "Cuba to Commit Large Health Corps to Ebola Fight." Dr. Chan emphasized the significance of the Cuban contribution, thanking other countries for supplies, but noting, "Money, materials are important, but those alone cannot stop Ebola transmission. . . . The thing we need most of all is people."

39. Cumming-Bruce, "Ebola Outpaces Global Response, W.H.O. Says."

40. Fitz, "The Latin American School of Medicine Today."

41. Porter, "Cuba-Trained Doctors Making Difference around the World."

42. "Alrededor de 5,500 profesionales prestan servicios en África."

43. Nusa Peñalver, "Más de 100 mil cubanos prestaron ayuda civil en pueblos de África."

44. Gleijeses, *Misiones en conflicto*, 457.

Chapter 2. ELAM, a School for All Nations

1. PAHO, "Impact of Hurricane Mitch in Central America."

2. The complex, 25 km west of Havana in the Santa Fe community, is built on 120 hectares and consists of 28 large buildings in which there are 130 classrooms, as well as many laboratories, dormitories, and cafeterias.

3. Vázquez García, "La escuela más avanzada del mundo."

4. "Décimo aniversario de la Escuela Latinoamericana de Medicina."

5. Huish, "How Cuba's Latin American School of Medicine Challenges the Ethics of Physician Migration."

6. Fawthrop, "Cuando La Habana forma gratuitamente médicos yanquis."

7. Huish, *Where No Doctor Has Gone Before*, 92.

8. "Matrícula de la Escuela Latinoamericana de Medicina en Cuba llega a los 10 000 estudiantes."

9. Mullan, "Affirmative Action, Cuban Style."

10. Remen and Holloway, "A Student Perspective on ELAM and Its Educational Program," 158.

11. De Araújo, "A Snapshot of the Medical School, Faculty of Health Sciences, National University of Timor Larosa'e, Democratic Republic of Timor-Leste," 3.

12. "Key Address by Dr. Fidel Castro Ruz, President of the Republic of Cuba, at the Inauguration of the Latin American School of Medicine, Havana, November 15, 1999."

13. Joanne Mae Souers, "Update from U.S. Student Joanne Mae Souers, Studying Medicine in Cuba."

14. "From Cuba to Martinez."

15. See "Graduados de medicina en Cuba tienen deficiencias en formación, afirma UCR."

16. Dougherty, "Doctor Diplomacy Requires Red Pledge?"

17. Daisy Valera, "ELAM Med School 10 Years After."

18. "WHO Praises Work of Cuban Health Specialists."

19. Gail Reed, "PAHO's Presence in Cuban Health: José Luis Di Fabio PhD."

20. The WHO has calculated that there is a shortage of 2.4 million medical personnel in the world. Unfortunately, this dire need for doctors, nurses, technicians, and midwives is not felt equally. In Africa, for instance, there are 2.3 healthcare workers for every 1,000 people, compared with 25 in the Americas. The exodus of badly needed physicians from developing countries continues unabated. In the continent of Africa there are some 16 countries where at least half of nationally trained doctors have left to work abroad. In Liberia and Burundi this has risen to 80 percent, while 75 percent of medical graduates from Mozambique have also left. Meanwhile in the UK, some 30 percent of the doctors working for the National Health Service are Indian-born, while half of Pakistan's 4,000 medical graduates leave annually to work in the United States and the UK. See Whellams, "Medical Migration: Options and Responsibilities for the 'Brain Drain.'"

21. "Cuba Answers the Call for Doctors."

22. Campion and Morrissey, "A Different Model—Medical Care in Cuba," 297.

23. Gorry, "Staying the Course in Haiti."

24. Gorry, "Interview with Dr. Patrick Dely: Part II."

25. Chan, "Remarks at the Latin American School of Medicine, October 27, 2009."

26. Frank and Reed, "Doctors for the (Developing) World."

27. Remen and Holloway, "A Student Perspective on ELAM and Its Educational Program," 160.

28. Kirk and Huish, "Cuban Medical Internationalism and the Development of the Latin American School of Medicine."

29. "Students study different type of disasters, their socio-economic and health consequences, and what preventive or preparatory steps should be taken. . . . They learn how to stage a disaster and determine the steps needed during each stage in order to minimize the damage. They learn everything from patient triage and treatment to the organization of medical personnel and supplies. Students study the history of various disasters and examine how each was dealt with and then discuss what was done, what should have been done, and what could be done to prevent a recurrence." Remen and Holloway, "A Student Perspective on ELAM and Its Educational Program," 161.

30. For a detailed study of this approach, see Huish, "Going Where No Doctor Has Gone Before: The Role of Cuba's Latin American School of Medicine in Meeting the Needs of Some of the World's Most Vulnerable Populations."

31. Gorry, "Cuba's Latin American School: Can Socially Accountable Medical Education Make a Difference?" 6.

32. Álvarez Sintes, ed., *Temas de Medicina General Integral*, vol. 1, *Salud y Medicina*, vii.

33. Ibid., 28.

34. Ibid., 72.

35. Ibid., 21.

36. Ibid., 72.

37. Fitz, "Cuba's Latin American School of Medicine—An 'Example of Internationalism and Human Solidarity.'" See also Sowa, "Living Communally in a Cuban University." Also useful are "From Cuba to Martinez," the Agence France Press report, "Cuba's ELAM—Making Dreams Come True," and "ELAM: Médicos pobres para los pobres."

38. In March 2013 a strike was launched by 187 of the 1,200 South African students studying medicine in Cuba. They demanded a 300 percent increase in their grant from the South African government (which was US$300 a month), as well as improved food. See Jenvey, "Strike of Medical Students in Cuba Sparks Controversy."

39. Ibid.

40. "Speech Delivered by Dr. Fidel Castro Ruz, President of the Republic of Cuba, at the Foundation Ceremony of the 'Henry Reeve' International Contingent of Doctors Specialized in Disaster Situations and Serious Epidemics, and the National Graduation of Students of Medical Sciences, in the Ciudad Deportiva, on September 19, 2005."

41. "The minimum average infant mortality rate for this age group in the four countries affected by the hurricane is 54. . . . We calculated what would be needed and the possibility to undertake a comprehensive program for reducing infant mortality which might be brought down to 20 if the program were properly implemented. Based on our own experience, we know how this goal can be achieved and even what the cost might be." See "Speech delivered by Commander in Chief Fidel Castro Ruz, First Secretary of the Central Committee of the Communist Party of Cuba and President of the Councils of State and of Ministers, at the Closing Session of the 12th National Science and Technology Forum, held at the International Conference Center on 21 November 1998."

42. "Key Address by Dr. Fidel Castro Ruz, President of the Republic of Cuba, at the Inauguration of the Latin American School of Medicine. Havana, November 15, 1999."

43. See "Speech Given by Dr. Fidel Castro Ruz, President of the Republic of Cuba, at the First Graduation of Students from the Latin American School of Medicine, Karl Marx Theatre, August 20, 2005."

44. Lamrami adds a useful contextual note: "In 2012 Cuba graduated 11,000 new doctors, who completed their six years of training in faculties of medicine recognized for their academic excellence. This was the largest graduating class in the history of Cuba. . . . Among the graduates, 5,315 were Cuban while 5,694 were from 59 countries of Latin America, Africa, Asia, and even the United States. The largest groups were from Bolivia (2,400), Nicaragua (429), Peru (453), Ecuador (308), Colombia (175), and Guatemala (170). And so in one year Cuba has trained almost twice the number of doctors as there were in the entire country in 1959." Salim Lamrami, "Cuba, la isla de la salud."

45. Francis Mexidor, "Vatican Secretary Lauds Cuba Med School."

46. "ELAM: Médicos pobres para los pobres."

47. Heidi Soca, academic vice rector of ELAM, noted that ELAM's resources were not limitless, and as a result, "in order to keep this project of humanitarian solidarity viable, financial support was needed." As a result, while the vast majority of students at ELAM receive their education at no charge to them, a minority are now being paid by their government. The website of ELAM has material from the parastatal company Servicios Médicos Cubanos SA, which provides material on charges for a medical degree. The total cost for a six-year program in medicine has been set at 85,000 CUC (roughly the same amount in US$). A five-year degree in nursing will cost 50,000 CUC, and a five-year degree in dentistry, 80,000 CUC.

48. This refers to one of the basic tenets of patient care in the Cuban approach to public healthcare. Rather than treat a medical condition in a curative approach, providing medicine to cure a pathology, the Cuban philosophy is to view patients as a product of their

environment, with their psychological health as well as their biological well-being also being assessed as key factors in the patient's condition.

49. Chan, "Remarks at the Latin American School of Medicine."

Chapter 3. Dealing with the "Handicapped" of ALBA: Setting the Balance Right

1. A complete definition of *disabilities* is found on the WHO website, http://www.who.int/topics/disabilities/en. The website emphasizes the medical limitations often faced by people in this situation: "People with disabilities have the same health needs as non-disabled people—for immunization, cancer screening, etc. They also may experience a narrower margin of health, both because of poverty and social exclusion, and also because they may be vulnerable to secondary conditions, such as pressure sores or urinary tract infections. Evidence suggests that people with disabilities face barriers in accessing the health and rehabilitation services they need in many settings." Recognition is appropriate here for Jessica Vorstermans and her experience researching this topic in Ecuador. Her support in helping me understand the approach employed by Cuba in these programs was extremely important. All interpretations of the data provided are my own.

2. Cobas Ruiz et al., "Caracterización epidemiológica de las personas con discapacidad en Cuba."

3. Rojas, "Misión José Gregorio Hernández: Un año de lucha y esperanza para los discapacitados."

4. Viñet Espinosa et al., "Misión José Gregorio Hernández, formadora de valores en los estudiantes de Medicina Integral Comunitaria," 132.

5. "Venezuela: Programa gubernamental cumple cinco años de atención a discapacitados."

6. Data found at "Misión José Gregorio Hernández saca a la luz a 334,018 venezolanos con discapacidad."

7. Carrasco Martín, "Andar seguro venezolano-cubano en la atención a la discapacidad en Venezuela."

8. Carrasco Martín, "Un proyecto convertido en hechos para bienestar de los venezolanos."

9. See "Misión José Gregorio Hernández brinda atención integral en todo el país."

10. It is important to recognize the influence of Fidel Castro on this program. President Rafael Correa noted this in an interview: "Since we are so grateful to Cuba, we could not ignore the collaboration of Comandante Fidel Castro in this program. Even though you might find it hard to believe, he calls us every day to see how things are progressing. When he discovers how things are, he assists us and collaborates." See "Vicepresidente de Ecuador destaca solidaridad de Fidel Castro en temas de salud."

11. Watts, "Ecuador's Lenín Moreno Gives Revolutionary Turn by Quitting While on Top."

12. "Lenín Moreno expuso Misión Manuela Espejo en la ONU."

13. Marco Fabricio Narváez Montenegro, "La investigación epidemiológica del programa 'Manuela Espejo' 2010–2011," 36.

14. Untitled report found on the website of the office of the vice president: http://www.vicepresidencia.gob.ec/el-diagnostico/.

15. Misión Solidaria Manuela Espejo data found at http://www.manuelaespejo.com.

16. "Misión Manuela Espejo atiende más de 180 mil ecuatorianos."

17. Data found at www.manuelaespejo.com.

18. Misión Joaquín Gallegos Lara report, found at http://www.presidencia.gob.ec/mision-joaquin-gallegos-lara/.

19. "Misión Manuela Espejo atiende más de 180 mil ecuatorianos."

20. "Ecuador y Cuba firman convenio para prevenir discapacidades."

21. "Seguimiento médico de casos de discapacidad se cumple a medias."

22. "'Manuela Espejo,' un plan para imitar."

23. Data found at www.manuelaespejo.com.

24. "Misión Espejo, con 236 médicos cubanos."

25. "Ecuador agradece la cooperación de Cuba y de Venezuela."

26. Information taken from Cuban government website with data on cooperation in Ecuador and was found at http://www.cubadiplomatica.cu/ecuador.Cooperación.aspx (now defunct). Accessed March 1, 2013.

27. All data in this section come from the press communiqué "Bolivia y Cuba celebran 30 años de restablecimiento de relaciones diplomáticas."

28. "Regresan a Bolivia centenares de médicos graduados en Cuba."

29. "Éxito de Misión Solidaridad Moto Méndez."

30. Data from the Bolivian government's Sistema de Información del Programa de Registro Único Nacional de la Persona con Discapacidad, 2011, located at http://siprunpcd.minsalud.gob.bo/.

31. Taboada Lugo et al., "Discapacidad intelectual: Aproximación a las principales causas en el Estado Plurinacional de Bolivia."

32. "Clausura de la Misión Solidaria Moto Méndez, La Paz." Press release of Bolivian government.

33. Osoria Ramírez, "Moto Méndez: misión de esperanza en Bolivia."

34. Grover Choque, "El 90 por ciento de la discapacidad es adquirida."

35. "Presidente uruguayo concluye visita oficial a Cuba."

36. While most of the press coverage was supportive of the mission, there were occasionally critical notes. In Santa Cruz, a representative of a group of *discapacitados* noted that not all of the work of the Moto Méndez brigade had been carried out for humanitarian reasons but rather had been done to gain political support: "We know that with this kind of activities nothing will be resolved . . . all that they are doing is to waste our money." See Escalante Salazar, "Gobierno inicia censo de discapacitados ante rechazo de dirigentes."

37. "Fidel y la brigada 'Moto Méndez': 'La felicidad de hacer el bien.'"

38. "Discurso Señor Vicepresidente en cumbre de vicepresidentes América sin barreras."

Chapter 4. Operación Milagro: Bringing Vision to Millions

1. See World Health Organization, Fact Sheet no. 282, "Visual Impairment and Blindness."

2. García Alcolea and Lahera Cabrales, "Influencia de la Misión Milagro en la salud visual latinoamericana," 382.

3. See, for example, some representative articles on this program: "Mujica Flies to Havana to Meet the Castro Brothers and Celebrate 60 Years of Cuba's Revolution"; "La

Operación Milagro, de Cuba, ha beneficiado a por lo menos 2.5 millones"; "Inauguran exposición sobre la Operación Milagro en Argentina"; "Venezuela supera el millón de cirugías por la Misión Milagro"; "Dominicans Continue to Benefit from Cuban Eye Care Program"; "Second Stage of Operation Miracle by Cuban Eye Doctors in Suriname a Success"; "Millions of People Treated in Operation Miracle in Venezuela"; "Más de 61,000 nicaraguenses atendidos por médicos cubanos"; "Operation Miracle: Five Years of Cuban Ophthalmology Services in Nicaragua"; "Health Minister Lauds Cuba's Kindness"; "Operación Milagro: Operados de la vista más de 15,000 paraguayos"; "Venezuela: 94 mil personas atendidas por la Misión Milagro en el 2012"; "Beneficiados miles de salvadoreños con la Operación Milagro"; "Operación Milagro concluye el 2011 con 90,000 operaciones"; and "Mexicanos agradecen a Cuba por Operación Milagro."

4. Conner Gorry, "Sight for Sore Eyes: Cuba's Vision Restoration Program," 49.

5. Strictly speaking, Operación Milagro and Operation Miracle are the same ophthalmology program devised by Cuba and practiced on the island and in a number of countries in Latin America, the Caribbean, and Africa. Misión Milagro refers to the program situated specifically in Venezuela, providing ophthalmology treatment both to Venezuelans and to others in Latin American and Caribbean regions who are operated on in Venezuela. Some confusion has set in, however, and the terms are often interchanged.

6. Kirk, "Operation Miracle: A New Vision of Public Health?" 369.

7. García Alcolea, "Influencia de la Misión Milagro en el desarrollo de la teleoftalmología cubana," 35.

8. To put this in a historical context, in 1959 there were 118 ophthalmologists in Cuba, of whom only 37 remained on the island. See Armas Padrino, "Third Anniversary of Operation Miracle."

9. Ibid., 50.

10. "Programa cubano ha salvado de ceguera a medio millón en AL."

11. McKinley, "Cuba, in a Campaign against Blindness, Uses Doctors to Bolster Its Image."

12. "Venezuela's 'Misión Milagro' Performs 5,000 Eye Surgeries Weekly."

13. Aguin, "Desarrollo de la Misión Milagro en Venezuela," 540.

14. García Alcolea and González Poveda, "La dirección de un centro oftalmológico en el extranjero: reto de la administración de salud."

15. "Hoy se conmemora el Día Mundial de la Salud Visual." The same article noted that so far that year 153,500 operations had been carried out in Venezuela. Some 444 flights bringing patients had arrived in Venezuela, and 30,998 patients had been treated.

16. Statistics found at http://www.cubacoop.com/CubaCoop/misionmilagros.htm. This site, now defunct, contained the official data of the Cuban government in terms of cooperation for the ophthalmology program.

17. Ramos Pereira et al., "Misión Milagro: Una tecnología social."

18. "Reconocen beneficios de la Operación Milagro."

19. Quoted in *Miami Herald* staff report, "Cuba, Venezuela Benefit from Surgeries."

20. Data found at http://www.cambios.bo/noticia.php?fecha=2011-09-028idn=53644.

21. Schipani, "Bolivia's Miracle of Sight."

22. Furtado et al., "Is Misión Milagro an Effective Program to Prevent Blindness in Latin America?" 397–98.

23. De la Osa, "Egresan 11 mil médicos de universidades cubanas."

24. Fidel Castro, "Lo que no dijo Notimex."

25. "Lanzan en Trujillo campaña 'Ver para Creer.'"

26. "Dispone Cuba retirada de brigada médica de Panamá."

27. Agence France Presse report, "Operación Milagro: Cuba lamenta 'intereses mezquinos.'"

28. Quoted in "Los ojos abiertos de América Latina."

29. "Cataratón Kiwanis 2013 devuelve visión 20–20 a un centenar de panameños."

30. Carballo Hechevarría, "Por Paraguay sentimos una gratitud infinita."

31. Lobo noted that it was an honor for him to congratulate the Cuban medical brigade on their work in the country since Hurricane Mitch. More than 246,000 lives had been saved through the work of the Cuban medical personnel, and President-elect Juan Orlando Hernández had asked Lobo to confirm his desire to continue working closely with the Cuban medical brigade. See "Presidente de Honduras condecora a brigada médica cubana."

32. "Venezuela's 'Mission Miracle' Performs 5,000 Eye Surgeries Weekly."

33. "Más de 1 millón 500 mil personas atendidas por la Misión Milagro."

34. Ibid.

35. Data found at the Venezuelan government website, http://ceims.mppre.gob.ve.

36. Castro Medel, "Milagro para tres millones de personas."

37. These qualities are outlined by Ladys Marlene León Corrales, "Valor social de la Misión Milagro en el contexto venezolano."

38. Buddan, "Miracle at Christmas."

39. Ibid.

40. "Más de tres millones de beneficiados con Operación Milagro en diez años."

41. Ibid.

42. "Cuba Helps 50,000 Bolivians to See."

43. Manzaneda, "Why You Will Not Be Told about This Miracle."

44. Fariñas Acosta, "Ban Ki-moon: La ELAM es la escuela médica más avanzada del mundo."

Chapter 5. Cuba's International Disaster Responses: From 1960s Chile to the 2005 Henry Reeve Brigade

1. "Antecedentes históricos de la asistencia de Cuba ante situaciones de desastre."

2. Reed, "Cuban Medical Teams in Global Disaster Relief."

3. Ibid.

4. "Mitch: The Deadliest Atlantic Hurricane since 1780."

5. Morgan, "Honduras Fights Back after Mitch."

6. "World Bank Releases $201 Million for Storm-Ravaged Central America."

7. "Castro: Cuban Aid Offer Is 'Revenge' against Mitch."

8. "Declaración del gobierno de Cuba a propósito del Huracán Mitch: El problema no es sólo llorar por los que han muerto, sino ocuparnos de salvar a aquellos que silenciosamente mueren cada año."

9. "Cooperación Cuba-Honduras."

10. Gorry, "Cuba-Guatemala Cooperation: Building Viable Models for Health."

11. Burghardt, "Guatemalans Hail Cuban Medical Workers."

12. "Asume nuevo jefe de brigada médica cubana en Guatemala."

13. Gorry, "Cuba's Response to Katrina Disaster"; "President Castro Reiterates Cuba's Offer of Medical Aid to the American People on the Round Table Program Aired on September 2, 2005."

14. Gorry, "Cuban Disaster Doctors in Guatemala, Pakistan"; "Remarks by Dr. Fidel Castro Ruz, President of the Republic of Cuba, Meeting with the Medical Doctors Assembled to Offer Assistance to the American People in the Areas Affected by Hurricane Katrina. Havana Convention Centre, September 4, 2005."

15. Gorry, "Cuban Disaster Doctors in Guatemala, Pakistan."

16. See the complete Executive Order (No. KBB 2005-33) issued by Kathleen Blanco at www.doa.la.gov/osr/other/kbb05-33.htm.

17. Gorry, "Cuban Disaster Doctors in Guatemala, Pakistan."

18. Ibid.

19. "32,000 Cuban Health Workers Bring Aid to 72 Countries, 'Support an Inspiration to Cuban People.'"

20. Akhtar, "Cuban Doctors in Pakistan: Why Cuba Still Inspires"; Gorry, "Touring Cuban Field Hospitals in Post-Quake Pakistan"; Clemons, "Cuba's Soft Power: Exporting Doctors Rather than Revolution"; "U.S. Says Goodbye to Last MASH."

21. "Statement of the First Deputy Minister of Foreign Affairs of the Republic of Cuba, His Excellency Mr. Bruno Rodríguez, 19 November, 2005."

22. "Se dedica a Fidel primera graduación de médicos de Pakistán."

23. Gorry, "Touring Cuban Field Hospitals in Post-Quake Pakistan."

24. Juvenal Balán Neyra, "Despide presidente de Paquistán a Misión Médica Cubana"; "32,000 Cuban Health Workers Bring Aid to 72 Countries, 'Support an Inspiration to Cuban People.'"

25. González Peña, "El Contingente Médico Cubano 'Henry Reeve.'"

26. Whitney, "Cuban Medic in Pakistan."

27. De La Hoz, "Tariq Ali on Cuba, Venezuela, Bolivia."

28. UNEP/OCHA, "Hurricane Stan: Environmental Impacts from Floods and Mudslides in Guatemala."

29. "Day-By-Day Recap"; "Central America, Mexico, and Haiti: Floods from Hurricane Stan—Appeal No. 05EA021 Final Report."

30. UNEP/OCHA, "Hurricane Stan"; "Additional €2.6m for Hurricane Stan Victims in Guatemala."

31. "Hurricane Stan Floods Coastal Guatemala—MSF Response"; Li, "Bettering Children's Lives Devastated by Hurricane Stan."

32. United Nations World Food Program, "Hurricane Stan: Humanitarian Update from Central America."

33. "IDB Grants $400,000 to Guatemala and El Salvador for Relief after Hurricane Stan."

34. "Hurricane Stan Floods Coastal Guatemala—MSF Response."

35. "Reconstruction of Water Systems after Hurricane Stan."

36. Gorry, "Cuban Disaster Doctors in Guatemala, Pakistan"; González Peña, "El Contingente Médico Cubano 'Henry Reeve'"; Riera, "In Two Months: Cuban Doctors Saved More than 1,000 Lives in Guatemala."

37. Fawthrop, "Cuba's Humanitarian Mission"; "Indonesian Earthquake Donations"; "Cuban Medical Brigade Returns from Helping Indonesia."

38. Recases, "Cuba's Doctors Help in Indonesia."

39. Fawthrop, "Cuba's Humanitarian Mission."

40. "Cuban Medical Brigade Returns From Helping Indonesia."

41. Recases, "Cuba's Doctors Help in Indonesia."

42. Fawthrop, "Cuba's Humanitarian Mission."

43. "Mexico Thanks Cuba for Medical Aid to Flood Victims."

44. "Red Bolivia Cuba puso a disposición 1,700 médicos y equipo logístico para atención de damnificados."

45. "400 médicos cubanos a damnificados por desastres naturales."

46. Rake, "Peru: How Cuba's Solidarity Make a Difference." Also see, "The Detachment Returns, Undefeated."

47. See the report, "Brigada Internacional Henry Reeve regresa de Chile."

48. "Reseña histórica de la brigada."

49. Gutiérrez Delgado, "Médico Cubano se une a brujo para asistir a la población de Guatemala."

50. Canales, "Cuba aporta a Guatemala 535 médicos para asistir damnificados."

51. "Reconoce Presidente de Guatemala internacionalismo de Cuba en la salud."

52. Burghardt, "Guatemalans Hail Cuban Medical Workers."

53. Reed, "Cuba and Guatemala: Innovations in Physician Training."

54. "Cuba's Medical Aid after Hurricane Mitch Recalled in Guatemala."

55. "Reconocida Brigada Médica Cubana en Guatemala como Personaje del Año."

56. "Cuba Receives Human Rights Prize for Medical Brigade."

57. "Guatemala Plans to Send More Medical Students to Cuba."

58. "Brigada Médica Cubana en Guatemala cumple 10 años." See also "Estructura de la BMC."

59. "Brigada Médica Cubana en Guatemala cumple 10 años."

60. "Asume nuevo coordinador de brigada médica en Guatemala."

61. "Cuba's Medical Missionaries Blanket Honduras"; "Cooperación Cuba-Honduras."

62. Gorry, "Innovative Project Brings Permanent Medical Services to Honduran Mosquitia."

63. Appelbaum and Bastian, "Honduras: Cuban-Trained Garifuna Doctors Supported in Hospital Expansion Drive."

64. "Cuban Doctors Make an Impact on Honduras Health Levels"; "Se rinde homenaje en Honduras al 11no. Aniversario de presencia de la brigada médica cubana."

65. "Impactos de las actividades de la BMC en Honduras."

66. "Cooperación Cuba-Honduras."

67. "Impactos de las actividades de la BMC en Honduras."

Chapter 6. South-South Cooperation in Biotechnology: Medicine for the Masses

1. "Cuba's Biotech Boom."

2. Lage Dávila, "Fidel o la inmediatez del futuro."

3. Heberprot-P is an injectable medicine that contains the human recombinant Epidermal Growth Factor as the active pharmaceutical ingredient. It supports the healing process in ulcers at later stages in diabetic patients.

4. "En Mérida redujeron las amputaciones en pacientes con diabetes." These figures seemed somewhat exaggerated. By contrast in Cuba, after a six-year period of study following 21,000 patients, it was found that there was a reduction in the risk of amputation by 71 percent. See "Miles de cubanos favorecidos con Heberprot-P para pie diabético."

5. "Reduce Cuba riesgos de amputación a pacientes de pie diabético."

6. Reid-Henry, *The Cuban Cure*, 168.

7. On September 19, 2005, Fidel Castro noted, "After more than forty years, and as the Special Period draws to an end, medical services have become the most important sector of our economy. And that is without Cuba ceasing medical cooperation—at no cost to the recipient countries—to over sixty countries in the Third World without economic resources. That's the way it has been, and always will be." Quoted in Garófalo Fernández and Gómez García, eds., *Pensamientos de Fidel sobre la salud pública*, 60.

8. UNESCO, "Science Policy for Sustainable Development: Cuba." Among the salient characteristics of the Cuban approach to biotechnology, the report highlights the role of the Cuban government as the source of investment, the close relationship between biotechnology and the national public health system, the "'closed cycle' from research to commercialization by fully integrated state institutions, with profits generated from sales in foreign markets, an important part of which is reinvested in R&D," the collaborative nature of research replacing individual competition as the "driving force" of Cuban biotechnology.

9. Cited in Scheye, "Cuban Healthcare and Biotechnology: Reform, a Bitter Pill to Swallow, or Just What the Doctor Ordered?"

10. Lage Dávila, "Fidel, o la inmediatez del futuro." He notes one of the important lessons from those early meetings: "We acquired a new perception of what we were capable of doing—since we ourselves had no idea what we were able to do. In that small laboratory in 1989 Fidel asked which company was the world leader in producing monoclonal antibodies, and how much they produced. We told him. His next question was: and you haven't thought of competing with those people? An amazing question for a small group of scientists in an underdeveloped country, victim of the U.S. embargo, and about to lose its greatest ally."

11. Mayte María Jiménez, "Productos biotecnológicos cubanos en 50 países."

12. Racotumomab (Vaxira) does not cure patients with lung cancer. It increases their life expectancy, stimulating the body's immune system so that the tumor stops growing or grows far more slowly. Cuban researchers were assisted by Argentine colleagues, and it is fitting that the first country outside Cuba where it became available is Argentina. A public/private consortium involved the Center for Molecular Immunology and, in Argentina, the Ángel Roffo Oncology Institute, the National Council of Scientific and Technical Research, and the University of Quilmes. See "Desarrollan cubanos y argentinos vacuna

contra cáncer de pulmón." CimavaxEGF is a therapeutic cancer vaccine that targets lung cancer, weakening the disease.

13. See Marc Caputo, "Rep. Garcia's Push for Cuba Drug Trials Tests Support for Embargo." In essence Miami congressman Joe García was seeking approval to test and market the diabetes treatment in the United States. This was opposed by several fellow Cuban Americans and would require a special license from the U.S. Department of the Treasury.

14. "Atendidos más de 34 mil pacientes con pie diabético a través del Ministerio de Salud."

15. "Firma Ecuador convenio para adquirir Heberprot."

16. See CIGB, "Portafolios de Negocios, 2012–13," 1.

17. Lage Dávila, "Fidel o la inmediatez del futuro."

18. For a good analysis of the research focus of these institutes, see Evenson, "Cuba's Biotechnology Revolution," 8–10.

19. Ibid., 3–4.

20. Reid-Henry, *The Cuban Cure*, 7.

21. Fidel Castro has explained the differences between the approaches: "In capitalism, for example, medicine represents merchandise, a form of business. Illness itself is part of that merchandise of capitalism. Indeed in capitalism both businesses and capitalist institutions need disease since it is simply one more means of doing business, making money through the sale of medicines. . . . [By contrast] in our country all the doctors who graduate go to work for the people. They don't exploit medicine as some form of private business. . . . So this commercial use of illness which we see in capitalism disappears in our system, and therefore our health program is not hindered by that limitation and so can advance to the best form of public health that humanity is capable of." This was taken from a speech at the opening of a polyclinic on January 8, 1969. See Garófalo Fernández and Gómez García, eds., *Pensamientos de Fidel Castro sobre la salud pública*, 17.

22. "Patricia Grogg entrevista a la científica cubana Concepción Campa."

23. Douglas Starr pointed out some of these differences between the biotechnology culture in Cuba and the developed world: "'They just don't get capitalism,' a diplomat tells me over coffee in Boston. 'The elite may watch American TV and read the *Wall Street Journal* on the Web, so they have a conversational familiarity. But on a fundamental level they don't get it and don't want to get it. They still think there's something immoral about profit.' . . . It's like Castro said: They don't really *like* patents. They like medicine. Cuba's drug pipeline is most interesting for what it lacks: grand-slam moneymakers, cures for baldness or impotence or wrinkles. It's all cancer therapies, AIDS medications, and vaccines against tropical diseases." Starr, "The Cuban Biotech Revolution."

24. Cárdenas, "The Cuban Biotechnology Industry: Innovation and Universal Health Care."

25. Fawthrop, "Cuba Ailing? Not Its Biomedical Industry."

26. Saénz, Thorsteinsdóttir, and de Souza, "Cuba and Brazil: An Important Example of South-South Collaboration in Health Biotechnology," 32.

27. "Alta demanda de monoclonal cubano en China."

28. Vives Romero, "China-Cuba: Colaboración biotecnológica con buena salud."

29. "Ampliarán en China presencia productos biotecnológicos cubanos."

30. Lu, Chen, and Gao, "Transcontinental Translational Medicine Collaboration: A Successful Sino-Cuban Joint B-to-B Program," 518.

31. "Vacunas cubanas consolidan su presencia en mercado vietnamita."

32. The product BioRat has been used in Cuba for over 25 years and is produced in Cuba and in Vietnam, from where it is exported to 22 countries in Africa, Latin America, and Asia.

33. Pierrat, "Inician en Nicaragua aplicación de rodenticida donado por Cuba."

34. This was part of a large Cuban presence in public health, the main goal of which was to reduce cases of malaria in Angola. According to official figures, the number of cases was reduced by approximately a million, with the number of fatalities falling 40 percent. See "Cuba promueve lucha contra la malaria en Angola."

35. González, "¿Empresa modelo o modelo de empresa?" 7.

36. Morales Valido, "Biorat: una pelea cubana contra las ratas."

37. "Reconoce Cuba significativa disminución de malaria en Angola." Two of the products used were Griselesf and Bactivec, which were designed to control various species of mosquitos.

38. See MINREX note, "Cuban Internationalists Fighting Malaria in Angola."

39. Peláez, "Valoran efectividad de biolarvicidas cubanos."

40. "Cuba y Ecuador consolidan cooperación en sector biofarmacéutico."

41. Sánchez Gutiérrez and Gorry, "Immunodiagnostics: The Convergence of Biotech and Public Health," 9.

42. Riera, "Cuba Exports Medical Equipment All Over the World."

43. Grogg, "Cuba, Brazil Unite for Africa's Health."

44. Ibid.

45. For an analysis of this example of collaboration, see Thorsteinsdóttir and Sáenz, "Tackling Meningitis in Africa," 1546–47.

46. Saénz et al., "Cuba and Brazil," 33.

47. Thorsteinsdóttir and Sáenz, "Tackling Meningitis in Africa," 1547.

48. Sáenz et al., "Cuba and Brazil," 33.

49. Ibid.

50. "Cuba to Access Global Pharmaceutical Markets via Brazil."

51. "Cuba impulsa comercialización productos biotecnológicos en Brasil."

52. Starr, "The Cuban Biotech Revolution."

53. See chapters 3–5 of Thorsteinsdóttir, ed., *South-South Collaboration in Health Technology*.

54. Gorry, "Biotech: The Magic Pill?"

55. "Cuba y Venezuela inauguran una de las plantas farmacéuticas más modernas de Latinoamérica."

56. Saénz et al., "Cuba and Brazil," 34.

57. "Cuba, Brazil in More Diplomacy for Closer Economic Ties."

58. ALBA members are Cuba, Venezuela, Bolivia, Ecuador, Dominica, Nicaragua, Antigua and Barbuda, and St. Vincent and the Grenadines. Haiti, Iran, and Syria hold observer status. The population of member countries is some 70 million people, with a GDP of $US 636 billion.

59. There remains the challenge of private pharmaceutical companies in the ALBA countries, since they are obviously concerned about losing their market share. This was seen clearly in the case of Ecuador, where President Rafael Correa sought to purchase $1.5 billion of Cuban-made drugs in 2011—only to have that plan shattered by the political opposition in Ecuador who claimed that the drugs were not officially registered there and also that the importation of Cuban products would take away employment from local pharmaceutical companies. As a result Correa had to reduce significantly his list of purchases.

60. See Cochetti, "ALBAmed: A New Regional Pharma Hub in the Americas?" The article goes on: "Although specific mechanisms by which savings will be realized have not yet been disclosed, one of the most effective ways for ALBA countries to successfully save on medical purchases would be by substituting the imports of costly international drugs with Cuban generic counterparts, whenever possible."

61. Reid-Henry, *The Cuban Cure*, 163.

62. Lage Dávila, "Socialism and the Knowledge Economy."

Chapter 7. The Cuba-Venezuela Medical Partnership: The Castro-Chávez Dream Lives On

1. I would like to express my gratitude to Dr. Arturo Menéndez Cabezas, a member of the Cuban medical team who worked for several years in Barcelona, Venezuela. He is a specialist in clinical biochemistry and public health administration. His insights, constructive criticism, and support have been extremely helpful to me in writing this chapter.

2. "Más de 60 mil personas ha atendido convenio de salud Cuba-Venezuela."

3. Jardim, "Prevention and Solidarity: Remedies for Democratizing Health in Venezuela."

4. D'Elia, ed., *Las misiones sociales en Venezuela*, 20.

5. Ibid., 28.

6. Jardim, "Prevention and Solidarity."

7. Brouwer, *Revolutionary Doctors*, 75.

8. Pan American Health Organization, *Mission Barrio Adentro*, 26.

9. Data provided in D'Elia, ed., *Las misiones sociales en Venezuela*, 36.

10. Figures taken from Brouwer, *Revolutionary Doctors*, 15.

11. A Cuban medical professor working in Venezuela noted that Cuban specialists are in charge in most of the CATs. In addition, increasingly Venezuelan physicians, trained in comprehensive community medicine, are filling positions in the local *consultorios* under the Barrio Adentro program. Many have undertaken their residency under the supervision of Cuban professors. In the *consultorios* some share responsibilities with a Cuban physician, while increasingly they are working alone. There is also a new position—that of the medical specialists known as *itinerantes*. These are highly qualified Cuban specialists, mainly with the teaching rank of associate professor or full professor, who come for a term of three months to work in the CATs or in some hospitals. Personal communication from Cuban medical school professor, December 3, 2013.

12. D'Elia, *Las misiones sociales en Venezuela*, 37.

13. Pan American Health Organization, "Venezuela."

14. D'Elia, ed., *Las misiones sociales en Venezuela,* 38.
15. "Venezuela y el drama del parto."
16. Mantiñán Búairambua, "Los cubanos están trayendo el cólera a Venezuela."
17. "Médicos cubanos estarán aquí hasta que Chávez decida."
18. D'Elia, *Las misiones sociales en Venezuela,* 39.
19. Wynter, "Venezuela: Cuban Doctors Helping the Poor."
20. Furtado et al., "Is Misión Milagro an Effective Program to Prevent Blindness in Latin America?" 398.
21. "Fact Sheet: Misión Milagro."
22. "Misión Milagro suma un millón de intervenciones en Venezuela."
23. "Venezuela supera el millón de cirugías por la Misión Milagro."
24. "Misión Milagro ha devuelto la visión a 2.5 millones de personas."
25. Ibid.
26. See, for example, "87 beneficiarios de Misión Milagro Chile ya fueron operados en Venezuela"; "90 salvadoreños viajaron a Venezuela en Operación Milagro"; "Primer grupo de pacientes de la Misión Milagro viaja a Venezuela"; "Ecuatorianos recuperan la visión gracias a 'Misión Milagro' en Venezuela"; and the poignantly titled "La Misión Milagro de Venezuela apoya a mexicanos *olvidados* por el Seguro Popular."
27. Cited in Brouwer, *Revolutionary Doctors,* 49.
28. "Federación Médica Venezolana: Aumento de salario de 75% es necesario pero insuficiente."
29. "Since the doctors and their students are operating within the context of radical social change, it has been possible to develop a unique medical curriculum and communicate scientific knowledge in brand-new ways. The new revolutionary doctors learn the same medical science that is taught throughout the world, only in a formulation that emphasizes the interrelatedness of the various traditional medical sciences and integrates them into broad courses of morphophysiology and morphopathology. In the course of their formal studies, their daily exposure to patients and practical questions of care have habituated them to integrate their growing scientific knowledge with the complexities of diagnosis and treatment. The fact that the students have daily access to extensive DVD material that relates to each formal class, often reviewed in study sessions with other students, gives them multiple opportunities to interpret or reinterpret the meaning of the scientific concepts and their social/medical applications. . . . The new Cuban-Venezuelan system of medical education, Medicina Integral Comunitaria, has taken the concept of apprenticeship and reconfigured it. By working half the day alongside a master/tutor, the apprentice/student learns not only the knowledge and techniques of the specialty, but also the social context and the ways the community can make use of this art." Brouwer, *Revolutionary Doctors,* 216–17.
30. Ibid., 216.
31. Gustavo Uzcategui, quoted in Robertson, "The 'Doctors of Socialism'? Meet Venezuela's Community Doctors." He continues, noting the difference between the traditional practice of medicine and that of MIC graduates: "I think that with a government of the opposition it would be very difficult for us to exercise community medicine, because we see medicine as a humanist vocation, and they [private sector doctors and the conservative

opposition] see medicine as a managerial vocation and as a means to make money. They see the patient as a commodity, that is, we squeeze them, we take everything that we can, and we leave them without mercy."

32. Robertson, "Attending Need, Not Profit: Venezuela's Experiment with Community Medicine."

33. Yanetzi Parades, quoted in Robertson, "The 'Doctors of Socialism'?"

34. As an example, see the Radio Martí article "Capriles y federación médica critican salud pública venezolana." In it the opposition leader, Henrique Capriles, and Douglas León Natera, president of the FMV, expressed identical sentiments about the state of the healthcare system.

35. "Venezuela supera el millón de cirugías por la Misión Milagro."

36. Janicke, "Venezuelan Doctors Step Up Protests against Government."

37. Pearson, "Venezuela's Community Doctors Gain Legal Recognition."

38. Brouwer, *Revolutionary Doctors*, 123.

39. "Destaca Nicolás Maduro labor de médicos cubanos en Venezuela."

40. Robertson, "Attending Need, Not Profit."

41. Brouwer, *Revolutionary Doctors*, 113.

42. "Venezuela y Cuba: nuevos convenios de la solidaridad."

43. Robertson, "Attending Need, Not Profit."

44. Castro Medel, "Reconocen logros de alianza Cuba-Venezuela."

45. "Destaca Nicolás Maduro labor de médicos cubanos en Venezuela."

46. "Maduro destaca ayuda 'incalculable' de Cuba en materia de salud."

47. "Elías Jaua niega que médicos cubanos cobren 200 mil dólares al año."

48. Tamayo, "Celebran 12 años del Convenio integral de cooperación Cuba-Venezuela."

49. "Chávez: Aportes de Cuba suman 10 veces más del costo del petróleo que envía Venezuela."

50. In late 2013, a summary of the impact of Cuban medical cooperation was provided. Since 2000 there had been 464 flights from Venezuela transporting 58,000 Venezuelans for medical treatment in Cuba. In addition, 1,900,000 Venezuelans had received ophthalmological operations, more than 700,000 Venezuelans had been saved from death through medical intervention in Misión Barrio Adentro (which had provided 780 million consultations), and almost 337,000 people with physical disabilities had been treated. Data provided by Castro Medel, "Vida que crece en tierra de Bolívar."

51. "Presidente Chávez anuncia relanzamiento de Convenio Cuba-Venezuela 2010."

52. Serrano, "Infiltrado en un avión de la Misión Milagro con destino a La Habana."

53. In November 2013, Venezuelan president Nicolás Maduro, commenting on Cuba's contribution to the developing world, proposed the creation of the Universidad de las Ciencias de la Salud Salvador Allende to train healthcare specialists for the countries of Latin America and the Caribbean, offering 1,000 scholarships annually for students. He reiterated his government's commitment to train 60,000 community doctors and 15,000 specialists for the Venezuelan people. See "Venezuela propone la creación de Universidad internacional de la salud."

Chapter 8. Cuba's Role in Haiti: Hurricanes, an Earthquake, and Cholera

1. In May 2013 *Prensa Latina* noted that since 1988, "nearly 11,000 collaborators have rendered their services, while nearly 700 Cubans remain in Haiti." Data found in "Haitian Premier Arrives in Cuba in Official Visit."

2. "Cuba to Send Doctors."

3. For an analysis of this stormy period in Haiti's period, see Paul Farmer, "Who Removed Aristide?" 28–31.

4. "Press Conference on Haiti Humanitarian Aid."

5. See the entry for "Haiti" on the Pan American Health Organization website, found at http://www.paho.org/english/dd/ais/cp_332.htm.

6. Chávez Alfonso and Marcelo Pentón, "Evaluación nutricional de niños menores de edad: Centro de Salud 'Soleil.' Departamento noroeste de Haití, 2005–06," 28–39. One of the saddest features of the health profile of Haiti was that HIV/AIDS killed 30,000 Haitians annually, with an estimated cumulative number of 196,000 deaths and 200,000 orphans by 2002. Castro and Farmer, "International Public Health Pitfalls and Economic Arguments: The Fight against AIDS in Cuba and Haiti."

7. See UNICEF, "At a Glance: Haiti," http://www.unicef.org/infobycountry/haiti_statistics.html.

8. Data provided in the "Declaración del Ministro de Relaciones Exteriores de Cuba en la Reunión de Donantes a Haití."

9. In an open letter to Secretary of State Colin Powell, Harvard medical professor Paul Farmer explained the situation of public health in Haiti: "In 2003 the budget of the entire Republic of Haiti, population 8 million, was less than $300 million. The 2003 budget of a single Harvard teaching hospital—and there are two dozen Harvard teaching hospitals—was pegged at $1.3 billion." See his letter, "U.S. Invasion of Haiti Deepens Health Crisis," in the April 2004 issue of *Peacework*.

10. Gorry, "Haiti One Year Later: Cuban Medical Team Draws on Experience and Partnerships," 53.

11. "Exitoso apoyo médico de Cuba en Haití."

12. Steif, "Cuban Doctors Aid Strife-Torn Haiti."

13. Eaton, "In Haiti, Cuban Doctors Stayed When No One Else Would." It is worth noting that in the midst of the violence (22 gunshot victims were treated on February 29 and March 1 by the Cubans), and with violence all around them, the Cuban medical staff were not bothered by looters or thieves. "The people have always protected us," noted Dr. Juan Carlos Chávez, the head of the Cuban mission. "We're here to take care of people's health."

14. As Havana radio correspondent Anna Kovac noted, Cuban medical personnel remained in Haiti despite tremendous political instability: "I think it's remarkable that the Cubans have stayed in spite of the February 29th coup, in spite of the fact that first you had a U.S. occupation, followed by a UN occupation, in spite of the fact that you had all these gangsters and ex-soldiers and criminals who practically took over Haiti. . . . The Cuban doctors stayed. . . . That just shows that Cuba is interested in helping the people. The Haitian people are number one, and governments are number two." See Kovac, "Cuban-Haitian Cooperation."

15. Steif, "Cuban Doctors Aid Strife-Torn Haiti."

16. Interview with Paul Farmer found at www.saludthefilm.net.

17. Kovac, "Cuban-Haitian Cooperation." The person interviewing Kovac, Roger Leduc, made a related comment: "The Haitians are really impressed by the attitude of the Cuban doctors, who really taught a lesson to the whole society in this way: the Haitian doctors tended to be very elitist and arrogant in their dealings with the poor masses in Haiti, and the Cuban doctors have shown that you can provide medical services while maintaining the dignity of the people you are servicing."

18. Data located at "At a Glance: Haiti."

19. Rodríguez Armas, "Cuba colabora en mejoría de indicadores de salud en Haití." A year later, the data suggested a continued improvement: "In the areas covered by the Cuban doctors, the infant mortality rate in children under 1 year of age has dropped from 80 to 28 per 1,000 live births—and in children under 5 years of age, the rate has fallen from 159 to 39 per 1,000 live births. The maternal mortality rate dropped from 523 deaths to 259 per 100,000 live births." See "Statement by Felipe Pérez Roque, Minister of Foreign Affairs of Cuba, at the Special Meeting of the Council of Ministers of the Association of Caribbean States. Panama City, 12 February 2004."

20. Davalos, "Cuban Vice President Meets with Haitian Foreign Minister."

21. See Morales Lugo et al., "Brigada Médica Internacionalista Cubana en Haití."

22. Steinsleger, "Haití, Cuba y la ley primera."

23. Quoted in Maltbie, "Haiti Earthquake: The Nations That Are Stepping Up to Help."

24. United Nations Office for the Coordination of Humanitarian Affairs, "Haiti, Earthquake Situation Report #14."

25. Data provided in the Merlin NGO report "Is Haiti's Health System Any Better?"

26. Gorry, "Haiti One Year Later," 54.

27. See "Haiti Earthquake Aid Pledged by Country."

28. The Voice of America news bulletin of January 22, 2010, noted how the Cuban government had allowed overflights of its territory by U.S. planes flying medical evacuation missions without any pre-clearance, thereby speeding up efforts. It also noted how relief efforts in Haiti had "received a boost from Cuba, which has more than 400 health workers, many of them doctors, working throughout the devastated country." See "Cuba Aids Haiti Relief."

29. Kirk and Kirk, "Cuban Medical Aid to Haiti: One of the World's Best-Kept Secrets."

30. See Harvard Medical School and NATO Joint Analysis and Lessons Learned Centre, *The Haiti Case Study*.

31. See "Haitian Medical Students in Cuba."

32. Data provided by Carriba, "Llama Cuba a cooperación con Haití y respetar principios."

33. Steif, "Cuban Doctors Aid Strife-Torn Haiti." See also the "Declaración del Ministro de Relaciones Exteriores de Cuba en la Reunión de Donantes a Haití."

34. Data provided a few days later by Dr. García illustrated how the Cuban medical delegation continued to expand: six rehabilitation theaters had been set up in Port-au-Prince, Cuban psychologists and psychiatrists had arrived to implement badly needed mental health services for the survivors, 20,000 Haitians had been vaccinated against disease, and the 938 members of the Cuban medical brigade had seen more than 50,000 patients. See "Prosiguen labores de brigada médica cubana en Haití."

35. Burnett, "Cuban Doctors Unsung Heroes of Haitian Earthquake."

36. Data in this section come from the address given by Ambassador Rodolfo Reyes Rodríguez on January 27, 2010, in Geneva at the 13th Special Session of the UN Human Rights Council on Haiti. It can be seen at "Cuba en Ginebra: 'Ante tan difícil situación humanitaria en Haití no puede haber titubeos ni indiferencia.'" See also Gómez Navia, "Médicos cubanos extienden sus labores en Haití."

37. See the Cubadebate report, "Médicos de Cuba han atendido más de 50,000 haitianos; comienzan servicios de rehabilitación." Also see Martínez Hernández and Balán, "Cuban Healthcare Continues in Haiti."

38. Castro, "Cooperation Spirit Is Put to the Test in Haiti."

39. Gorry, "Once the Earth Stood Still (Part II): Mental Health Services in Post-Quake Haiti," 44. The participants had been trained at the Latin American Center for Disaster Medicine (CLAMED), based in Havana.

40. For a detailed analysis of Cuba's role in fighting cholera, see Somarriba López et al., *Cólera en Haití.*

41. Data from Gorry, "Haiti One Year Later: Cuban Medical Team Draws on Experience and Partnerships," 52.

42. See Llanes et al., "Did the Cholera Epidemic in Haiti Really Start in the Artibonite Department?" 753–55.

43. Merlin, "Is Haiti's Health System Any Better?"

44. Centers for Disease Control and Prevention, "Cholera in Haiti."

45. Archibold, "Cuba Takes Lead Role in Haiti's Cholera Fight."

46. Ibid.

47. Barzilay et al., "Cholera Surveillance during the Haiti Epidemic," 599.

48. See Kirk and Kirk, "Cuban Medical Aid to Haiti."

49. Martínez Hernández and Balán, "Cuba fue el primer país que nos ayudó."

50. Barbosa León, "Cuba and Haiti."

51. Data provided in the "Declaración del Ministro de Relaciones Exteriores de Cuba en la Reunión de Donantes a Haití."

52. Maceo Leyva, "Quince años de batas blancas."

53. See the final communiqué of the conference, available at http://www.haiticonference.org/communique.html.

54. For an analysis of the funding pledged, see "International Conference Raises Almost $10 Billion as More than 130 Donors Contribute 'Towards a New Future for Haiti.'" United Nations press release (GA/10932) of March 31, 2010. For a report on the amount disbursed to the government, see Vijaya Ramachandan and Julie Walz, "Haiti: Where Has All the Money Gone?" A Report by the Center for Global Development, CGD Policy Paper 004, May 2012. Available at www.cgdev.org/files/1426185_file_Ramachandan_Walz_haiti_FINAL.pdf.

55. Data provided in Humanitarian Response Index 2011, "Focus on Haiti," 8.

56. "This was especially problematic in the second cholera epidemic. The resurgence of cholera in the spring and summer of 2011 became the biggest scandal between NGOs and institutional donors. NGOs vocally criticized the donors for the abrupt termination of cholera funding at a point when the attack rate of cholera was increasing, in the spring and summer of 2011," "Focus on Haiti," 10.

57. All information on Cuba's pledge for the reconstruction of Haiti comes from the speech given at the United Nations by Cuban foreign minister Bruno Rodríguez Parrilla. See "Declaración del Ministro de Relaciones Exteriores de Cuba en la Reunión de Donantes a Haití." It is worth noting that a subject analysis of the coverage of the Haiti Donor Conference by five major U.S. media (CNN, the *Miami Herald*, the *Washington Post*, the *New York Times*, and the *Boston Globe*) shows 38 posts in the 10 days following the conference. Despite Cuba's major contribution, Cuba was mentioned only once and then briefly.

58. Carpineta, "Habla el jefe de los 744 médicos cubanos instalados en Haití desde hace doce años."

59. Martínez Hernández, "Nuestros compromisos con Haití continúan inalterables."

60. See the *Huffington Post* report of January 27, 2010, "Quebec Doctors Want Pay for Haiti Volunteer Work."

61. Burnett, "Cuban Doctors Unsung Heroes of Haitian Earthquake."

62. See Cuban Foreign Minister Bruno Rodríguez's statement to the Haiti Donor Conference, overseas.blogpost.ca/2010/04/statement-of-cuban-foreign-minister-at.html.

63. "Haiti-Cuba Cooperation Is in the Agenda of Prime Minister Laurent Lamothe."

64. Barbosa León, "Cuba and Haiti: A History of Solidarity."

65. "Raúl Castro asegura ayuda cubana para Haití el tiempo que sea necesario."

Chapter 9. Cuba's Medical Internationalism in the South Pacific

1. Ministry of Public Health, Timor-Leste, *Human Resources for Health: Country Profile—Timor-Leste*, 5.

2. Ibid., 15, 18.

3. De Araújo, "A Snapshot of the Medical School, Faculty of Health Sciences, National University of Timor Lorosa'e, Democratic Republic of Timor-Leste."

4. Anderson, "Cuban Health Cooperation in Timor-Leste and the South West Pacific," 82. Anderson notes that by 2008 there were 350 Cuban healthcare workers in the region. For further analysis, see 77–86.

5. Ministry of Public Health, Timor-Leste, *Human Resources for Health,* 6.

6. De Araújo, "A Snapshot of the Medical School," 4.

7. Kirk, "Cuban Medical Internationalism under Raúl Castro," 83.

8. Ministry of Public Health, Timor-Leste, *Human Resources for Health,* 38.

9. More details, including videos of recent medical graduates in Timor-Leste, can be found at http://www.youtube.com/watch?v=eOLmUIGdYjE&feature=plcp. Also worth noting are the video of South Pacific students at ELAM (http://www.youtube.com/watch?v=AhMAncnEDQQ&feature=plcp) and other material found in Tim Anderson's YouTube recording, http://www.youtube.com/user/timand2037/videos?sort=dd&flow=grid&view=0&page=2.

10. Anderson, "Social Medicine in Timor Leste," 186.

11. Ministry of Public Health, Timor-Leste, *SISCa Health Service*, n.d.

12. Tim Anderson, "Social Medicine in Timor Leste," 188.

13. De Araújo, "A Snapshot of the Medical School," 2.

14. Ibid., 1.

15. Kirk, "Cuban Medical Internationalism under Raúl Castro," 82–83.

16. De Araújo, "A Snapshot of the Medical School," 1.

17. Cabral et al., "Scaling Up the Medical Workforce in Timor-Leste: Challenges of a Great Leap Forward," 2.

18. Tim Anderson, "Social Medicine in Timor-Leste," 187.

19. Ibid.

20. Ministry of Public Health, Timor-Leste, *Human Resources for Health*, 6.

21. Marce Cameron, "East Timorese Doctor: 'Cuban Medicine Is about Human Values.'"

22. Fawthrop, "Cuban Doctors Popular in Quake-Stricken Java."

23. Negin, "Cuba in the Pacific: More than Rum and Coke."

24. Countries included besides Australia were Fiji, Kiribati, Nauru, Papua New Guinea, Solomon Islands, Tuvalu, and Vanuatu. The choice of these countries is also significant in that they either have existing medical cooperation agreements with Cuba or are working toward one. Much of the research in this next section on Pacific Island countries was undertaken by Chris Walker, of the International Development Studies program at Saint Mary's University, to whom the author expresses his profound gratitude.

25. Asante et al., "Analysis of Policy Implications and Challenges of the Cuban Health Assistance Program Related to Human Resources for Health in the Pacific," 3.

26. Anderson, "Social Medicine in Timor Leste."

27. Asante et al., "Analysis of Policy Implications," 4.

28. Ibid., 6.

29. The Cuban News Agency notes that by 2010 there were 23 Cuban health professionals working in Kiribati who had given 308,712 consultations since 2006. See "President of Kiribati Pays Tribute to José Martí." Asante et al. also highlight that in 2008 six Cuban medical personnel had arrived in Vanuatu. See their "Analysis of Policy Implications," 4.

30. Data taken from several articles by Tim Anderson, "Solidarity Aid: The Cuban-Timor Leste Health Programme," "Cuban Health Cooperation in Timor-Leste and the South-West Pacific," and "Social Medicine in Timor-Leste" and also from Asante et al., "Analysis of Policy Implications."

31. Assante et al., "Analysis of Policy Implications," 1.

32. Negin puts the number of Solomon Island students at 90. See "Cuba in the Pacific: More than Rum and Coke."

33. The Cuban News Agency article of 2010, "President of Kiribati Pays Tribute to José Martí," notes that 33 scholarships had been given to Kiribati youth to study at ELAM, with 31 for students to become physicians.

34. Some other sources including Asante el al. and Negin record the number to be around 20 Tuvaluans as of 2009.

35. According to Anderson there were 18 medical scholarships for Nauru as of 2009. See Anderson, "Cuban Health Cooperation in Timor-Leste and the South-West Pacific," 77–86.

36. Government of Vanuatu, "Health Sector Strategy," September 29, 2011. It is worth noting that they sent the first 17 students to Cuba in 2008 and followed up with another 10 in 2009. They estimate that there should be 24 new medical graduates by 2015/2016.

37. Six medical scholarships were offered by Cuba, and three were utilized by Tonga, although it was thought that in the future 10 might be accepted. See Anderson "Cuban

Health Cooperation in Timor-Leste and the South-West Pacific," and Tonga Ministry of Information and Communications, "Prime Minister Visits Cuba."

38. See Fiji Government, "Fiji Benefits from Additional Cuban Scholarships."

39. "Cuban Doctors Reduce Kiribati Mortality Rate by 80 Percent."

40. See "Cuban Solidarity with Kiribati."

41. In an April 25, 2012, report from the Permanent Mission of Fiji to the United Nations, it was noted that Fijian first secretary Khatri met with the "13 Kiribati students currently on medical studies, as well as a representative of the 3 sports and 18 medical students based in the Provinces." See "Fijian Medical Students Faring Well in Cuba."

42. Asante et al., "Analysis of Policy Implications," 3.

43. Wasuka, "Cuban Doctors to Fill Shortage."

44. Asante, Roberts, and Hall, "A Review of Health Leadership and Management Capacity in the Solomon Islands," 166–67.

45. Asante et al., "Analysis of Policy Implications," 4.

46. Wasuka, "Cuban Doctors to Fill Shortage."

47. Asante, Roberts, and Hall, "A Review of Health Leadership and Management Capacity in the Solomon Islands," 171.

48. See Negin, "Australia and New Zealand's Contribution to Pacific Island Health Worker Brain Drain," 507.

49. The most recent data indicate that 14 students are currently in Fiji. See Fiji Government, "Fiji Benefits from Additional Cuban Scholarships."

50. "Fijian Medical Students Faring Well in Cuba."

51. Loanakadavu, "Cuba Seeks Deal."

52. "Australia Looks to Work with Cuba on Pacific Aid."

53. Loanakadavu, "Cuba Seeks Deal."

54. Anderson believes that there were 18 medical scholarships for Nauru as of 2009. See "Cuban Health Cooperation in Timor-Leste and the South-West Pacific," 77–86, for a detailed analysis of the Cuban role.

55. Hopper, "Nauru's Health Crisis: 661 Patients per Doctor."

56. Feinsilver, "Fifty Years of Cuba's Medical Diplomacy: From Idealism to Pragmatism," 93. As noted previously, since 2010 five Cuban doctors have been working there. See Asante et al., "Analysis of Policy Implications," 5.

57. See "Cuban Doctors Inaugurated New Health Services in Tuvalu, a Small Pacific Island."

58. Tuvalu Ministry of Health, "Tuvalu Ministry of Health Strategic Health Plan, 2009–2018."

59. Asante et al., "Analysis of Policy Implications," 3.

60. Government of Vanuatu report of September 29, 2011, "Health Sector Strategy"; Asante et al., "Analysis of Policy Implications," 5.

61. Cook Islands Government report of June 2012, "Medical Scholarships to Cuba."

62. Data from Anderson, "Unlikely Partners: Challenges for Australian-Cuban Collaboration in Public Health."

63. Hodal, "Cuban Infusion Remains the Lifeblood of Timor-Leste's Health Service."

64. Australian Parliament, "Cuban Aid to East Timor, Kimberley Development."

65. Wasuka, "Cuban Doctors to Fill Shortage."

66. Australian Parliament, "Cuban Aid to East Timor, Kimberley Development."

67. Cameron, "East Timorese Doctor: 'Cuban Medicine Is about Human Values.'"

68. Anderson, "Latin America, the Caribbean, and the South-West Pacific: Opportunities for South-South Cooperation."

69. "Presidente de Timor Leste agradece postura ejemplar de Cuba."

70. Hodal, "Cuban Infusion Remains the Lifeblood of Timor-Leste's Health Service."

Chapter 10. The Children of Chernobyl: 25,000 Treated

1. See the report by the International Federation of Red Cross and Red Crescent Societies for 2010–11, "Chernobyl Humanitarian Assistance and Rehabilitation Programme (CHARP)."

2. Information concerning the technical aspects of the Chernobyl accident is taken from http://www.world-nuclear.org/info/chernobyl/inf07.html.

3. See "Annan Urges Continued International Support for Victims of Chernobyl Disaster."

4. Grogg, "Chernobyl Kids Keep Arriving in Cuba."

5. See the report of April 2006 issued by the World Health Organization (WHO), "Ionizing Radiation: Health Effects of the Chernobyl Accident, an Overview." See also WHO report of September 5, 2005, "Chernobyl: The True Scale of the Accident."

6. "Hundreds of thousands of people still live in an informational limbo, not knowing if the radiation they were exposed to in 1986 (radioactive iodine-131) and later permanently living on territories polluted by caesium-137, caused cancers and other diseases in their bodies. Women are especially at risk, double so when pregnant or planning a family. These fears and following depression very often trigger unhealthy lifestyles such as alcohol and drug abuse or heavy smoking." International Federation of Red Cross and Red Crescent Societies, "Chernobyl Humanitarian Assistance and Rehabilitation Programme (CHARP)," 5.

7. See "New York, 26 April 2012—Statement Attributable to the Spokesperson for the Secretary-General on the 26th Anniversary of the Chernobyl Disaster."

8. See "UN Experts: Socio-economic Recovery of Chernobyl-Affected Areas Requires Regular Governmental Interventions."

9. See "Largest-Ever International Stamp Issue to Aid Chernobyl Children."

10. See "550 Million Euros New Contributions to International Chernobyl Projects."

11. See the "News Alerts" reports for the Chernobyl Children's Project International for May 2005.

12. International Federation of Red Cross and Red Crescent Societies, "Chernobyl Humanitarian Assistance and Rehabilitation Programme (CHARP)," 1.

13. "Palabras del Dr. Carlos Dotres, Ministro de Salud Pública, en el Acto de Conmemoración del VII Aniversario de la llegada a Cuba del primer grupo de niños ucranianos procedentes de Chernobil, 29/3/97."

14. Dotres Martínez et al., "Programa para la atención médica integral a niños expuestos a contaminación ambiental por sustancias radiactivas."

15. Data from this section come from the report on Chernobyl found at the Infomed website, http://www.sld.cu/sitios/chernobil.

16. McQuaid, "Chernobyl Kids: Thousands of Soviet Children Find Help, Tropical Fun in Cuba."

17. Luque Álvarez, "Cuba constituye una esperanza para los niños de Chernobil."

18. See "Programa cubano de atención médica integral a niños relacionados con el accidente de Chernobil" (no date), received on January 23, 2012, from Dr. Julio Medina, medical director of the Tarará medical program. The detailed data in this section come from this analysis. In terms of the adults treated, it is worth noting that mainly these had come to Cuba to accompany their children but were also given medical treatment during their time there. In total 2,226 Ukrainian adults were examined; 5,478 consulted with specialists, and 9,130 tests were done.

19. Gorry, "Cuba Marks 15 Years Treating Chernobyl Victims."

20. Ibid.

21. Ukrainian News Agency, "Ukraine to Finance Treatment and Rehabilitation of Ukrainian Children, Victims."

22. "Ratifica Presidente de Ucrania colaboración médica con Cuba."

23. Luque Álvarez, "Leonid Kuchma: Unos mostraron lástima, pero Cuba nos ayudó."

24. Schipani, "Revolutionary Care: Castro's Doctors Give Hope to the Children of Chernobyl."

25. Ibid.

Chapter 11. Cuba's Medical Internationalism in El Salvador since Hurricane Ida

1. Forteza, "Canciller cubano: No damos lo que nos sobra. Compartimos lo que tenemos."

2. "Some of the worst damage was in Verapaz, where mudslides covered cars, and boulders two cars wide blocked streets. The rain loosened a flow of mud and rocks that descended from the nearby Chichontepec volcano and buried homes and streets in Verapaz, a town of about 3,000 located 30 miles east of San Salvador, the capital." See "El Salvador Floods, Mudslides Kill 124." In all, some 300 homes in Verapaz were destroyed.

3. Cárdenas, "Médicos cubanos se instalan en San Vicente."

4. See López, "La función de la medicina cubana no es para que los salvadoreños abracen otra bandera."

5. For a thorough study of the extensive role of the Cuban medical brigade in 2000 (which consisted of 53 Cuban specialists), see Lemus Lago et al., *Campaña por la esperanza*. Of particular note is the chapter titled "El recuento de lo acontecido," where a detailed analysis of the strategy and results of the Cuban brigade are provided (231–52). In 2009, President Mauricio Funes spoke about the significance of the Cuban cooperation: "Cuba has shown solidarity with El Salvador . . . in the contingents of Cuban doctors who have helped us—not the government, but rather our people as they fought the [dengue epidemic]. With an adequate preventive policy we could decrease its impact, but it was only with the experience of the Cuban doctors, experience gained through their years of practice in the field, that we were able to reduce the levels of dengue in our countries. And this at a time when there were no diplomatic relations." See "Discurso, Sr. Mauricio Funes, Presidente de la República."

6. Solórzano, "Médicos cubanos atienden más de 20 mil personas."

7. In February 2010 I visited this community and met with the mayor of Verapaz and members of the town council to discuss both the extent of the tragedy and the role of the Cuban medical brigade. All were fulsome in their praise of the Cubans, emphasizing their willingness to do all that was requested of them, their hands-on practical approach to the medical challenges facing the community, their energy (since they slept only a few hours in rudimentary conditions before continuing their health functions on a daily basis), and their down-to-earth approach with the people affected by the tragedy. They also stressed that the Cubans made no attempt to discuss political matters and instead focused entirely on their humanitarian mission.

8. "Canada Offers Condolences and Support after El Salvador Floods."

9. "Floods, Mudslides Kill Scores in El Salvador."

10. Thompson, "U.S. Military Team Delivers 370,000 Lbs. of Aid, Begins Medical Treatments in El Salvador."

11. Thompson, "U.S. Military Docs Treat Nearly 3,000 People in Storm-Ravaged El Salvador."

12. "Brigadas médicas de Cuba y EEUU atienden a damnificados en El Salvador."

13. Lemus Lago et al., *Campaña por la esperanza*, 16.

14. From my own experiences in El Salvador in February 2010, visiting communities affected by Hurricane Ida—the Platanillos cantón in Quezaltepeque, Las Moras community in the southern coastal area, Verapaz, San Vicente, and San Ildefonso—it was obvious that Cuban and Salvadoran medical teams were extremely comfortable working together and that there was a natural confluence of shared ideas and effort. For the purposes of this research project I interviewed members of all these communities, as well as Salvadoran health promoters (with whom I participated in an anti-dengue project, visiting members of the San Ildefonso community), doctors (including graduates from both the National University of El Salvador and ELAM), public health directors, and elected government officials, including the minister of public health and social assistance.

15. Presentation by health promoter, San Ildefonso, El Salvador, February 23, 2010.

16. See Menéndez Quintero, "La salud, una prioridad para El Salvador"; Díaz Ruiz, "Canciller salvadoreño orgulloso de formación de médicos de su país en Cuba"; and "Coro infantil y estudiantes de medicina dan bienvenida a Vicepresidente Sánchez Cerén en Cuba."

17. Several interviews were carried out with 20 ELAM graduates in El Salvador, and all spoke about the gradual acceptance of their qualifications and experience by the medical establishment. In one interview, the minister of public health and social assistance, Dr. María Isabel Rodríguez, criticized the "mechanical" nature of medical training in her country and the advantages of training at the ELAM, where the ability to relate to patients, to develop a "truly humanitarian" spirit of communication, was consciously developed.

18. Information provided in the document "Brigada Médica Cubana en El Salvador."

19. Interview with Dr. Eduardo Ojeda, interim director of the Cuban medical brigade, San Vicente, El Salvador, February 21, 2010.

20. It is important to bear in mind the depth of Cuban support for the entire gamut of their activities—from providing medical treatment to public health education, from visits to homes to the fumigation of mosquito breeding grounds and destruction of rodents. Dr.

Ojeda calculated that by mid-March 2010, more than 250,000 Salvadorans had benefited from Cuban medical support. This has continued to grow, as Cuban activities in public health have increased.

21. Interview with Dr. Elsy Guadalupe Brizuela, NEFROLEMPA, Lower Lempa, February 25, 2010.

22. PowerPoint presentation of the Brigada Médica Cubana in Guatemala, "Cooperación cubana en Guatemala. Misión Milagro: Un pueblo saliendo de la oscuridad. Cuarto trimestre 2009."

23. "Beneficiados miles de salvadoreños con la Operación Milagro."

24. "Cooperación técnica Cuba–El Salvador fortalece el proceso de reforma en salud."

25. In an earlier interview, the minister noted that the Cuban public health system was one of the best in the world, ensuring medical coverage of the entire population and at no cost to patients. She praised the advanced level of scientific research and technology, the production of vaccines and quality pharmaceutical products, and the excellent quality of medical training found in Cuba. She concluded, "We have much to learn from Cuba, and indeed we can take inspiration from the Cuban public health experience." Solórzano, "El Ministro de Salud Pública retomará las buenas experiencias del sistema de salud de Cuba para la próxima reforma de salud de 2010."

26. Interview with Dr. María Isabel Rodríguez, San Salvador, February 25, 2010.

27. Confidential correspondence with Salvadoran authorities, April 12, 2010.

Conclusion: No Longer the World's Best-Kept Secret

1. Baine, "How Can Health Research Help to Save 500,000 Mothers?"

2. Nullis-Kapp, "Efforts Underway to Stem the 'Brain Drain' of Doctors and Nurses."

3. Ibid.

4. Abdu Misau, Al-Sadat, and Bakari-Gerei, "Braindrain and Health Care Delivery in Developing Countries."

5. Ibid. The authors provide some useful data to illustrate the awkward distribution of medical personnel and the imbalance between developing and developed countries in this regard. Zambia, for instance, needed 15,000 physicians for its healthcare system to function adequately, yet had only 800. Malawi had just 100 doctors and 2,000 nurses to serve a population of 12 million people. Uganda had only 1 doctor for 24,700 inhabitants, and in Africa as a whole the physician-to-patient ratio was 13/100,000, compared with 280/100,000 in the United States. Another indicator of the brain drain was the situation in Asia where in 2001 alone 13,536 Filipino nurses left the country.

6. See U.S. Department of State, "Cuban Medical Professional Parole Program."

7. See, for example, "Cubano que abandonou Mais Médicos posta foto em Miami."

8. "Cubanos sao minoria entre desistentes do Mais Medicos, diz ministro."

9. Ianoni, "A populacao quer 'Mais Médicos.'"

10. Nublat, "A um mes das eleicoes, governo divulga pesquisa favorável ao Mais Médicos."

11. "U.S. Embassy Cables: U.S. Seeks Out Bad News about Cuban Healthcare."

12. Erisman, "Brain Drain Politics: The Cuban Medical Professional Parole Programme," 286.

13. "Las bondades de la solidaridad."

14. This section draws on the analysis of Debra Evenson, "The Right to Health Care and the Law."

15. The medical federations, critical of the arrival of Cuban physicians, often claim that there are local doctors who could fill these positions. This is often a false argument, since the local doctors are generally loath to go to work in underserved communities, far from the cities, where living conditions are inferior and salaries are not as lucrative. But this is exactly where they are most needed. The president of Ecuador, Rafael Correa, has defended his decision to import Cuban medical staff to work in the jungle and mountainous areas of the country, noting that "if [Ecuadoran specialists] are not prepared to work where they are most needed, we will bring doctors from Cuba and other parts of the world." He added that he would not sacrifice the population of his people and hoped that in time Ecuadoran doctors would fulfill their mission to their people. See the Prensa Latina report, "Resalta presidente Correa estado de las relaciones con Cuba."

Another complaint raised by several medical federations in countries where the Cuban medical staff are working is that the doctors are of poor quality. The president of the Ecuadoran Medical Federation, Alberto Narváez, has called upon Correa "not to commit this antipatriotic act of replacing Ecuadoran professionals with Cuban doctors." The Cubans are "doctors of just average training in family medicine, they are not the best, and we have grave doubts about their quality." (He was quoted in Solano, "Médicos en Ecuador se oponen a servicios de doctores cubanos.") What Narváez fails to understand is the pragmatic nature of the training provided at Cuban medical schools and the commitment of their graduates. He also seems to prefer the status quo, with masses of underserved Ecuadorans waiting for medical treatment from graduates of their own universities—treatment which to date has been sorely lacking. For further information on the nature of medical training and the approach to public healthcare, see Whiteford and Branch, *Primary Health Care in Cuba*, Pérez, *Caring for Them from Birth to Death*, and Mason, Strug, and Beder, eds., *Community Health Care in Cuba*.

16. Quoted in Gorry, "Cuban Disaster Doctors in Guatemala, Pakistan."

17. In 1978 Fidel Castro touched upon the possibility of exporting medical services "for the economic development of our country." At the start of the 1978/79 academic year he noted, "We are thinking not only about our own needs but also about the extraordinary request for our doctors that we are receiving from abroad. The exportation of technical services is becoming an important factor for the economic development of our country. And so, with regard to the question of healthcare matters, we are working to increase and improve our medical services both in terms of quantity and quality. These technical services can be exported, and in addition we can donate these services to countries with fewer financial resources." Cited in Garófalo Fernández and Gómez García, eds., *Pensamientos de Fidel sobre la salud pública*, 20.

18. Cited in Kirk and Erisman, *Cuban Medical Internationalism*, 186.

19. "Speech delivered by Dr. Fidel Castro Ruz, President of the Republic of Cuba, at the foundation ceremony of the 'Henry Reeve' International Contingent of Doctors Specialized in Disaster Situations and Serious Epidemics, and the National Graduation of Students of Medical Sciences, in the Ciudad Deportiva, on September 19, 2005."

20. Werlau, "Cuba's Cash-for-Doctors Program."

21. Werlau, "Cuba's Partners in Human Exploitation."

22. Werlau, "Cuba's Health-Care Diplomacy: The Business of Humanitarianism."

23. Ibid. "Havana realized it had stumbled onto a winning strategy: the state could mobilize Health workers at very short notice and send them practically anywhere, including hardship locations, make them work under unique terms, and have them stay as long as necessary. The care they provided was an advertisement for socialism, especially the Cuban brand."

24. Marquis, "Medical School for Latins Earns Cuba Goodwill."

25. Montaner, "Slaves in White Coats." He continues: "His kind, revolutionary internationalism is based on the sacrifice of the Cuban medics. Sometimes he uses them to foment political dependence, as in his wealthy Venezuelan colony; others, to promote propaganda or exert diplomatic pressure on the country that receives his poisoned present."

26. Cooper, Kennelly, and Ordúñez-García, "Health in Cuba," 821.

27. Ibid., 821–22. They refer in cautious terms to the polarized nature of discussion on medical personnel serving abroad: "Offhand dismissal by observers in industrialized countries of the Cuban medical aid programme, which has such a powerful impact on these marginalized communities, is a clear indication of how perilously divided the discourse over global development has become" (822).

28. Martínez Hernández and Puig Meneses, "Aprobó Consejo de Ministros incremento salarial para el sector de la Salud."

29. A glance at the website of Servicios Médicos Cubanos SA is instructive. Foreigners can be treated in any of 54 hospitals for dozens of medical conditions, from colorectal cancer and Hodgkin's disease to macular degeneration and plastic surgery. See http://smcsalud.cu/smc/servlet/wpinicio . A good overview of these services can be seen in Sosin Martínez, "Exportando salud: Servicios Médicos Cubanos."

30. Dr. Yiliam Jiménez, then deputy foreign minister and in charge of Cuba's medical programs abroad, noted that MI was "an integral part of Cuban politics. . . . Our goal is to develop solidarity bridges with African, Caribbean, and Latin American countries." Cited in Kirk and Erisman, *Cuban Medical Internationalism*, 179.

31. "Unos 132,000 médicos cubanos cumplieron misiones en el exterior desde 1963."

32. Cited in Garófalo Fernández and Gómez García, eds., *Pensamientos de Fidel sobre la salud pública*, 10. This is from Fidel Castro's address at the graduation of 90 dentists that took place in the Chaplin Theater on June 18, 1965.

33. Kirk and Walker, "Moral Medicine, the Cuban Way," 27.

Bibliography

"32,000 Cuban Health Workers Bring Aid to 72 Countries, 'Support an Inspiration to Cuban People.'" *Scotland Unison*, June 22, 2007. http://www.unison-scotland.org.uk/conf2007/story1.htm.

"400 médicos cubanos a damnificados por desastres naturales." *Agencia Boliviana de Información*, February 21, 2007.

"550 Million Euros New Contribution to International Chernobyl Projects." *Pollution Solutions* online, April 19, 2011. http://www.pollutionsolutions-online.com/news/hazardous-waste/20/ebrd/550_million_new_contribution_to_international_chernobyl_projects/14991/.

"87 beneficiarios de Misión Milagro Chile ya fueron operados en Venezuela." *El Ciudadano*, June 17, 2006. http://www.elciudadano.cl/2010/06/17/23604/87-beneficiarios-de-mision-milagro-chile-ya-fueron-operados-en-venezuela/.

"90 salvadoreños viajaron a Venezuela en Operación Milagro." *Chichicaste*. Blog. February 13, 2011. http://chichicaste.blogcindario.com/2011/02/01706-90-salvadorenos-viajaron-a-venezuela-en-operacion-milagro.html.

Abdu Misau, Yusuf, Nabilia Al-Sadat, and Adamu Bakari-Gerei. "Braindrain and Health Care Delivery in Developing Countries." *Journal of Public Health in Africa* 1, no. 1 (2010). http://www.publichealthinafrica.org/index.php/jphia/article/view/jphia.2010.e6/html_5.

"Additional €2.6m for Hurricane Stan Victims in Guatemala." European Commission, July 18, 2006. http://eu-un.europa.eu/articles/en/article_6118_en.htm.

Aguin, Víctor. "Desarrollo de la Misión Milagro en Venezuela." *Revista Cubana de Salud Pública* 37, no. 4 (2011): 537–41.

Akhtar, Aasim Sajjad. "Cuban Doctors in Pakistan: Why Cuba Still Inspires." *Monthly Review* 58, no. 6 (2006). http://www.monthlyreview.org/2006/11/01/cuban-doctors-in-pakistan-why-cuba-still-inspires.

"Alrededor de 5,500 profesionales prestan servicios en África." *Cubadebate*, June 5, 2012. http://www.cubadebate.cu/noticias/2012/06/05/alrededor-de-5-500-profesionales-cubanos-prestan-servicios-en-africa/#.VFO2Pld_Qcs.

"Alta demanda de monoclonal cubano en China." *Juventud Rebelde*, February 24, 2012.

Álvarez Sintes, Roberto. *Salud Familiar: Manual del Promotor*. Valencia, Venezuela: Ministerio de Salud y Desarrollo Social, 2004.

———, ed. *Temas de Medicina General Integral.* Vol. 1, *Salud y Medicina.* Havana: Editorial Ciencias Médicas, 2001.

"Ampliarán en China presencia productos biotecnológicos cubanos." *Granma*, July 1, 2013.

Anderson, Tim. "Cuban Health Cooperation in Timor-Leste and the South-West Pacific." In *South-South Cooperation: A Challenge to the Aid System?* 77–86. Quezon City, Philippines: IBON Books, 2012.

———. "Latin America, the Caribbean, and the South West Pacific: Opportunities for South-South Cooperation." Unpublished paper, provided by the author.

———. Recent medical graduates in Timor-Leste. Video. http://www.youtube.com/watch?v=eOLmUIGdYjE&feature=plcp.

———. "Social Medicine in Timor-Leste." *Social Medicine* 5, no. 4 (2010): 182–91. http://www.socialmedicine.info/socialmedicine/index.php/socialmedicine/article/view/480/1028.

———. "Solidarity Aid: The Cuba–Timor-Leste Health Programme." *International Journal of Cuban Studies* 1, no. 2 (2008): 53–65.

———. South Pacific students at ELAM. Video. http://www.youtube.com/watch?v=AhMAncnEDQQ&feature=plcp.

———. "Unlikely Partners: Challenges for Australian-Cuban Collaboration in Pacific Health." Unpublished paper, provided by the author.

"Annan Urges Continued International Support for Victims of Chernobyl Disaster." Press release of the UN News Centre, April 26, 2004. http://www.un.org/apps/news/story.asp?NewsID=10515&Cr=chernobyl&Crl=#VZRdvFLLq-g.

"Antecedentes históricos de la asistencia de Cuba ante situaciones de desastre." Internal report of the Cuban Ministry of Foreign Relations, n.d.

Appelbaum, Diane, and Hope Bastian. "Honduras: Cuban-Trained Garifuna Doctors Supported in Hospital Expansion Drive." *Cuba Health Reports, MEDICC Review,* September 2008.

Archibold, Randal C. "Cuba Takes Lead Role in Haiti's Cholera Fight." *New York Times*, November 7, 2011.

Armas Padrino, Iris. "Third Anniversary of Operation Miracle." Agencia de Información Nacional report, July 9, 2007.

Asante, Augustine, John Negin, John Hall, John Dewdney, and Anthony Zwi. "Analysis of Policy Implications and Challenges of the Cuban Health Assistance Program Related to Human Resources for Health in the Pacific." *Human Resources for Health* 10, no. 1 (2012): 1–9.

Asante, Augustine, Graham Roberts, and John Hall. "A Review of Health Leadership and Management Capacity in the Solomon Islands." *Pacific Health Information Network: Progressing HIS in the Region* 18, no. 1 (2012): 166–77.

"Asume nuevo coordinador de brigada médica en Guatemala." Prensa Latina report of February 27, 2014.

"Asume nuevo jefe de brigada médica cubana en Guatemala." *Prensa Latina*, November 15, 2013.

"At a Glance: Haiti." http://www.unicef.org/infobycountry/haiti_statistics.html.

"Atendidos más de 34 mil pacientes con pie diabético a través del Ministerio de Salud." *Correo del Orinoco*, November 19, 2011.

"Australia Looks to Work with Cuba on Pacific Aid." ABC Radio Australia, July 27, 2011. http://www.radioaustralia.net.au/international/radio/onairhighlights/australia-looks-to-work-with-cuba-on-pacific-aid.

Australian Parliament. "Cuban Aid to East Timor, Kimberley Development." Hansard proceedings online, March 10, 2009. http://www.parliament.nsw.gov.au/prod/parlment/hansard.nsf/86ca1d5c167e46c8ca2571ca000080c8/bb45da8da1e3baf7ca25757f001745ab!OpenDocument.

Baine, Theresa. "How Can Health Research Help to Save 500,000 Mothers?" *Bulletin of the World Health Organization* 83, no. 2 (February 2005).

Balán Neyra, Juvena. "Despide presidente de Paquistán a Misión Médica Cubana." *Granma,* May 25, 2006.

Barbosa León, Nuria. "Cuba and Haiti: A History of Solidarity." *Granma International,* February 28, 2013.

"Barrio Adentro llega a su noveno aniversario." *Cubadebate,* June 12, 2014. http://www.cubadebate.cu/noticias/2014/06/12/barrio-adentro-llega-a-su-noveno-aniversario/#.VF548xYXEXw.

Barzilay, Ezra J., Nicolas Schaad, Roc Magloire, Kam S. Mung, Jacques Boncy, Georges A. Dahourou, Eric D. Mintz, Maria W. Steenland, John F. Vertefeuille, and Jordan W. Tappero. "Cholera Surveillance during the Haiti Epidemic: The First Two Years." *New England Journal of Medicine* 368, no. 7 (February 14, 2013): 599–609.

"Beneficiados miles de salvadoreños con la Operación Milagro." *Juventud Rebelde,* March 20, 2010.

Blanco, Kathleen. Executive Order KBB 2005-33. Issued by Kathleen Blanco, Governor of Louisiana, September 12, 2005. http://www.doa.la.gov/osr/other/kbb05-33.htm.

"Bolivia y Cuba celebran 30 años de restablecimiento de relaciones diplomáticas." *ANF: Agencia de Noticias Fides,* January 11, 2013. http://www.noticiasfides.com/g/politica/bolivia-y-cuba-celebran-30-anos-del-restablecimiento-de-.relaciones-diplomaticas-8744/.

"Brigada Internacional Henry Reeve regresa de Chile." *CubaMinrex: Ministerio de Relaciones Exteriores de Cuba,* November 21, 2010. http://anterior.cubaminrex.cu/Cooperacion/2010/brigada7.html.

"Brigada Médica Cubana en El Salvador." Internal report produced by the Henry Reeve medical brigade in El Salvador, February 22, 2010.

"Brigada Médica Cubana en Guatemala cumple 10 años." *CubaMinrex: Ministerio de Relaciones Exteriores de Cuba,* July 7, 2008. http://anterior.cubaminrex.cu/Actualidad/2008/Julio/Brigada1. html. Document of the Cuban Ministry of Foreign Relations.

Brigada Médica Cubana en Haití, Coordinación General. "Comportamiento de enfermedades transmisibles, Haití. Febrero 2008." Mimeo, provided to author by members of the Cuban medical brigada in Haiti.

"Brigadas médicas de Cuba y EEUU atienden a damnificados en El Salvador." *Economista,* November 14, 2009. http://ecodiario.eleconomista.es/internacional/noticias/1695922/11/09/Brigadas-medicas-de-Cuba-y-EEUU-atienden-a-damnificados-en-El-Salvador.html#.Kku8ESoaQY78yXx.

Brooke, James. "Cuban Doctors and Builders Also Aid Angola." *New York Times,* February 15, 1989.

Brouwer, Steve. *Revolutionary Doctors: How Venezuela and Cuba Are Changing the World's Conception of Health Care*. New York: Monthly Review Press, 2011.

Buddan, Robert. "Miracle at Christmas." *Jamaica Gleaner*, December 18, 2005.

Burghardt, Leo. "Guatemalans Hail Cuban Medical Workers." *People's Weekly World Newspaper*, March 6, 2004. http://peoplesworld.org/guatemalans-hail-cuban-medical-workers/.

Burnett, John. "Cuban Doctors Unsung Heroes of Haitian Earthquake." *National Public Radio*, January 24, 2010. http://www.npr.org/templates/story/story.php?storyId=122919202.

Cabral, Jorge, Gilles Dussault, James Buchan, and Paulo Ferrinho. "Scaling Up the Medical Workforce in Timor-Leste: Challenges of a Great Leap Forward." *Social Science and Medicine* 30 (2013): 1–5.

Cameron, Marce. "East Timor: Cuba 'Taught Me to Love People and Be Independent.'" *Green Left Weekly*, November 6, 2011. https://www.greenleft.org.au/node/49355.

———. "East Timorese Doctor: 'Cuban Medicine Is about Human Values.'" *Green Left Weekly*, May 6, 2013. https://www.greenleft.org.au/node/54008.

Campion, Edward W., and Stephen Morrissey. "A Different Model—Medical Care in Cuba." *New England Journal of Medicine* 368 (January 24, 2013): 297–99.

"Canada Offers Condolences and Support after El Salvador Floods." News release 342, November 12, 2009, Foreign Affairs and International Trade Canada. http://www.international.gc.ca/media/state-etat/news-communiques/2009/342.aspx?lang=eng.

Canales, Ulises. "Cuba aporta a Guatemala 535 médicos para asistir damnificados." *Cubadebate*, October 13, 2005. http://visionesalternativas.com/index.php?option=com_content&view=article&id=14584:emplazados-en-los-departamentos-maaacutes-afectados-por-la-tormenta-stan&catid=2.

"Capriles y federación médica critican salud pública venezolana." Radio Martí, August 21, 2013. http://www.martinoticias.com/articleprintview/26612.html.

Caputo, Marc. "Rep. Garcia's Push for Cuba Drug Trials Tests Support for Embargo." *Miami Herald*, October 7, 2013. http://www.miamiherald.com/news/politics-government/article1955994.html.

Carballo Hechevarría, Héctor. "Por Paraguay sentimos una gratitud infinita." *Juventud Rebelde*, July 10, 2012.

Cárdenas, Andrés. "The Cuban Biotechnology Industry: Innovation and Universal Health Care." White paper. Institute of Institutional and Innovation Economics, University of Bremen, Germany, November 2009. http://www.theairnet.org/files/research/cardenas/andres-cardenas_cubab_biotech_paper_2009.pdf.

Cárdenas, Leonor. "Médicos cubanos se instalan en San Vicente." *DiarioCoLatino*, November 14, 2009. http://www.argenpress.info/2009/11/el-salvador-medicos-cubanos-se-instalan.html.

Carpineta, María Laura. "Habla el Jefe de los 744 médicos instalados en Haití desde hace doce años." *Página 12*, February 4, 2010.

Carrasco Martín, Juana. "Andar seguro venezolano-cubano en la atención a la discapacidad en Venezuela." *Juventud Rebelde*, September 26, 2011.

———. "Un proyecto convertido en hechos para bienestar de los venezolanos." *Juventud Rebelde*, October 13, 2011.

Carriba, Victor M. "Llama Cuba a cooperación con Haití y respetar principios." *Prensa Latina*, January 22, 2010.

Castro, Arachu, and Paul Farmer. "International Public Health Pitfalls and Economic Arguments: The Fight against AIDS in Cuba and Haiti." *MEDICC Review* 8, no. 1 (2006).

"Castro: Cuban Aid Offer Is 'Revenge' against Mitch." *Cubanet* report, November 23, 1998.

Castro Medel, Osviel. "Milagro para tres millones de personas." *Juventud Rebelde*, August 6, 2013.

———. "Reconocen logros de alianza Cuba-Venezuela." *Juventud Rebelde*, October 31, 2013.

———. "Vida que crece en tierra de Bolívar." *Juventud Rebelde*, November 30, 2013.

Castro Ruz, Fidel. "Cooperation Spirit Is Put to the Test in Haiti." January 16, 2010. http://www.cuba.cu/gobierno/reflexiones/2010/ing/f160110i.html.

———. "Key Address by Dr. Fidel Castro Ruz, President of the Republic of Cuba, at the Inauguration of the Latin American School of Medicine, Havana, November 15, 1999." http://www.cuba.cu/gobierno/discursos/1999/ing/i151199i.html.

———. "Lo que no dijo Notimex." *Granma*, April 2, 2009.

———. "Remarks by Dr. Fidel Castro Ruz, President of the Republic of Cuba, Meeting with the Medical Doctors Assembled to Offer Assistance to the American People in the Areas Affected by Hurricane Katrina. Havana Convention Centre, September 4, 2005." http://www.cuba.cu/gobierno/discursos/2005/ing/f040905i.html.

———. "Speech delivered by Commander in Chief Fidel Castro Ruz, First Secretary of the Central Committee of the Communist Party of Cuba and President of the Councils of State and of Ministers, at the Closing Session of the 12th National Science and Technology Forum, held at the International Conference Center on 21 November 1998, Year of the 40th Anniversary of the Decisive Battles of the Liberation Year." http://www.cuba.cu/gobierno/discursos/1998/ing/f211198i.html.

———. "Speech Delivered by Dr. Fidel Castro Ruz, President of the Republic of Cuba, at the Foundation Ceremony of the 'Henry Reeve' International Contingent of Doctors Specialized in Disaster Situations and Serious Epidemics, and the National Graduation of Students of Medical Sciences, in the Ciudad Deportiva, on September 19, 2005." www.cuba.cu/gobierno/discursos/2005/ing/f190905i.html.

———. "Speech Given by Dr. Fidel Castro Ruz, President of the Republic of Cuba, at the Celebration of the 40th Anniversary of INDER and the Dedication of the International School of Physical Education and Sports, on February 23, 2001." http://www.cuba.cu/gobierno/discursos/2001/ing/f230201i.html.

———. "Speech Given by Dr. Fidel Castro Ruz, President of the Republic of Cuba, at the First Graduation of Students from the Latin American School of Medicine, Karl Marx Theatre, August 20, 2005." http://www.cuba.cu/gobierno/discursos/2005/ing/f200805i.html.

Castro Ruz, Raúl. "Cuba no teme a la mentira ni se arrodilla ante presiones." *Cubadebate*, April 4, 2010. http://www.cubadebate.cu/opinion/2010/04/04/cuba-no-teme-a-la-mentira-ni-se-arrodilla-ante-presiones-fotos/.

———. "Intervención del General de Ejército Raúl Castro Ruz, Presidente del Consejo de Estado y de Ministros en la sesión plenaria de la Cumbre de América Latina y el Caribe, el 23 de febrero de 2010." http://cuba.cu/gobierno/rauldiscursos/2010/esp/r230210e.html.

"Cataratón Kiwanis 2013 devuelve visión 20–20 a un centenar de panameños." Club Kiwanis de Panamá online, February 26, 2013. http://www.clubkiwanispanama.com/act/cataraton-kiwanis-2013-devuelve-vision-20-20-a-un-centenar-de-panamenos/.

Centers for Disease Control and Prevention. "Cholera in Haiti." http://wwwnc.cdc.gov/travel/notices/watch/haiti-cholera.

"Central America, Mexico, and Haiti: Floods from Hurricane Stan—Appeal No. 05EA021 Final Report." Report from International Federation of Red Cross And Red Crescent Societies, December 31, 2006. ReliefWeb, August 3, 2007, http://www.reliefweb.int/rw/rwb.nsf/db900SID/KHII-75T2WJ?OpenDocument.

Chan, Margaret. "Remarks at the Latin American School of Medicine Havana, Cuba, October 27, 2009." World Health Organization. http://www.who.int/dg/speeches/2009/cuba_medical_20091027/en/.

Chávez Alfonso, María del Carmen, and Juan Luis Marcelo Pentón. "Evaluación nutricional de niños menores de edad: Centro de Salud 'Soleil.' Departamento noroeste de Haití, 2005–06." *Panorama Cuba y Salud* 2, no. 2 (May–August 2007): 28–39.

"Chávez: Aportes de Cuba suman 10 veces más del costo del petróleo que envía Venezuela." Portal ALB-TCP, April 20, 2010. http://www.partealta.ec/america/venezuela/11317-chavez-aportes-de-cuba-suman-10-veces-mas-del-costo-del-petroleo-que-envia-venezuela.

CIA. *World Factbook*. https://www.cia.gov/library/publications/the-world-factbook/.

CIGB. "Portafolios de Negocios, 2012–13." Havana: Center for Genetic Engineering and Biotechnology catalog.

"Clausura de la Misión Solidaria Moto Méndez, La Paz." August 13, 2010. Press release of the Bolivian Ministry of Health.

Clemons, Steve. "Cuba's Soft Power: Exporting Doctors Rather than Revolution." *Huffington Post*, November 12, 2009. http://www.huffingtonpost.com/steve-clemons/cuba-soft-power-exportin_b_355373.html.

Cobas Ruiz, Marcia, Eduardo Zacca Peña, Francisco Morales Catalayud, Emilia Icart Pereira, Aida Jordán Hernández, and Mitchel Valdés Sosa. "Caracterización epidemiológica de las personas con discapacidad en Cuba." *Revista Cubana de Salud Pública* 36, no. 4 (2010). http://www.scielosp.org/scielo.php?script=sci_arttext&pid=S0864-34662010000400004.

Cochetti, Chiara. "ALBAmed: A New Regional Pharma Hub in the Americas?" http://healthcare.blogs.ihs.com/2013/08/28/albamed-a-new-regional-pharma-hub-in-the-americas/.

Collazo Montano, Vivian. "Cuba, por incrementar los servicios médicos." *Prensa Latina*, March 25, 2014.

"Con Más Médicos, una revolución en la salud que cumple un año." *Cubadebate*, July 9, 2014. http://www.cubadebate.cu/noticias/2014/07/09/con-mas-medicos-una-revolucion-en-la-salud-que-cumple-un-ano/#.VFuEGWd_Qcs.

Cook Islands Government, Foreign Affairs and Immigration. "Medical Scholarships to Cuba." News section, June 1, 2012. http://www.mfai.gov.ck/index.php/news/19-general/191-medical-scholarships-to-cuba.html.

Cooper, Richard S., Joan F. Kennelly, and Pedro Ordúñez-García. "Health in Cuba." *International Journal of Epidemiology* 35, no. 4 (2006): 817–24.
"Cooperación Cuba-Honduras." *Colaboración*, October 2006. Report of the Cuban Ministry of Foreign Relations.
"Cooperación cubana en Guatemala. Misión Milagro—Un pueblo saliendo de la oscuridad. Cuatro trimestre 2009." PowerPoint of the Brigada Médica Cubana in Guatemala, provided to author by head of Cuban medical delegation in Guatemala.
"Cooperación técnica Cuba–El Salvador fortalece el proceso de reforma de salud." Ministerio de Salud, El Salvador, July 4, 2009. http://www.salud.gob.sv/novedades/noticias/noticias-ciudadanosas/150-julio-2011/969—04-07-2011-cooperacion-tecnica-cuba-el-salvador-fortalece-el-proceso-de-reforma-de-salud.html.
"Coro infantil y estudiantes de medicina dan bienvenida a Vicepresidente Sánchez Cerén en Cuba." Press release from the Office of the Vice President, Government of El Salvador, December 5, 2009.
"Cuba Aids Haiti Relief." *Voice of America*, January 22, 2010.
"Cuba Answers the Call for Doctors." *Bulletin of the World Health Organization* 88, no. 5 (May 1, 2010): 325–26.
"Cuba, Brazil in More Diplomacy for Closer Economic Ties." *Xinhua*, May 8, 2013. http://news.xinhuanet.com/english/world/2013-05/09/c_132369932.htm.
"Cuba en Ginebra: 'Ante tan difícil situación humanitaria en Haití no puede haber titubeos ni indiferencia.'" *Cubadebate*, January 27, 2010. http://www.cubadebate.cu/especiales/2010/01/27/cuba-en-ginebra-sobre-reconstruccion-haiti/#.VFuFm2d_Qcs.
"Cuba ha colaborado en Salud con 120 países del mundo." *Cubadebate*, May 22, 2014. http://www.cubadebate.cu/noticias/2014/05/22/cuba-ha-colaborado-en-salud-con-120-paises-del-mundo/#.VFuF4Gd_Qcs.
"Cuba Helps 50,000 Bolivians to See." *Prensa Latina*, December 20, 2006.
"Cuba impulsa comercialización productos biotecnológicos en Brasil." *Público.es*, October 10, 2011.
"Cuba llega a Ginebra para unirse a esfuerzos de la ONU contra el ébola." *Cubadebate*, September 11, 2014." http://www.cubadebate.cu/noticias/2014/09/11/cuba-llega-a-ginebra-para-unirse-a-esfuerzos-de-la-onu-contra-el-ebola/#.VFuGK2d_Qcs.
"A Cuban Brain Drain, Courtesy of the U.S." *The New York Times*, November 16, 2014.
"Cuban Doctors Inaugurated New Health Services in Tuvalu, a Small Pacific Island." *Cuban Daily News*, June 14, 2009. http://www.cubaheadlines.com/2009/06/14/17664/cuban_doctors_have_inaugurated_a_series_new_health_services_tuvalu_a_small_island_nation_pacific.html.
"Cuban Doctors Make an Impact on Honduras Health Levels." Agencia de Información Nacional, September 7, 2007.
"Cuban Doctors Reduce Kiribati Mortality Rate by 80 Percent." Radio New Zealand International, July 19, 2007. http://www.radionz.co.nz/international/pacific-news/171387/cuban-doctors-reduce-kiribati-infant-mortality-rate-by-80-percent.
"Cuban Hospital in Qatar Achieves JCI Accreditation." *Prensa Latina*, March 17, 2014.
"Cuban Internationalists Fighting Malaria in Angola." Note. MINREX (Ministry of Foreign Relations), January 28, 2011.
"Cuban Medical Brigade Returns from Helping Indonesia." *Granma*, September 7, 2006.

"Cubano que abandonou Mais Médicos posta foto em Miami." *Veja*, February 20, 2014.

"Cubanos sao minoría entre desistentes do Mais Médicos, diz ministro." Agencia Brasil, June 4, 2014. http://agenciabrasil.ebc.com.br/geral/noticia/2014-06/cubanos-sao-minoria-entre-desistentes-do-mais-medicos-diz-ministro.

"Cuban Solidarity with Kiribati." *CubaMinrex: Ministerio de Relaciones Exteriores de Cuba*, April 7, 2012. http://www.cubaminrex.cu/en/cuban-solidarity-kiribati.

"Cuba promueve lucha contra la malaria en Angola." *Granma*, February 2, 2011.

"Cuba Receives Human Rights Prize for Medical Brigade." *Granma*, December 8, 2007.

"Cuba's Biotech Boom." Editorial. *Nature* 457, no. 130 (January 8, 2009). www.nature.com/nature/journal/v457/n7226/full/457130a.html.

"Cuba's ELAM—Making Dreams Come True." *Arab News*, October 31, 2013. http://www.arabnews.com/print/470026.

"Cuba's Medical Aid after Hurricane Mitch Recalled in Guatemala." *Prensa Latina*, November 17, 2006.

"Cuba's Medical Missionaries Blanket Honduras." *Prensa Latina*, February 18, 2005.

"Cuba's Tower of Babel Gives Free Medical Education." Agence France-Press, October 30, 2013. http://www.globalpost.com/dispatch/news/afp/131030/cubas-tower-babel-gives-free-medical-education.

"Cuba to Access Global Pharmaceutical Markets via Brazil." *Cuba Standard*, September 24, 2011.

"Cuba to Send Doctors." *New York Times*, November 12, 1998.

"Cuba, Venezuela Benefit from Surgeries." *Miami Herald*, January 20, 2007.

"Cuba y Ecuador consolidan cooperación en sector biofarmacéutico." *Prensa Latina*, September 3, 2013.

"Cuba y Venezuela acuerdan nuevos proyectos para atención al pueblo." *Cubadebate*, February 21, 2014. http://www.cubadebate.cu/noticias/2014/02/21/cuba-y-venezuela-acuerdan-nuevos-proyectos-para-atencion-del-pueblo/#.VFuJk2d_Qcs.

"Cuba y Venezuela inauguran una de las plantas farmacéuticas más modernas de Latinoamérica." *Cubadebate,* June 24, 2014. http://www.cubadebate.cu/noticias/2014/06/24/cuba-y-venezuela-inauguran-una-de-las-plantas-farmaceuticas-mas-modernas-de-latinoamerica/#.VFuJ7Wd_Qcs.

Cumming-Bruce, Nick. "Ebola Outpaces Global Response, W.H.O. Says." *New York Times*, September 12, 2014.

Davalos, Gabriel. "Cuban Vice President Meets with Haitian Foreign Minister." *Granma International*, April 26, 2007.

de Araújo, Rui Maria. "A Snapshot of the Medical School, Faculty of Health Sciences, National University of Timor Lorosa'e, Democratic Republic of Timor Leste." Paper presented at the Expert Group Meeting on Finalization of Regional Guidelines on Institutional Quality Assurance Mechanism for Undergraduate Medical Education held in New Delhi by WHO/SEARO, 2009.

"Décimo aniversario de la Escuela Latinoamericana de Medicina." *Agencia Rodolfo Walsh*, November 15, 2009. http://www.agenciawalsh.org/c/educacion/3874-decimo-aniversario-de-la-escuela-latinoamericana-de-medicina.html.

"Declaración del gobierno de Cuba a propósito del Huracán Mitch: El problema no es sólo llorar por los que han muerto, sino ocuparnos de salvar a aquellos que silenciosamente mueren cada año." Government of Cuba Press Release, November 20, 1998. http://www.eroj.org/entero10/item13.htm.

"Declaración del Ministro de Relaciones Exteriores de Cuba en la Reunión de Donantes a Haití." *Juventud Rebelde*, April 1, 2010.

de La Hoz, Pedro. "Tariq Ali on Cuba, Venezuela, Bolivia." *Granma*, November 29, 2005.

de la Osa, José. "A las aulas casi 86 mil estudiantes de Ciencias Médicas." *Granma*, August 30, 2013.

———. "Egresan 11 mil médicos de universidades cubanas." *Granma*, July 11, 2012.

Delgado Legón, Elio. "Massive Graduation of Doctors in Cuba." *Havana Times*, July 29, 2013.

D'Elia, Yolanda, ed. *Las misiones sociales en Venezuela: Una aproximación a su comprensión y análisis*. Caracas: Instituto Latinoamericano de Investigaciones Sociales, 2006.

"Desarrollan cubanos y argentinos vacuna contra cáncer de pulmón." *La Jornada*, June 1, 2013.

"Destaca Nicolás Maduro labor de médicos cubanos en Venezuela." *Cubadebate*, March 10, 2014. http://www.cubadebate.cu/noticias/2014/03/10/destaca-nicolas-maduro-labor-del-medicos-cubanos-en-venezuela/#.VFuLomd_Qcs.

"The Detachment Returns, Undefeated." Cuban embassy report. *CubaMinrex: Ministerio de Relaciones Exteriores de Cuba*, March 29, 2008. http://www.voltairenet.org/article156231.html.

Díaz Ruiz, Olga. "Canciller salvadoreño orgulloso de formación de médicos de su país en Cuba." *Granma*, March 13, 2010.

"Directora de la OMS reconoce rápida respuesta de Cuba ante el ébola." *Prensa Latina*, September 12, 2014.

"Discurso Señor Vicepresidente en cumbre de vicepresidentes América sin barreras." Press release, Office of the Vice-President, Government of Ecuador, December 10, 2011. http://www.vicepresidencia.gob.ec/discurso-senor-vicepresidente-en-cumbre-de-vicepresidentes-america-sin-barreras/.

"Discurso, Sr. Mauricio Funes, Presidente de la República, Firma del acuerdo de restablecimiento de las relaciones diplomáticas entre El Salvador y Cuba." June 1, 2009. Document available through *La Prensa Grafica*. http://especiales.laprensagrafica.com/2011/funes2doaniversario/wp-content/uploads/2011/05/2-Restablecimiento-relaciones-con-Cuba.pdf.

"Dispone Cuba retirada de brigada médica de Panamá." *Cubadebate*, February 1, 2010. http://www.cubadebate.cu/noticias/2010/02/01/dispone-cuba-retirada-de-brigada-medica-de-panama/#.VFuNSWd_Qcs.

Domínguez, Jorge. *To Make a World Safe for Revolution: Cuba's Foreign Policy*. Cambridge: Harvard University Press, 1989.

"Dominicans Continue to Benefit from Cuban Eye Care Program." *CaribbeanNetNews*, July 27, 2006. http://www.caribbeannewsnow.com/caribnet/cgi-script/csArticles/articles/000025/002522.htm.

Dotres Martínez, Carlos, Oscar Grandío Zequeira, Raciel Llanes Pérez, Antonio González Fernández, José Piñon Vega, and Patricia Puig Anzorandía. "Programa para la atención médica integral a niños expuestos a contaminación ambiental por sustancias radiactivas." *Revista Cubana de Pediatría*, 67, no. 1 (January–April 1995). http://scielo.sld.cu/scielo.php?script=sci_arttext&pid=S0034-75311995000100002.

Dougherty, Jon. "Doctor Diplomacy Requires Red Pledge?" *CubaNet*, February 20, 2001. http://www.cubanet.org/htdocs/CNews/y01/feb01/21e6.htm.

"East Timor Rebuilds Health Infrastructure from Ashes." *Jakarta Post*, September 16, 2002.

Eaton, Tracey. "In Haiti, Cuban Doctors Stayed When No One Else Would." *Dallas Morning News*, March 10, 2004.

"Ecuador agradece la cooperación de Cuba y de Venezuela." *Telesur*, December 29, 2010.

"Ecuadoran President Thanks Cuba's Assistance in the Public Health Sector." November 23, 2011. http://www.cuba-solidarity.org/news.asp?ItemID=2117.

"Ecuador y Cuba firman convenio para prevenir discapacidades." http://www.medular-digital.com/main.php?act=dnews&s=24&n=1943.

"Ecuatorianos recuperan la visión gracias a 'Misión Milagro' en Venezuela." March 6, 2007. http://www.elnuevosiglo.com.co/video/11-2011-ecuatorianos-recuperan-la-visi%C3%B3n-gracias-misi%C3%B3n-milagro-en-venezuela.html.

Edmonds, Kevin. "Cuba's Other Internationalism: Angola 25 Years Later." *NACLA Report on the Americas*, September 27, 2013. https://nacla.org/blog/2013/9/27/cubas-other-internationalism-angola-25-years-later.

ELAM. (Escuela Latinoamericana de Medicina). Historia de La ELAM. http://instituciones.sld.cu/elam/historia-de-la-elam/.

———. Primeros años de estudio e ingreso en la ELAM. http://instituciones.sld.cu/elam/primeros-anos-de-estudio-e-ingreso-en-la-elam/.

"ELAM: Médicos pobres para los pobres." *Cubadebate*, October 31, 2013. cubadebate.cu/especiales/2013/10/31/elam-medicos-pobres-para-los-pobres/#U75kv7Hb6AI.

"Elías Jaua niega que médicos cubanos cobren 200 mil dólares al año." July 8, 2011. http://informe21.com/print/96338.

"El Salvador Floods, Mudslides Kill 124." *USA Today*, November 8, 2009.

"En Mérida redujeron las amputaciones en pacientes con diabetes." *Correo del Orinoco*, August 26, 2012.

Erisman, H. Michael. "Brain Drain Politics: The Cuban Medical Professional Parole Programme." *International Journal of Cuban Studies* 4 (Autumn/Winter 2012): 269–90.

———. *Cuba's Foreign Relations in a Post-Soviet World*. Gainesville: University Press of Florida, 2009.

Escalante Salazar, Jaime. "Gobierno inicia censo de discapacitados ante rechazo de dirigentes." *El Mundo*, February 4, 2009.

"Estructura de la BMC," Internal report of the Ministry of Foreign Relations, Government of Cuba, n.d.

"Estudio psicosocial, pedagógico y clínico-genético de personas con discapacidad." N.d., unpublished report. Provided to the author by the Ministry of Public Health (MINSAP) in Cuba, February 2013.

Evenson, Debra. "Cuba's Biotechnology Revolution." *MEDICC Review* 9, no. 1 (Fall 2007): 8–10.

———. "The Right to Health Care and the Law." *MEDICC Review* 7, no. 9 (November/December 2005).

"Éxito de Misión Solidaridad Moto Méndez." *Tarija*, August 15, 2010. http://tarijalibre.tarijaindustrial.com/exito-de-mision-solidarid.

"Exitoso apoyo médico de Cuba en Haití." *La Jornada*, February 12, 2007.

"Fact Sheet: Misión Milagro." Embassy of the Bolivarian Republic of Venezuela to the UK and Ireland, n.d.

Fariñas Acosta, Lisandra. "Ban Ki-moon: La ELAM es la escuela médica más avanzada del mundo." *Granma*, January 28, 2014.

———. "Cuba ha demostrado que es posible tener salud y bienestar para todos." *Granma*, July 14, 2014.

Farmer, Paul. *Pathologies of Power: Health, Human Rights, and the New War on the Poor*. Berkeley: University of California Press, 2003.

———. "U.S. Invasion of Haiti Deepens Health Crisis."*Peacework*, April 4, 2011. http://www.peaceworkmagazine.org/pwork/0404/040411.htm.

———. "Who Removed Aristide?" *London Review of Books* 26, no. 8 (April 15, 2004): 28–31.

Fawthrop, Tom. "Cuando La Habana forma gratuitamente médicos yanquis." *Granma*, March 19, 2007.

———. "Cuba Ailing? Not Its Biomedical Industry." *Straits Times*, January 26, 2004. http://yaleglobal.yale.edu/print/1427.

———. "Cuba Doctors Popular in Quake-Stricken Java." *BBC News*, August 18, 2006. http://news.bbc.co.uk/2/hi/americas/4792071.stm.

———. "Cuba's Humanitarian Mission." *Guardian*, August 16, 2006. http://www.theguardian.com/commentisfree/2006/aug/16/tomfawthropcubandocs.

"Federación Médica Venezolana: Aumento de salario de 75% es necesario pero insuficiente." *Confirmado*, September 11, 2013. http://confirmado.com.ve/federacion-medica-venezolana-aumento-de-salario-de-75-es-necesario-pero-insuficiente/.

Feinberg, Richard E. "Reaching Out: Cuba's New Economy and the International Response." Washington, D.C.: Brookings Institution, 2011.

———. "Soft Landing in Cuba? Emerging Entrepreneurs and Middle Classes." Washington, D.C.: Brookings Institution, 2013.

Feinsilver, Julie M. "Fifty Years of Cuba's Medical Diplomacy: From Idealism to Pragmatism." *Cuban Studies* 41 (2010): 85–104.

———. *Healing the Masses: Cuban Health Politics at Home and Abroad*. Berkeley: University of California Press, 1993.

"Fidel y la brigada 'Moto Méndez': 'La felicidad de hacer el bien.'" *Cubadebate*, August 18, 2010. http://www.cubadebate.cu/noticias/2010/08/18/fidel-y-la-brigada-moto-mendez-la-felicidad-de-hacer-el-bien/#.VF-cP8kXEXw.

"Fijian Medical Students Faring Well in Cuba." http://www.fijiprun.org/index.php?option=com_content&view=articles&id=84:fijian-medical-students-faring-well-in-cuba&catid=13&Itemid=178. Accessed June 1, 2014.

Fiji Government. "Fiji Benefits from Additional Cuban Scholarships." May 18, 2012. http://www.foreignaffairs.gov.fj/media-resources/media-release/108-fiji-benefits-from-additional-cuban-scholarships.

"Final Communiqué." International Donors' Conference Towards a New Future for Haiti (2010). http://www.haiticonference.org/communique.html.

"Firma Ecuador convenio para adquirir Heberprot." *Granma*, June 21, 2012.

Fitz, Don. "Cuba's Latin American School of Medicine—An 'Example of Internationalism and Human Solidarity.'" *Links*, May 18, 2011. http://links.org.au/node/2325.

———. "The Latin American School of Medicine Today." *Monthly Review* 62, no. 10 (March 2011). http://monthlyreview.org/2011/03/01/the-latin-american-school-of-medicine-today.

"Floods, Mudslides Kill Scores in El Salvador." CNN.com, November 9, 2009. http://www.cnn.com/2009/WORLD/americas/11/09/el.salvador.mudslides/index.html?_s=PM:WORLD.

Fonticoba, Onaisys. "Cuba tiene médicos por todo el mundo." *Granma*, March 25, 2014.

Forteza, Francisco. "Canciller cubano: No damos lo que nos sobra. Compartimos lo que tenemos." World Data Service Report, June 27, 2007.

Francis Mexidor, Deisy. "Vatican Secretary Lauds Cuba Med School." *Granma*, February 27, 2008.

Frank, Michele, and Gail A. Reed. "Doctors for the (Developing) World." *MEDICC Review* 7, no. 8 (August/September 2005).

"From Cuba to Martinez." *Martinez Gazette*, December 4, 2012. http://martinezgazette.com/from-cuba-to-martinez.

Furtado, Joao Marcello, Fabiano Cade, Van C. Lansingh, Andrea Zin, Carlos Eduardo Arieta, Jerónimo Fabiani, Cristián Luco, and Serge Reskinoff. "Is Misión Milagro an Effective Program to Prevent Blindness in Latin America?" *Arquivos Brasileiros de Oftalmologia* 73, no. 5 (September/October 2010): 397–98.

García Alcolea, Eglis Esteban. "Influencia de la Misión Milagro en el desarrollo de la teleoftalmología cubana." *Panorama Cuba y Salud* 4, no. 2 (May–August 2009): 31–37.

García Alcolea, Eglis Esteban, and Diana González Poveda. "La dirección de un centro oftalmológico en el extranjero: reto de la administración de salud." *Revista de Oftalmología: Misión Milagro* 3, no. 3 (July–September 2009). http://www.misionmilagro.sld.cu/vol3no3/inv3303.php.

García Alcolea, Eglis Esteban, and Rebeca Lahera Cabrales. "Influencia de la Misión Milagro en la salud visual latinoamericana." *Revista Cubana de Salud Pública* 36, no. 4 (2010): 382–84.

García Domínguez, Carlos, and José Miguel Ceruto Machado. "Cooperación internacional para el desarrollo de un nuevo modelo de atención primaria de salud (APS) en Haití." *Revista Cubana de Salud Pública Internacional* 1, no. 1 (2010): 76–91.

Garófalo Fernández, Nicolás, and Ana María Gómez García, eds. *Pensamientos de Fidel sobre la salud pública*. Havana: Editorial Ciencias Médicas, 2011.

Gleijeses, Piero. *Misiones en Conflicto: La Habana, Washington y África, 1959–1976*. Havana: Ciencias Sociales, 2002.

Gleijeses, Piero, Jorge Risquet, and Fernando Remírez. *Cuba y África: Historia común de lucha y sangre*. Havana: Editorial de Ciencias Sociales, 2007.

Gómez Navia, Raymundo. "Médicos cubanos extienden sus labores en Haití." *Juventud Rebelde*, January 21, 2010.

González, Ana Margarita. "¿Empresa modelo o modelo de empresa?" *Labiofam* 2, no. 3 (2011): 7.

González Peña, Mayreth. "El Contingente Médico Cubano 'Henry Reeve.'" *Nuestros Médicos* 4 no. 3 (September–December 2009): 55–59.

Gorry, Conner. "Biotech: The Magic Pill?" *Scientific American Worldview* (2012): 68–69 (top of pages). http://www.saworldview.com/archive/2012/download-the-2012-issue/.

———. "Cuba-Guatemala Cooperation: Building Viable Models for Health." *MEDICC Review* 11, no. 3 (Summer 2009): 48–51.

———. "Cuba Marks 15 Years Treating Chernobyl Victims." *MEDICC Review* 7, no. 5 (May 2005).

———. "Cuban Disaster Doctors in Guatemala, Pakistan." *MEDICC Review* 7, no. 9 (November/December 2005).

———. "Cuba's Latin American School: Can Socially Accountable Medical Education Make a Difference?" *MEDICC Review* 14, no. 3 (July 2012): 5–11.

———. "Cuba's Response to Katrina Disaster." *MEDICC Review* 7, no. 8 (August/September 2005).

———. "Haiti One Year Later: Cuban Medical Team Draws on Experience and Partnerships." *MEDICC Review* 13, no. 1 (January 2011): 52–55.

———. "Innovative Project Brings Permanent Medical Services to Honduran Mosquitia." *MEDICC Review*, November 30, 2006.

———. "Interview with Dr. Patrick Dely: Part II." *Field Notes from MEDICC*, July 9, 2010.

———. "Joining Forces to Develop Human Resources for Health." *MEDICC Review* 7, no. 8 (August/September 2005).

———. "Once the Earth Stood Still (Part II): Mental Health Services in Post-Quake Haiti." *MEDICC Review* 12, no. 3 (July 2010): 44–47.

———. "Sight for Sore Eyes: Cuba's Vision Restoration Program." *MEDICC Review* 10, no. 2 (Spring 2008): 49–51.

———. "Staying the Course in Haiti." *Field Notes from MEDICC*, July 9, 2010.

———. "Touring Cuban Field Hospitals in Post-Quake Pakistan." *MEDICC Review* 8, no. 1 (March/April 2006).

Government of Bolivia. Sistema de Información del Programa de Registro Único Nacional de la Persona con Discapacidad, 2011. http://siprunpcd.minsalud.gob.bo/.

Government of Vanuatu, Ministry of Health. "Moving Health Forward: Health Sector Strategy, 2010–2016. http://www.wpro.who.int/health_services/vanuatu_nationalhealthplan.pdf.

"Graduados de medicina en Cuba tienen deficiencias en formación, afirma UCR." *El País*, August 22, 2012.

Grogg, Patricia. "Chernobyl Kids Keep Arriving in Cuba." Inter Press Service, May 7, 2009. http://www.ipsnews.net/2009/05/health-chernobyl-kids-keep-arriving-in-cuba/.

———. "Cuba, Brazil Unite for Africa's Health." Inter Press Service, October 25, 2010. http://www.ipsnews.net/2010/10/cuba-brazil-unite-for-africas-health/.

Grover Choque, Freddy. "El 90 por ciento de la discapacidad es adquirida." *La Prensa*, October 23, 2011.

"Guatemala Plans to Send More Medical Students to Cuba." *Granma*, February 1, 2008.

Gutiérrez Delgado, Yuliet. "Médico cubano se une a brujo para asistir a la población de Guatemala." *Juventud Rebelde*, February 13, 2009.

"Haiti." Pan American Health Organization website. http://www.paho.org/english/dd/ais/cp_332.htm.

"Haitian President Arrives in Cuba in Official Visit." *Prensa Latina*, May 15, 2013.

"Haiti-Cuba Cooperation Is in the Agenda of Prime Minister Laurent Lamothe." October 14, 2012. http://hispaniolainfo.com/2012/10/?p=936.

"Haiti Earthquake Aid Pledged by Country." *Guardian*, January 14, 2010.

Harvard Medical School and NATO Joint Analysis and Lessons Learned Centre. *The Haiti Case Study: Working Paper of the Collaborative NATO-Harvard Project: Towards A Comprehensive Response to Health System Strengthening in Crisis-Affected Fragile States.* Cambridge, Mass.: Harvard/NATO, 2012.

"Health Minister Lauds Cuba's Kindness." *Jamaica Star*, June 25, 2012.

Heritage Foundation. "The Cuban Economy." http://www.heritage.org/index/country/cuba.

Hodal, Kate. "Cuban Infusion Remains the Lifeblood of Timor-Leste's Health Service." *Guardian*, June 25, 2012.

Hopper, Jonathan. "Nauru's Health Crisis: 661 Patients per Doctor." *3rd Degree* 13, no. 9 (May 2012). http://3degree.ecu.edu.au/articles/4554.

"Hoy se conmemora el Día Mundial de la Salud Visual." *Correo del Orinoco*, October 13, 2011.

Huish, Robert. "Going Where No Doctor Has Gone Before: The Role of Cuba's Latin American School of Medicine in Meeting the Needs of Some of the World's Most Vulnerable Populations." *Public Health* 122, no. 6 (2008): 552–57.

———. "How Cuba's Latin American School of Medicine Challenges the Ethics of Physician Migration." *Social Science and Medicine* 69, no. 3 (2009): 301–4.

———. *Where No Doctor Has Gone Before: Cuba's Place in the Global Health Landscape.* Waterloo, Ont.: Wilfred Laurier University Press, 2013.

Humanitarian Response Index. *Focus on Haiti*." http:// daraint.org/wp-content/uploads/2012/02/HRI2011-FocusOnHaiti.pdf.

"Hurricane Stan Floods Coastal Guatemala—MSF Response." *Médecins sans Frontieres*, October 14, 2005. http://www.msf.org/article/hurricane-stan-floods-coastal-guatemala-msf-response.

Ianoni, Marcus. "A populacao quer 'Mais Médicos.'" *Jornal do Brasil*, May 20, 2014.

"IDB Grants $400,000 to Guatemala and El Salvador for Relief after Hurricane Stan." *Port of Entry*, October 12, 2005.

"Inauguran exposición sobre la Operación Milagro en Argentina." *LAinformation.com*, November 5, 2013. http://noticias.lainformacion.com/noticias/inauguran-exposicion-sobre-operacion-milagro-en-argentina_4AInFnrI2MCnaKfTtYKkK3/.

"Indonesian Earthquake Donations." *Virtual Information Center*, June 6, 2006.

"Información sobre el resultado del Debate de los Lineamientos de la Política Económica y Social del Partido y la Revolución." *Cubadebate*, May 2011. www.cubadebate.cu/wp-content/uploads/2011/05/tabloide_debate_lineamientos.pdf.

"In Just One Month, Cubans Save More than 1,000 Lives in Guatemala." *Granma*, November 16, 2005.

"International Conference Raises Almost $10 Billion as More than 130 Donors Contrib-

ute 'Towards a New Future for Haiti,'' March 31, 2010, United Nations Press Release GA/10932.
International Federation of Red Cross and Red Crescent Societies. "Chernobyl Humanitarian Assistance and Rehabilitation Programme (CHARP)." 2010–11.
Janicke, Kiraz. "Venezuelan Doctors Step Up Protests against Government." *Venezuelanalysis.com*, September 22, 2007. http://venezuelanalysis.com/print/2631.
Jardim, Claudia. "Prevention and Solidarity: Remedies for Democratizing Health in Venezuela." *Venezuelanalysis.com*, October 13, 2004. http://venezuelanalysis.com/print/735.
Jenvey, Nicola. "Strike of Medical Students in Cuba Sparks Controversy." *University World News*, no. 261 (March 2, 2013). http://www.universityworldnews.com/article.php?story=20130228161900444.
Jiménez, Mayte María. "Productos biotecnológicos cubanos en 50 países." *Juventud Rebelde*, December 18, 2012.
"Jorge Rodríguez: 'Cuba no exporta armas, exporta salud, un servicio para el planeta,'" *El Universo*, January 12, 2015.
Kirk, Emily J. "Operation Miracle: A New Vision of Public Health?" *International Journal of Cuban Studies* 3, no. 4 (Winter 2011): 366–81.
Kirk, Emily J., and John M. Kirk. "Cuban Medical Aid to Haiti: One of the World's Best-Kept Secrets." *Counterpunch*, April 1, 2010. http://www.counterpunch.org/2010/04/01/cuban-medical-aid-to-haiti/.
Kirk, John M. "Cuban Medical Internationalism and Its Role in Cuban Foreign Policy." *Diplomacy and Statecraft* 20 (2009): 275–90.
———. "Cuban Medical Internationalism: Development and Rationale." *Bulletin of Latin American Research* 28, no. 3 (2009): 497–511.
———. "Cuban Medical Internationalism under Raúl Castro." *Bulletin of Latin American Research* 31 (2012): 77–90.
———. "El internacionalismo médico de Cuba: ¿dónde está el secreto?" *Temas* 74 (July–September 2012): 84–91.
Kirk, John M., and H. Michael Erisman. *Cuban Medical Internationalism: Origins, Evolution, and Goals*. New York: Palgrave Macmillan, 2009.
Kirk, John M., and Robert Huish. "Cuban Medical Internationalism and the Development of the Latin American School of Medicine." *Latin American Perspectives* 34, no. 6 (November 2007): 77–92.
Kirk, John M., and Marguerite Jiménez. "Cuban Medical Internationalism: Central America, a Decade after Hurricane Mitch." *Journal of Iberian and Latin American Studies* 15, no. 2 (December 2009): 83–101.
Kirk, John M., and Chris Walker. "Moral Medicine, the Cuban Way." *New Internationalist* 457 (November 2012): 24–27.
Kovac, Anna. "Cuban-Haitian Cooperation: An Interview with Radio Havana's Anna Kovac." *Political Affairs*, April 24, 2006. http://www.politicalaffairs.net/cuban-haitian-cooperation-an-interview-with-radio-havana-s-anna-kovac/.
———. "Cuba Trains Hundreds of Haitian Doctors to Make a Difference." *Medicc Review*, August 6, 2007. http://www.medicc.org/publications/cuba_health_reports/documents/018_000.pdf.

Kupferschmeidt, Kai. "Cuba to Commit Large Health Corps to Ebola Fight." *Science*, September 12, 2014. http://sciencemag.org/africa/2014/09/cuba-commit-karge-health.

Lage Dávila, Agustín. "Fidel o la inmediatez del futuro." *Cubadebate*, February 27, 2007. http://www.cubadebate.cu/opinion/2007/02/27/fidel-o-la-inmediatez-del-futuro-2/print/.

———. "Socialism and the Knowledge Economy: Cuban Biotechnology." *Monthly Review* 58, no. 7 (December 2006). www.monthlyreview.org/2006/12/01/socialism-and-the-knowledge-economy-cuban-biotechnology.

"La Misión Milagro de Venezuela apoya a mexicanos *olvidados* por el Seguro Popular." *La Jornada*, March 6, 2007. http://www.jornada.unam.mx/2007/03/06/index.php?section=sociedad&article=039n1soc.

Lamrami, Salim. "Cuba, la isla de la salud." *La pupila insomne*. Blog. August 4, 2012. http://lapupilainsomne.wordpress.com/2012/08/04/cuba-la-isla-de-la-salud.

"Lanzan en Trujillo campaña 'Ver para Creer.'" Video. Uploaded by El Congresso de la República del Perú, May 27, 2010. https://www.youtube.com/watch?v=zTGeoDI4vd4.

"La Operación Milagro, de Cuba, ha beneficiado a por lo menos 2.5 millones." *La Jornada*, June 1, 2013.

"La participación cubana en el enfrentamiento al ébola en África Occidental no es un hecho aislado." *Juventud Rebelde*, September 12, 2014.

"Largest-Ever International Stamp Issue to Aid Chernobyl Children." *UNESCO.org*, April 7, 1997. http://www.unesco.org/bpi/eng/unescopress/hebdo97e/stamp.htm.

"La Salud Pública cubana apuesta a más calidad y más eficiencia." *Cubadebate*, March 28, 2014. http://www.cubadebate.cu/especiales/2014/03/28/la-salud-publica-cubana-apuesta-a-mas-calidad-y-mas-eficiencia/#.VF-0I8kXEXw.

"Las bondades de la solidaridad." *Granma*, November 11, 2013.

Lemus Lago, Elia Rosa, Gonzalo Estévez Torres, and Juan Carlos Velázquez Acosta. *Campaña por la esperanza: La lucha contra el dengue.* Havana: Editora Política, 2002.

"Lenín Moreno expuso Misión Manuela Espejo en la ONU." *El Telégrafo*, September 12, 2012.

León Corrales, Ladys Marlene. "Valor social de la Misión Milagro en el contexto venezolano." *Revista Cubana de Salud Pública* 35, no. 4 (October–December 2009). http://scielo.sld.cu/scielo.php?pid=S0864-34662009000400006&script=sci_arttext.

Li, Kun. "Bettering Children's Lives Devastated by Hurricane Stan." UNICEF, October 12, 2005. http://www.unicef.org/infobycountry/guatemala_28728.html?q=printm.

Llanes, Rafael., Lorenzo Somarriba, PlácidoPedroso, Emiliano Mariscal, Carlos Fuster and Yamila Zayas. "Did the Cholera Epidemic in Haiti Really Start in the Artibonite Department?" *Journal of Infection in Developing Countries* 15, no. 7 (2013): 753–55.

Loanakadavu, N. "Cuba Seeks Deal." *Fiji Sun*, April 9, 2012.

López Blanch, Hedelberto. *Historias secretas de médicos cubanos.* Havana: Centro Cultural Pablo de la Corriente Brau, 2005.

López, Ernesto. "La función de la medicina cubana no es para que los salvadoreños abracen otra bandera." *La Prensa Gráfica*, November 27, 2009.

"Los ojos abiertos de América Latina." *Granma*, February 2, 2010.

Lu, Kai, Tao Chen, and George F. Gao. "Transcontinental Translational Medicine Collaboration: A Successful Sino-Cuban Joint B-to-B Program." *Biomedical and Environmental Sciences* 26, no 7 (July 2013): 517–19.

Luque Álvarez, Luis. "Cuba constituye una esperanza para los niños de Chernobil." *Juventud Rebelde*, March 26, 2010.

———. "Leonid Kuchma: Unos mostraron lástima, pero Cuba nos ayudó." *Juventud Rebelde*, March 29, 2010.

Maceo Leyva, Leandro. "Quince años de batas blancas." *Granma*, December 4, 2013.

"Maduro destaca ayuda 'incalculable' de Cuba en materia de salud." *El Nuevo Herald*, March 10, 2014.

Maltbie, Tyler. "Haiti Earthquake: The Nations That Are Stepping Up to Help." *Christian Science Monitor*, January 14, 2010.

Mantiñán Búairambua, Iara. "Los cubanos están trayendo el cólera a Venezuela." *ABC*, May 9, 2013.

"'Manuela Espejo,' un plan para imitar." *Los Tiempos*, May 15, 2011.

Manzaneda, José. "Why You Will Not Be Told about This Miracle." *Meeting Point*. Blog. November 21, 2008. http://nuestrosricos.blogspot.com/2008/11/why-you-will-not-be-told-of-this.html.

Marquis, Christopher. "Medical School for Latins Earns Cuba Goodwill." *Miami Herald*, March 13, 2000.

Martínez Hernández, Leticia. "Nuestros compromisos con Haití continúan inalterables." *Granma*, March 31, 2010.

Martínez Hernández, Leticia, and Juvenal Balán. "Cuba fue el primer país que nos ayudó." *Granma*, January 29, 2010.

———. "Cuban Healthcare Continues in Haiti." *Granma*, February 2, 2010.

Martínez Hernández, Leticia, and Yaima Puig Meneses. "Aprobó Consejo de Ministros incremento salarial para el sector de la Salud." *Granma*, March 21, 2014.

"Más de 1 millón 500 mil personas atendidas por la Misión Milagro." *Cubadebate*, July 8, 2012. http://www.cubadebate.cu/noticias/2012/07/08/mas-de-1-millon-500-mil-personas-han-sido-atendidas-por-la-mision-milagro/#.VF-2fskXEXw.

"Más de 37000 cubanos y 10000 extranjeros estudian medicina." *El Nuevo Herald*, August 30, 2013.

"Más de 60 mil personas ha atendido convenio de salud Cuba-Venezuela." *Correo del Orinoco*, March 28, 2014.

"Más de 61,000 nicaraguenses atendidos por médicos cubanos." *Economista*, February 8, 2010.

"Más de tres millones de beneficiados con Operación Milagro en diez años." *Cubadebate*, July 1, 2014. http://www.cubadebate.cu/noticias/2014/07/01/mas-de-tres-millones-de-beneficiados-con-operacion-milagro-en-diez-anos/#.VF-3fckXEXw.

Mason, Susan E., David L. Strug, and Joan Beder, eds. *Community Health Care in Cuba*. Chicago: Lyceum Books, 2010.

"Matrícula de la Escuela Latinoamericana de Medicina en Cuba llega a los 10 000 estudiantes." *Cubadebate*, March 16, 2010. http://www.cubadebate.cu/noticias/2010/03/16/matricula-de-la-escuela-latinoamericana-de-medicina-en-cuba-llega-a-los-10-000-estudiantes/#.VF-3zMkXEXw.

McKinley, James C., Jr. "Cuba, in a Campaign against Blindness, Uses Doctors to Bolster Its Image." *International Herald Tribune*, November 19, 2007.

McQuaid, John. "Chernobyl Kids: Thousands of Soviet Children Find Help, Tropical Fun in Cuba." Newhouse News Service, February 8, 1991. http://community.seattletimes.nwsource.com/archive/?date=19910208&slug=1265090.

"Medical Education: Inspired by Cuba, Students Hope to Overhaul Pakistani Health Care." *Express Tribune*, September 3, 2011.

"Médicos cubanos estarán aquí hasta que Chávez decida." *Últimas Noticias*, March 25, 2010.

"Médicos de Cuba han atendido más de 50,000 haitianos; comienzan servicios de rehabilitación." *Cubadebate*, February 1, 2010. http://www.cubadebate.cu/noticias/2010/02/01/medicos-cubanos-han-atendido-mas-de-50-000-haitianos/.

"Médicos graduados en Cuba reprueban exámenes en Chile." *La Patilla*, January 1, 2011. http://cafefuerte.com/cuba/csociedad/1531-medicos-graduados-en-cuba-reprueban-examenes-en-chile/.

Menéndez Cabezas, Arturo. "Experience of Cuban Faculty in Establishing a Medical School in the Republic of The Gambia." *MEDICC Review* 7, no. 8 (August/September 2005).

Menéndez Quintero, Marina. "La salud, una prioridad para El Salvador." *Juventud Rebelde*, December 4, 2009.

Merlin NGO. "Is Haiti's Health System Any Better?" Global Health Workforce Alliance. http://www.who.int/workforcealliance/knowledge/resources/merlinhaiti2011/en/.

"Mexicanos agradecen a Cuba por Operación Milagro." *Juventud Rebelde*, May 8, 2011.

"Mexico Thanks Cuba for Medical Aid to Flood Victims." Agencia de Información Nacional, January 4, 2008.

"Miles de cubanos favorecidos con Heberprot-P para pie diabético." *Prensa Latina*, June 25, 2013.

"Millions of People Treated in Operation Miracle in Venezuela." Infomed, Centro Nacional de Información de Ciencias Médicas, May 11, 2012. http://articulos.sld.cu/desastres/2012/05/14/millions-of-people-treated-in-operation-miracle-in-venezuela/.

Millman, Joel. "New Prize in Cold War: Cuban Doctors." *Wall Street Journal*, January 15, 2011.

Ministry of Public Health, Timor-Leste. *Human Resources for Health: Country Profile—Timor-Leste*. N.d.

———. *SISCa Health Service*. N.d. http://www.moh.gov.tl/?q=node/82.

"Misión Barrio Adentro ha fortalecido la salud pública de Venezuela." *Cubadebate*, April 9, 2014. http://www.cubadebate.cu/noticias/2014/04/09/mision-barrio-adentro-ha-fortalecido-la-salud-publica-de-venezuela/#.VF-9JskXEXw.

"Misión Espejo, con 236 médicos cubanos." *Hoy*, September 21, 2009.

"Misión Joaquín Gallegos Lara" report, http://www.presidencia.gob.ec/mision-joaquin-gallegos-lara/.

"Misión José Gregorio Hernández brinda atención integral en todo el país." Gobierno Bolivariano de Venezuela, March 17, 2011. http://www.mpcomunas.gob.ve/misiann-josao-gregorio-hernaendez-brinda/. Accessed July 24, 2013.

"Misión José Gregorio Hernández saca a la luz a 334,018 venezolanos con discapacidad."

ReporteConfidencial, October 31, 2008. http://www.reporteconfidencial.info/noticia/2194/mision-jose-gregorio-hernandez-saca-a-la-luz-a-334018-venezolanos-con-discapacidad/.
"Misión Manuela Espejo atiende más de 180 mil ecuatorianos." IPS: Inter Press Service in Cuba, August 13, 2012. http://www.ipscuba.net/index.php?option=com_k2&view=item&id=4990:misi%C3%B3n-manuela-espejo-atiende-m%C3%A1s-de-180-mil-ecuatorianos&Itemid=7.
"Misión Milagro cumple su décimo aniversario." *Juventud Rebelde*, July 8, 2014.
"Misión Milagro ha devuelto la visión a 2.5 millones de personas." Television report on Telesur channel in Latin America, May 31, 2013.
"Misión Milagro ha devuelto la visión a miles de salvadoreños." *Granma*, July 8, 2014.
"Misión Milagro suma un millón de intervenciones en Venezuela." *Cubadebate*, May 29, 2010. http://www.cubadebate.cu/noticias/2010/05/29/mision-milagro-suma-un-millon-de-intervenciones-en-venezuela/#.VF_A28kXEXw.
"Misión Solidaria Manuela Espejo" data. http://www.manuelaespejo.com.
"Mitch: The Deadliest Atlantic Hurricane since 1780." National Climatic Data Center, August 26, 2006. http://lwf.ncdc.noaa.gov/oa/reports/mitch/mitch.html.
Montaner, Carlos Alberto. "Slaves in White Coats." *Miami Herald*, September 13, 2005.
Morales Lugo, Mérida, Osvaldo Segura Sardiñas, Eliades González Pérez, and Aida Sánchez Rodríguez. "Brigada Médica Internacionalista Cubana en Haití, Boletín Epidemiológico." April 2008. Mimeo, provided to author by officials of Cuban Ministry of Public Health.
Morales Valido, Charly. "Biorat: una pelea cubana contra las ratas." *Prensa Latina*, May 15, 2011.
Morgan, Peter. "Americas: Honduras Fights Back after Mitch." BBC News, February 11, 1999. http://news.bbc.co.uk/2/hi/americas/276122.stm.
"Mujica Flies to Havana to Meet the Castro Brothers and Celebrate 60 Years of Cuba's Revolution." *MercoPress*, July 24, 2013. http://en.mercopress.com/2013/07/24/mujica-flies-to-havana-to-meet-the-castro-brothers-and-celebrate-60-years-of-cuba-s-revolution.
Mullan, Fitzhugh. "Affirmative Action, Cuban Style." *New England Journal of Medicine* 351, no. 26 (December 23, 2004): 2682.
Narváez, Marco Fabricio. "La investigación epidemiológica del programa 'Manuela Espejo' 2010–2011." Master's thesis, Universidad Técnica Particular de Loja, Quito, 2012.
Negin, Joel. "Australia and New Zealand's Contribution to Pacific Island Health Worker Brain Drain." *Australian and New Zealand Journal of Public Health* 32, no. 6 (2008): 507–11.
———. "Cuba in the Pacific: More than Rum and Coke." Development Policy Blog. February 24, 2012. http://devpolicy.org/cuba-in-the-pacific-more-than-rum-and-coke-2-20120224/.
"Nelson Mandela on How Cuba 'Destroyed the Myth of the Invincibility of the White Oppressor.'" *Democracy Now!.org*. http://www.democracynow.org/blog/2013/12/11/nelson_mandela_on_how_cuba_destroyed.
"News Alerts." Reports for the Chernobyl Children's Project International for May 2005. http://www.chernobyl-international.org/news2.html.
"New York, 26 April 2012—Statement Attributable to the Spokesperson for the Secretary-

General on the 26th Anniversary of the Chernobyl Disaster." http://www.un.org/sg/statements/?nid=6024.

Nichter, Mark. *Global Health: Why Cultural Perceptions, Social Representations, and Biopolitics Matter*. Tucson: University of Arizona Press, 2008.

Nublat, Johanna. "A um mes das eleicoes, governo divulga pesquisa favorável ao Mais Médicos." *Folha de S. Paulo*, September 4, 2014.

Nullis-Kapp, Clare. "Efforts Underway to Stem the 'Brain Drain' of Doctors and Nurses." *WHO Bulletin*, February 2005. www.who.int/bulletin/volumes/83/2/news.pdf.

Nusa Peñalver, Juan Diego. "Más de 100 mil cubanos prestaron ayuda civil en pueblos de África." *Granma*, June 26, 2008.

Obama, Barack. Closing press conference of President Barack Obama. Summit of the Americas, Trinidad and Tobago, April 19, 2009. www.c-spanvideo.org/videoLibrary/clip.php?transchunkid=202172.

"OMS reconoce labor de colaboración de médicos cubanos." *Juventud Rebelde*, May 23, 2014.

ONE. Data from www.one.cu/aec2011/esp/19_tabla_cuadro.htm.

"Operación Milagro concluye el 2011 con 90,000 operaciones." January 18, 2012. Report of the Cuban Ministry of Foreign Relations.

"Operación Milagro: Cuba lamenta 'intereses mezquinos.'" Agence France Presse, February 3, 2010.

"Operación Milagro: Operados de la vista más de 15,000 paraguayos." *Juventud Rebelde*, April 5, 2012.

"Operation Miracle: Five Years of Cuban Ophthalmology Services in Nicaragua." *La Demajagua*, May 17, 2012.

Osoria Ramírez, Pablo. "Moto Méndez: misión de esperanza en Bolivia." Bolpress, November 11, 2009. http://www.bolpress.com/art.php?Cod=2009111305.

"Palabras del Dr. Carlos Dotres, Ministro de Salud Pública, en el Acto de Conmemoración del VII Aniversario de la llegada a Cuba del primer grupo de niños ucranianos procedentes de Chernobil, 29/3/97." http://www.infomed.sld.cu/discursos/chernobi.html.

Pan American Health Organization. "Haiti." Regional Core Health Data Initiative: Health Profiles by Country. http://www.paho.org/saludenlasamericas/index.php?option=com_docman&task=doc_view&gid=134&Itemid=.

———. "Impact of Hurricane Mitch in Central America." *Epidemiological Bulletin* 19, no. 4 (December 1998). http://www1.paho.org/english/sha/epibul_95-98/be984mitch.htm.

———. *Mission Barrio Adentro: The Right to Health and Social Inclusion in Venezuela*. Caracas: PAHO, 2006.

———. "Venezuela." Regional Core Health Data Initiative: Health Profiles by Country. http://www.paho.org/saludenlasamericas/index.php?option=com_docman&task=doc_view&gid=154&Itemid=.

"Patricia Grogg entrevista a la científica cubana Concepción Campa." Inter Press Service, September 1, 2010.

Pearson, Tamara. "Venezuela's Community Doctors Gain Legal Recognition." *Venezuelanalysis*, November 2, 2011. http://www.venezuelanalysis.com/print/6601.

Peláez, Orfilio. "Valoran efectividad de biolarvicidas cubanos." *Granma*, September 29, 2012.

Pérez, Christina. *Caring for Them from Birth to Death: The Practice of Community-Based Medicine*. Lanham, Md.: Lexington Books, 2008.

Pierrat, Alfredo. "Inician en Nicaragua aplicación de rodenticida donado por Cuba." *Prensa Latina*, October 23, 2010.

Porter, Catherine. "Cuba-Trained Doctors Making Difference around the World." *Toronto Star*, June 2, 2012.

"President Castro Reiterates Cuba's Offer of Medical Aid to the American People on the Round Table Program aired on September 2, 2005." Portal Cuba.cu. http://www.cuba.cu/gobierno/discursos/2005/ing/f020905i.html.

"Presidente Chávez anuncia relanzamiento de Convenio Cuba-Venezuela 2010–2020." *Cubadebate*, November 7, 2010. http://www.cubadebate.cu/noticias/2010/11/07/presidente-chavez-anuncia-relanzamiento-de-convenio-cuba-venezuela-2010-2020/#.VF_MGskXEXw.

"Presidente de Honduras condecora a brigada médica cubana." *Cubadebate*, January 17, 2014, http://www.cubadebate.cu/noticias/2014/01/17/presidente-de-honduras-condecora-a-brigada-medica-cubana.

"Presidente de Timor Leste agradece postura ejemplar de Cuba." *Prensa Latina*, September 27, 2013.

"Presidente uruguayo concluye visita oficial a Cuba." *Prensa Latina*, July 27, 2013.

"President of Kiribati Pays Tribute to José Martí." Radio Rebelde, December 14, 2010. http://www.radiorebelde.cu/english/news/president-of-kiribati-pays-tribute-to-jose-marti-20101214/.

Press Conference on Haiti Humanitarian Aid. United Nations, March 23, 2004. http://www.un.org/News/briefings/docs/2004/CanadaPressCfc.doc.htm.

"Primer grupo de pacientes de la Misión Milagro viaja a Venezuela." *Agencia Prensa Rural*, March 23, 2007. http://prensarural.org/spip/spip.php?article305.

"Programa cubano de atención médica integral a niños relacionados con el accidente de Chernobil." N.d. Mimeo, provided to author by medical staff at Tarará hospital.

"Programa cubano ha salvado de ceguera a medio millón en AL." *La Jornada*, December 5, 2006.

"Prosiguen labores de brigada médica cubana en Haití." *Juventud Rebelde*, February 1, 2010.

"Quebec Doctors Want Pay for Haiti Volunteer Work." *Huffington Post*, January 27, 2010. http://www.huffingtonpost.com/2010/01/27/quebec-doctors-want-pay-f_n_438934.html.

Rake, Damian. "Peru: How Cuba's Solidarity Make a Difference." *Green Left*, September 27, 2007. https://www.greenleft.org.au/node/38360.

Ramachandran, Vijaya and Julia Walz. "Haiti: Where Has All the Money Gone?" A Report by the Center for Global Governance, CGD Policy Paper 004, May 2012. www.cgdev.org/files/1426185_file_Ramachandran_Walz_haiti_FINAL.pdf.

Ramos Pereira, Yanay, Eglis Esteban García Alcolea, María Sánchez Miranda, Arianna Hernández Pérez, Raúl Reynaldo Leyva, and Liliana María Batista Hernández. "Misión Milagro: Una tecnología social." *Revista Oftalmológica: Misión Milagro* 2, no. 2 (2009). http://www.misionmilagro.sld.cu/vol2no2/orig8.php.

"Ratifica Presidente de Ucrania colaboración médica con Cuba." *Juventud Rebelde*, October 23, 2011.
"Raúl Castro asegura ayuda cubana para Haití el tiempo que sea necesario." *La Jornada*, February 3, 2010.
Recasens, Maricela. "Cuba's Doctors Help in Indonesia." *Canadian Network on Cuba*, 2006. http://www.canadiannetworkoncuba.ca/Documenta/Java-2006.shtml.
"Reconoce Cuba significativa disminución de malaria en Angola." *Granma*, September 20, 2010.
"Reconocen beneficios de la Operación Milagro." *Granma*, May 27, 2014.
"Reconocen logros de alianza Cuba-Venezuela." *Juventud Rebelde*, November 1, 2013.
"Reconoce Presidente de Guatemala internacionalismo de Cuba en la salud." *Granma*, December 1, 2004.
"Reconocida Brigada Médica Cubana en Guatemala como Personaje del Año." *Granma*, December 29, 2006. http://cubasi.mforos.com/28304/5365570-reconocida-brigada-medica-cubana-en-guatemala/.
"Reconstruction of Water Systems after Hurricane Stan." Embassy of the United States press release, March 30, 2006. http://guatemala.usembassy.gov/pbe20060330.html.
"Red Bolivia Cuba puso a disposición 1,700 médicos y equipo logístico para atención de damnificados." *Prensa Latina*, February 26, 2007.
"Reduce Cuba riesgos de amputación a pacientes de pie diabético." *Cubadebate*, April 2, 2014. http://www.cubadebate.cu/noticias/2014/04/02/reduce-cuba-riesgos-de-amputacion-a-pacientes-de-pie-diabetico/#.VF_P4MkXEXw.
Reed, Gail A. "Cuba and Guatemala: Innovations in Physician Training." *MEDICC Review* 7, no. 6 (June 2005).
———. "Cuban Medical Teams in Global Disaster Relief." *MEDICC Review*, n.d. http://www.medicc.org/publications/medicc_review/1204/pages/international_cooperation_report.html.
———. "PAHO's Presence in Cuban Health: José Luis Di Fabio PhD." *MEDICC Review* 14, no. 4 (October 2012): 10–13.
"Regresan a Bolivia centenares de médicos graduados en Cuba." *Cubadebate*, August 8, 2013. http://www.cubadebate.cu/noticias/2013/08/08/regresan-a-bolivia-centenares-de-medicos-graduados-en-Cuba.
Reid-Henry, Simon M. *The Cuban Cure: Reason and Resistance in Global Science*. Chicago: University of Chicago Press, 2010.
Remen, Razel, and Lillian Holloway. "A Student Perspective on ELAM and Its Educational Program." *Social Medicine* 3, no. 2 (July 2008): 158–64.
"Resalta presidente Correa estado de las relaciones con Cuba." *Prensa Latina*, January 22, 2014.
"Reseña histórica de la brigada, Colaboración Médica Cubana." Internal report of Cuban Ministry of Foreign Relations, n.d.
Riera, Lilliam. "Cuba Exports Medical Equipment All Over the World." *Granma International*, January 18, 2008.
———. "In Two Months: Cuban Doctors Saved More than 1,000 Lives in Guatemala." *Cubainsideout*. http://www.cubainsideout.org/international/missions/medguat.shtml.
Riverry, T. J. "Misión Milagro de dos fronteras." *Granma*, May 9, 2006.

Robertson, Ewan. "Attending Need, Not Profit: Venezuela's Experiment with Community Medicine." *Venezuelanalysis.com*, October 14, 2013. http:/venezuelanalysis.com/print/10092.

———. "The 'Doctors of Socialism'? Meet Venezuela's Community Doctors." *Venezuelanalysis.com*, October 16, 2013. http://www.forumdesalternatives.org/en/the-doctors-of-socialism-meet-venezuelas-community-doctors.

Rodríguez, Ilsa. "Científico cubano promueve en Beijing Zona de Desarrollo." *Prensa Latina*, April 24, 2014.

Rodríguez Armas, Gisela. "Cuba colabora en mejoría de indicadores de salud en Haití." World Data Service report, March 15, 2003.

Rodríguez Guevara, Víctor Manuel. *Haití querido*. Havana: Pablo de la Torriente Editorial, 2003.

Rojas, Isis. "Misión José Gregorio Hernández: Un año de lucha y esperanza para los discapacitados." SiBCI: Sistema Bolivariano de Comunicación e Información, March 17, 2009. http://www.alopresidente.gob.ve/informacion/6/1115/misiuen_josugregorio_hernandezun.

Saénz, Tirso W., Halla Thorsteinsdóttir, and María Carlota de Souza. "Cuba and Brazil: An Important Example of South-South Collaboration in Health Biotechnology." *MEDICC Review* 12, no. 3 (July 2010): 32–35.

¡Salud! Documentary film. http://saludthefilm.net/. Accessed November 22, 2011.

Sánchez Gutiérrez, Aramís, and Conner Gorry. "Immunodiagnostics: The Convergence of Biotech and Public Health." *MEDICC Review* 15, no. 1 (January 2013): 7–10.

Scheye, Elaine. "Cuban Healthcare and Biotechnology: Reform, a Bitter Pill to Swallow, or Just What the Doctor Ordered?" *Cuba in Transition*, vol. 21. Papers and Proceedings of the Twenty-First Annual Meeting, Miami, August 4–6, 2011. http://www.ascecuba.org/c/wp-content/uploads/2014/09/v21-scheye.pdf.

Schipani, Andrés. "Bolivia's Miracle of Sight." *Guardian*, October 22, 2008.

———. "Revolutionary Care: Castro's Doctors Give Hope to the Children of Chernobyl." *Guardian*, July 2, 2009.

"Second Stage of Operation Miracle by Cuban Eye Doctors in Suriname a Success." *Havana Journal.com*, February 13, 2010. http://havanajournal.com/culture/print/8914.

"Se dedica a Fidel primera graduación de médicos de Pakistán en Cuba." *Cubadebate*, March 2, 2014. www.cubadebate.cu/noticias/2014/03/02/se-dedica-a-fidel-primera-graduacion-de-medicos-de-pakistan-en-cuba/#U76b-7Ht.

"Seguimiento médico de casos de discapacidad se cumple a medias." *El Universo*, June 17, 2012.

"Se rinde homenaje en Honduras al 11no. Aniversario de presencia de la brigada médica cubana." *CubaMinrex: Ministerio de Relaciones Exteriores de Cuba*, November 6, 2009. Note. http://anterior.cubaminrex.cu/Actualidad/2009/Noviembre/SeRinde.html.

Serrano, Pascual. "Infiltrado en un avión de la Misión Milagro con destino a La Habana." *Rebelion.org*, February 7, 2006. www.rebelion.org/noticia.php?id=26464.

Servicios Médicos Cubanos SA. Website. http://smcsalud.cu/smc/servlet/wpinicio.

Solano, Gonzalo. "Médicos en Ecuador se oponen a servicios de doctores cubanos." *El Nuevo Herald*, September 26, 2013.

Solórzano, Claudia. "El Ministro de Salud Pública retomará las buenas experiencias del sistema de salud de Cuba para la próxima reforma de salud de 2010." *Diario Co Latino*, December 9, 2009. http://www.simpatizantesfmln.org/blog?p=4358. Accessed January 3, 2010.

———. "Médicos cubanos atienden más de 20 mil personas." *Diario Co Latino*, December 17, 2009.

Somarriba López, Lorenzo, Rafael A. Llanes Caballero, and María de Jesús Sánchez Pérez. *Cólera en Haití: Lecciones aprendidas por la Brigada Médica Cubana*. Havana: Editorial Ciencias Médicas, 2013.

Sosin Martínez, Eileen. "Exportando salud: Servicios Médicos Cubanos." *OnCuba*, November 7, 2013. http://oncubamagazine.com/economia-negocios/exportando-salud-servicios-medicos-cubanos/.

Souers, Joanne Mae. "Cuba Leads the World in Lowest Patient per Doctor Ratio: How Do They Do It?" *Social Medicine Portal*, July 30, 2012. http://www.socialmedicine.org/2012/07/30/about/cuba-leads-the-world-in-lowest-patient-per-doctor-ratio-how-do-they-do-it/.

———. "Update from U.S. Student Joanne Mae Souers, Studying Medicine in Cuba." *Social Medicine Portal*, October 25, 2009. http://www.socialmedicine.org/2009/10/25/cuba/update-from-us-student-joanne-mae-souers-studying-medicine-in-cuba/.

Sowa, Graham. "Living Communally in a Cuban University." *Havana Times*, May 23, 2011. http://www.havanatimes.org/?p=71020.

Spiegel, Jerry M., and Annalee Yassi. "Lessons from the Margins of Globalization: Appreciating the Cuban Health Paradox." *Journal of Public Health Policy* 25, no. 1 (2005): 85–110.

Starr, Douglas. "The Cuban Biotech Revolution." *Wired* 12, no. 12 (December 2004). http://www.wired.com/wired/archive/12.12/cuba_pr.html.

Statement by Felipe Pérez Roque, Minister of Foreign Affairs of Cuba, at the Special Meeting of the Council of Ministers of the Association of Caribbean States. Panama City, 12 February 2004. *HNet:Humanities and Social Sciences Online*. http://h-net.msu.edu/cgi-bin/logbrowse.pl?trx=vx&list=h-caribbean&month=0402&week=c&msg=nUL7nup2kTelmFOOZvPDzg&user=&pw=.

Statement of the First Deputy Minister of Foreign Affairs of the Republic of Cuba, His Excellency Mr. Bruno Rodríguez. Islamabad, November 19, 2005. http://www.canadiannetworkoncuba.ca/Documents/Pakistan05.shtml.

Steif, William. "Cuban Doctors Aid Strife-Torn Haiti." *State*, April 26, 2004. http://havanajournal.com/culture/entry/cuban_doctors_aid_strife_torn_haiti.

Steinsleger, José. "Haití, Cuba y la ley primera." *La Jornada*, February 3, 2010.

Taboada Lugo, Noel, Odalys Bravo Téllez, María Amanda Licea Rodríguez, Odelinda Acosta Camacho, Osvaldo Pérez Estévez, Rosario Díaz Serraniega, Luis José Rodríguez Vivar, Antonio Bacallao Bell, Keiler Arnaldo González Torres, and Nélson Morales del Castillo. "Discapacidad intelectual: Aproximación a las principales causas en el Estado Plurinacional de Bolivia." http://bvs.sld.cu/revistas/rcgc/v5n2-2/rcgc060111.html.

Tamayo, René. "Celebran 12 años del Convenio integral de cooperación Cuba-Venezuela." *Juventud Rebelde*, October 30, 2012.

Thompson, SSgt. Chad. "U.S. Military Team Delivers 370,000 Lbs. of Aid, Begins Medical

Treatments in El Salvador." *United States Southern Command News Bulletin*, November 19, 2009.

———. "U.S. Military Docs Treat Nearly 3,000 People in Storm-Ravaged El Salvador." *United States Southern Command News Bulletin*, November 25, 2009.

Thorsteinsdóttir, Halla, ed. *South-South Collaboration in Health Technology*. New Delhi: Academic Foundation; Ottawa: International Development Research Centre, 2012.

Thorsteinsdóttir, Halla, and Tirso W. Sáenz. "Tackling Meningitis in Africa." *Science* 338 (December 21, 2012): 1546–47.

Tonga Ministry of Information and Communications. "Prime Minister Visits Cuba." December 9, 2009. http://www.mic.gov.to/ministrydepartment/14-govt-ministries/prime-ministers-office/1112-prime-minister-visits-cuba.

Tuvalu Ministry of Health. "Tuvalu Ministry of Health Strategic Health Plan, 2009–2018." World Health Organization report. http://www.wpro.who.int/health_services/tuvalu_nationalhealthplan.pdf.

Ubieta Gómez, Enrique. *Venezuela Rebelde: Solidaridad vs. Dinero*. Havana: Casa Editora Abril, 2006.

Ukrainian News Agency. "Ukraine to Finance Treatment and Rehabilitation of Ukrainian Children, Victims." October 23, 2011.

UNEP (United Nations Environment Program) and OCHA (United Nations Office for the Coordination of Humanitarian Affairs (OCHA). "Hurricane Stan: Environmental Impacts from Floods and Mudslides in Guatemala." October 26, 2005.

UNESCO. "Science Policy for Sustainable Development: Cuba." http://www.unesco.org/new/fileadmin/MULTIMEDIA/HQ/SC/pdf/sc_usrl0_cuba_EN.pdf.

"UN Experts: Socio-economic Recovery of Chernobyl-Affected Areas Requires Regular Governmental Interventions." UNICEF, April 19, 2011. http://www.unicef.org/ceecis/media_17014.html.

UNICEF. "At a Glance: Haiti." http://www.unicef.org/infobycountry/haiti_statistics.html.

United Nations Office for the Coordination of Humanitarian Affairs. "Haiti, Earthquake Situation Report #14." January 27, 2010.

United Nations World Food Program. "Hurricane Stan: Humanitarian Update from Central America." October 14, 2005. https://www.wfp.org/stories/hurricane-stan-humanitarian-update-central-america.

"Unos 132,000 médicos cubanos cumplieron misiones en el exterior desde 1963." *El Nuevo Herald*, March 25, 2014.

U.S. Department of State. "Cuban Medical Professional Parole Program." http://www.state.gov/p/wha/rls/fs/2009/115414.htm.

"U.S. Embassy Cables: U.S. Seeks Out Bad News about Cuban Healthcare." *Guardian*, December 17, 2010.

"U.S. Says Goodbye to Last MASH." MSNBC Associated Press, February 16, 2006. http://www.msnbc.msn.com/id/11385413/print/1/displaymode/1098/.

"U.S. Spearheads Global Response to Haiti Earthquake." *Fox News*, January 13, 2010. http://www.foxnews.com/politics/2010/01/13/spearheads-global-response-haiti-earthquake/.

"Vacunas cubanas consolidan su presencia en mercado vietnamita." *Prensa Latina*, December 12, 2011.

Valera, Daisy. "ELAM Med School 10 Years After." *Havana Times*, November 30, 2009.

Vázquez García, Nyliam. "La escuela médica más avanzada del mundo." *Juventud Rebelde*, January 28, 2014.

"Venezuela: 94 mil personas atendidas por la Misión Milagro en el 2012." *Cubadebate*, June 15, 2012. http://www.cubadebate.cu/noticias/2012/06/15/94-mil-personas-atendidas-por-la-mision-milagro-en-el-2012/#.VF_k6ckXEXw.

"Venezuela: Programa gubernamental cumple cinco años de atención a discapacitados." *Cubadebate*, March 15, 2013. http://www.cubadebate.cu/noticias/2013/03/15/venezuela-programa-cumple-cinco-anos-de-atencion-a-discapacitados/#.VF_lHckXEXw.

"Venezuela propone la creación de Universidad internacional de la salud." *Granma*, November 26, 2013.

"Venezuela's 'Misión Milagro' Performs 5,000 Eye Surgeries Weekly." Bulletin from the Embassy of the Bolivarian Republic of Venezuela in the United States, July 6, 2012.

"Venezuela supera el millón de cirugías por la Misión Milagro." *Juventud Rebelde*, July 6, 2012.

"Venezuela y Cuba: nuevos convenios de la solidaridad." *Cubadebate*, April 28, 2013. http://www.cubadebate.cu/noticias/2013/04/28/venezuela-y-cuba-nue.

"Venezuela y el drama del parto." *BBC Mundo*, August 18, 2009. http://www.bbc.co.uk/mundo/america_latina/2009/08/090817_2359_sanidad_venezuela_irm.shtml.

"Vicepresidente de Ecuador destaca solidaridad de Fidel Castro en temas de salud." *Cubadebate*, October 31, 2009. http://www.cubadebate.cu/noticias/2009/10/31/vice-presidente-de-ecuador-destaca-solidaridad-de-fidel-castro-en-temas-de-salud/#.VF_mQ8kXEXw.

Viñet Espinosa, Luisa Marlen, Alicia Rodríguez González, Carmen María Sayu Cisneros, Doris María Prieto Ramírez, and Guadalupe Quesada Pita. "Misión José Gregorio Hernández, formadora de valores en los estudiantes de Medicina Integral Comunitaria." *Pedagogía Universitaria* 17, no. 1 (2012): 126–36.

Vives Romero, Teresita de J. "China-Cuba: Colaboración biotecnológica con buena salud." *Prensa Latina*, March 3, 2012.

Wasuka, E. "Cuban Doctors to Fill Shortage." *Island Business*, May 3, 2007.

Watts, Jonathan. "Ecuador's Lenín Moreno Gives Revolutionary Turn by Quitting While on Top." *Guardian*, February 19, 2013.

Weaver, Matthew, and Paul Owens. "Nelson Mandela's Memorial Service, as It Happened." *Guardian*, December 10, 2013.

Werlau, María C. "Cuba's Cash-for-Doctors Program." *Wall Street Journal*, August 16, 2010.

———. "Cuba's Health-Care Diplomacy: The Business of Humanitarianism." *World Affairs*, March/April 2013. http://www.worldaffairsjournal.org/article/cuba%E2%80%99s-health-care-diplomacy-business-humanitarianism.

———. "Cuba's Partners in Human Exploitation." *Miami Herald*, December 5, 2012.

Whellams, Diana. "Medical Migration: Options and Responsibilities for the 'Brain Drain.'" Master of Public Health thesis, Simon Fraser University, 2009.

Whiteford, Linda M., and Laurence G. Branch. *Primary Health Care in Cuba*. Lanham, Md.: Rowman and Littlefield, 2008.

Whitney, W. T. "Cuban Medic in Pakistan." *Guardian*, April 5, 2006.

"WHO Praises Work of Cuban Health Specialists." *Havana Reporter*, November 8, 2012.

World Bank Data. "Physicians per 1,000 People." http://data.worldbank.org/indicator/SH.MED.PHYS.ZS.

"World Bank Releases $201 Million for Storm-Ravaged Central America." CNN.com, November 11, 1998.

World Health Organization. "Chernobyl: The True Scale of the Accident." September 5, 2005. http://www.who.int/mediacentre/news/releases/2005/pr38/en/index.html.

———. "Health Topics: Disabilities." http://www.who.int/topics/disabilities/en.

———. "Ionizing Radiation. Health Effects of the Chernobyl Accident: An Overview." April 2006. www.who.int/ionizing_radiation/chernobyl/backgrounder/en/index.html.

———. "Visual Impairment and Blindness." Fact Sheet No. 282. June 2012. Updated August 2014. http://www.who.int/mediacentre/factsheets/fs282/en/.

World Nuclear Association. "Chernobyl Accident 1986." http://www.world-nuclear.org/info/chernobyl/inf07.html.

Wynter, Coral. "Venezuela: Cuban Doctors Helping the Poor." Global Research, April 19, 2010. http://www.globalresearch.ca/venezuela-cuban-doctors-helping-the-poor/18730.

Index

Page numbers in *italics* indicate tables.

John M. Kirk is professor of Latin American Studies at Dalhousie University in Canada. His research interests focus on contemporary Cuba, its foreign policy, and the country's development model. He lives in Halifax, Nova Scotia.

CONTEMPORARY CUBA

Edited by John M. Kirk

Afro-Cuban Voices: On Race and Identity in Contemporary Cuba, by Pedro Pérez-Sarduy and Jean Stubbs (2000)

Cuba, the United States, and the Helms-Burton Doctrine: International Reactions, by Joaquín Roy (2000)

Cuba Today and Tomorrow: Reinventing Socialism, by Max Azicri (2000)

Cuba's Foreign Relations in a Post-Soviet World, by H. Michael Erisman (2000)

Cuba's Sugar Industry, by José Alvarez and Lázaro Peña Castellanos (2001)

Culture and the Cuban Revolution: Conversations in Havana, by John M. Kirk and Leonardo Padura Fuentes (2001)

Looking at Cuba: Essays on Culture and Civil Society, by Rafael Hernández, translated by Dick Cluster (2003)

Santería Healing: A Journey into the Afro-Cuban World of Divinities, Spirits, and Sorcery, by Johan Wedel (2004)

Cuba's Agricultural Sector, by José Alvarez (2004)

Cuban Socialism in a New Century: Adversity, Survival, and Renewal, edited by Max Azicri and Elsie Deal (2004)

Cuba, the United States, and the Post–Cold War World: The International Dimensions of the Washington-Havana Relationship, edited by Morris Morley and Chris McGillion (2005)

Redefining Cuban Foreign Policy: The Impact of the "Special Period," edited by H. Michael Erisman and John M. Kirk (2006)

Gender and Democracy in Cuba, by Ilja A. Luciak (2007)

Ritual, Discourse, and Community in Cuban Santería: Speaking a Sacred World, by Kristina Wirtz (2007)

The "New Man" in Cuba: Culture and Identity in the Revolution, by Ana Serra (2007)

U.S.-Cuban Cooperation Past, Present, and Future, by Melanie M. Ziegler (2007)

Protestants, Revolution, and the Cuba-U.S. Bond, by Theron Corse (2007)

The Changing Dynamic of Cuban Civil Society, edited by Alexander I. Gray and Antoni Kapcia (2008)

Cuba in the Shadow of Change: Daily Life in the Twilight of the Revolution, by Amelia Rosenberg Weinreb (2009)

Failed Sanctions: Why the U.S. Embargo against Cuba Could Never Work, by Paolo Spadoni (2010)

Sustainable Urban Agriculture in Cuba, by Sinan Koont (2011)

Fifty Years of Revolution: Perspectives on Cuba, the United States, and the World, edited by Soraya M. Castro Mariño and Ronald W. Pruessen (2012)

Cuban Economists on the Cuban Economy, edited by Al Campbell (2013)

Cuban Revelations: Behind the Scenes in Havana, by Marc Frank (2013)

Cuba in a Global Context: International Relations, Internationalism, and Transnationalism, edited by Catherine Krull (2014)

Healthcare without Borders: Understanding Cuban Medical Internationalism by John M. Kirk (2015)

Rescuing Our Roots: The African Anglo-Caribbean Diaspora in Contemporary Cuba by Andrea Queeley (2015)

www.ingramcontent.com/pod-product-compliance
Ingram Content Group UK Ltd.
Pitfield, Milton Keynes, MK11 3LW, UK
UKHW040612030426
469645UK00004B/53

9 780813 0610